SECOND EDITION

Using the ELECTRONIC HEALTH RECORD

In the Health Care Provider Practice

Shirley Eichenwald Maki
MBA, RHIA, FAHIMA

Bonnie J. Petterson
PhD, RHIA

e-Medsys® Educational Edition 2.0
Software Exercises
prepared by

Janelle Wapola
MA, RHIA

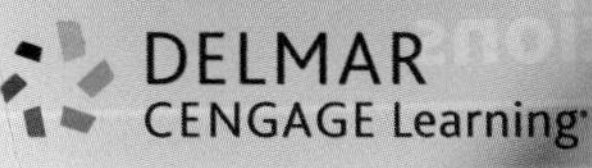

Australia • Brazil • Japan • Korea • Mexico • Singapore • Spain • United Kingdom • United States

DELMAR
CENGAGE Learning

Using the Electronic Health Record in the Health Care Provider Practice, Second Edition
Shirley Eichenwald Maki, Bonnie J. Petterson

Vice President, Careers & Computing: Dave Garza

Publisher: Stephen Helba

Executive Editor: Rhonda Dearborn

Director, Development-Career and Computing: Marah Bellegarde

Product Development Manager: Juliet Steiner

Senior Product Manager: Sarah Prime

Product Manager: Lauren Whalen

Editorial Assistant: Courtney Cozzy

Executive Brand Manager: Wendy Mapstone

Senior Market Development Manager: Nancy Bradshaw

Senior Production Director: Wendy Troeger

Production Manager: Andrew Crouth

Content Project Manager: Brooke Greenhouse

Senior Art Director: Jack Pendleton

Media Editor: William Overocker

Cover image(s): © Cengage Learning

Library of Congress Control Number: 2012949134

ISBN-13: 978-1-1116-4560-1

ISBN-10: 1-111-64560-4

Delmar
5 Maxwell Drive
Clifton Park, NY 12065-2919
USA

Cengage Learning is a leading provider of customized learning solutions with office locations around the globe, including Singapore, the United Kingdom, Australia, Mexico, Brazil, and Japan. Locate your local office at:
international.cengage.com/region

Cengage Learning products are represented in Canada by Nelson Education, Ltd.

To learn more about Delmar, visit **www.cengage.com/delmar**

Purchase any of our products at your local college store or at our preferred online store **www.cengagebrain.com**

Printed in the United States of America
1 2 3 4 5 6 7 17 16 15 14 13

Dedication

We dedicate this work to those health care professionals who take on, as their life's work, the education of the future generations of our nation's health care workforce. They actively engage in assessing the profession's challenges today and also look ahead to the opportunities of tomorrow. Most notably, they devote themselves to the important work of translating the evolving workforce requirements of the health care industry into curriculum to ensure professional competence and relevance.

Shirley Eichenwald Maki

Bonnie Petterson

Contents

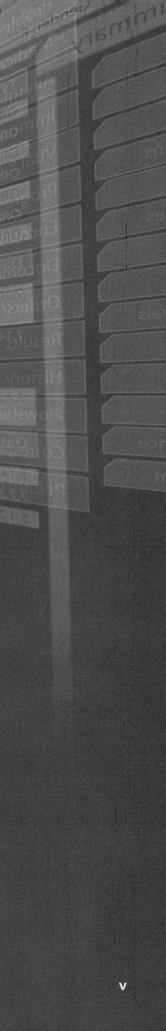

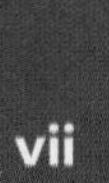

CHAPTER 13

LIST OF TABLES

Preface

The nation's health care delivery system is being transformed rapidly by the introduction of computer-based health information systems—specifically, by electronic health records (EHRs). There are a significant number of activities at the national, regional, and state levels aimed at encouraging adoption of these systems, with a special emphasis on implementation in health care provider practices.

As you prepare for a career in the health care workplace, it is important that you develop a clear understanding of the significant impact an EHR system has on the work processes in that setting. When you begin your career, you either will immediately or very soon be using an EHR system as a primary tool to support your work and the office workflow. The EHR knowledge and experience gained through your educational program will be a valuable component of the full set of competencies and skills you bring to your workplace.

Using the Electronic Health Record in the Health Care Provider Practice is focused on providing you with:

- The foundational knowledge of EHR systems.
- A practical perspective on how an EHR system affects the work and workflow in a provider office practice.
- Directed hands-on experiences using an educational version of an EHR product designed for use in an ambulatory health care setting.

ORGANIZATION OF THE TEXT

The text is divided into 13 chapters:

- Chapters 1–4 present foundational knowledge about the EHR: what it is, how it benefits the health care industry and workplace, what is required to implement it in the provider office, what its basic structural components are, and how its content is determined.
- Chapters 5–12 present a detailed discussion of the specific ways that an EHR supports the variety of tasks and communications that are associated with the normal clinical workflow in a health care provider practice.
- Chapter 13 introduces the personal health record and the continuity of care record, two concepts that are receiving considerable attention and increasing support as potentially efficient vehicles for electronically communicating relevant and accurate patient health information between health care providers in support of a seamless transfer of care.
- Appendices A and B focus on providing practical hands-on EHR experience using e-Medsys® Educational Edition 2.0 software from TriMed Technologies.
- A list of acronyms translates each acronym used in the text.
- A glossary defines all key terms.

SOFTWARE SUPPORT

The **Premium Website** includes support documentation for e-Medsys® Educational Edition 2.0 software. Follow the directions on the printed access card to access the Premium Website at www.cengagebrain.com.

INSTRUCTOR SUPPORT

An **Instructor Resources CD-ROM** is available for instructor support in and out of the classroom. Deliver powerful lectures, create total lesson plans, customize exams, and monitor student progress throughout the course, including:

- Complete electronic **Instructor's Manual** files, which include lecture outlines with objectives, answer keys for Review Questions, screenshot solutions for the CareTracker Computer Exploration exercises, and additional references.
- Instructor slides in **Microsoft PowerPoint** for each chapter that cover key concepts presented in the text.
- A **Computerized Test Bank** in ExamView with more than 550 questions and answers, organized by chapter.

Additionally, the Instructor's Manual and Instructor Slides in Microsoft PowerPoint are accessible on the **Instructor Companion Site**. Go to http://login.cengage.com/cb/ and log in with your Cengage instructor account. If you are a first-time user, click "Create a New Faculty Account" and follow the prompts.

REVIEWERS

The authors and publisher would like to thank the following reviewers, whose comments, suggestions, and feedback were instrumental to the development of this book.

Katherine E. Baus, RHIA, CCS-P
Program Manager, Health Information Management
Southwest Florida College
Ft. Myers, FL

Charlene A. Crump, CPC, AHI, CMAS
Medical Billing and Coding Instructor
Remington College
North Olmsted, OH

Jazmine Cunningham
Medical and Business Instructor
Ridley-Lowell Business & Technical Institute
Poughkeepsie, NY

Laurie Dennis, CBCS
Allied Health Team Leader
Florida Career College
Clearwater, FL

Dr. Thomas F. Finnegan IV, DC, FABDA, DAAIM, DAAETS
Dunwoody College of Technology
Minneapolis, MN

Mary F. Koloski, CBCS, CHI
Health Insurance Billing & Coding, Program Coordinator
Florida Career College
Clearwater, FL

Stephanie Hollan
Allied Health Chair
Remington College
Webster, TX

Loreen W. MacNichol, CMRS, RMC, CCS-P
Professor
Andover College
South Portland, ME

Tracey A. McKethan, MBA, CCA
Department Chair/Associate Professor
Springfield Technical Community College
Springfield, MA

Frank J. Miranda
Computer Instructor
Health Care Training Services
Fall River, MA

Latrina Mitchell, MA, NCMOA
Medical Office Administrative Specialist Program Coordinator
Platt College
Dallas, TX

Krista Moloney, RHIA
Instructor/Trainer
Trident Technical College
Charleston, SC

Linda Scarborough, NSHA, BSM, RN, CPC, CMA (AAMA)
Healthcare Management Technology Instructor
Lanier Technical College
Oakwood, GA

Marilyn Turner, RN, CMA (AAMA)
Medical Assisting Program Director
Ogeechee Technical College
Statesboro, GA

Michael Weinard, BA
Program Manager
Kaplan Higher Education
Chicago, IL

Stacey Wilson, CMA (AAMA), MT/PBT(ASCP), MHA, AHI
Program Chair and Assistant Professor
Carrabus College of Health Sciences
Concord, NC

Acknowledgments

To my husband, Duane, whose encouragement, patience, and gentle nature are a constant presence in my life. To my adult children, Jill and Scott, to the grandchildren they have gifted to us, and to our entire blended family, who provide us with such joy and sustain us with their constant loving attention in the midst of busy and sometimes challenging days. To Bonnie Petterson, who has been a perfect partner in this collaborative writing project, a highly respected educator, professional colleague, and longtime friend. To Janelle Wapola, who is the best professional "tech-savvy sidekick" ever; an energetic, dedicated, and talented young educator; an admired colleague; and forever a friend. Thank you!

Shirley Eichenwald Maki, MBA, RHIA, FAHIMA

First a special thanks to all of my family, especially my sons Brian and Matthew and my four sisters, for supporting me through my professional adventures, graduate school, and this continuing project. Throughout my career, your belief in me and what I can do has not wavered. A very special thank you also is sent to my colleagues in this adventure. Shirley, you provided research guidance early in my career and continued to be a mentor and friend throughout the years. Your vision of health information in the future has been the catalyst for change in the profession. You have challenged me and made me grow—thank you for encouraging me to become involved in this book. Janelle, it has been my pleasure to share your enthusiasm, energy, and technical expertise—and to gain a new friend. Finally, my appreciation goes to my professional colleagues in the Phoenix College health information management programs. Your wholehearted commitment to students and support for whatever it takes to prepare them for the future allowed me the freedom to explore and made my work at Phoenix College a real pleasure.

Bonnie Petterson PhD, RHIA

To my mentor, Shirley Eichenwald Maki, whose personal and professional support allows me to try new things, and whose love for health information never wants. You are an incredible inspiration and a special person in my life. Thank you, Shirley. Thank you Bonnie and Shirley for allowing me to be a part of this textbook journey; I have learned from each of you. To Mike, who continually pushes me to try different things. And to my boys, Tyler and Daniel: may you have many adventures and see the world!

Janelle Wapola, MA, RHIA

Together we acknowledge Sarah Prime, our senior product manager, for her guidance and support throughout the revision process. She kept us on course and patiently brought us through the revision effort. Our sense of accomplishment and satisfaction with the revised text is a testimony to her interpersonal and technical talents.

Shirley, Bonnie, and Janelle

About the Authors and Contributor

Shirley Eichenwald Maki is an Assistant Professor in the Department of Health Informatics and Information Management at the College of St. Scholastica in Duluth, Minnesota, and a Fellow of the American Health Information Management Association. From 2002–2008 she was the project director for The ATHENS Project, a U.S. Department of Education, Title III grant-funded initiative—the first of its kind in the nation—to implement a state-of-the-art electronic health-record system and integrate it as a teaching/learning tool in the health professions' curricula of the College's physical therapy, nursing, occupational therapy, athletic training, medical social work, and health information management programs. From 2008–2011 Shirley was engaged as an HIM and EHR subject-matter expert in three HRSA-funded projects focused on supporting the implementation of health information technologies in rural health care facilities. In 2010–2011 she served as an HIT Consultant within the Regional HIT Extension Center serving Minnesota and North Dakota.

Bonnie Petterson founded HIM Education Consulting in 2011 after retiring as the Director of Health Information Programs at Phoenix College, part of the Maricopa Community College District (MCCD) in Phoenix, Arizona. During her tenure at Phoenix College, Bonnie worked with students in many health care-related programs, and saw the enrollment in health information programs grow exponentially. Her career also included full-time employment and consulting in a wide variety of health care settings including hospitals and clinics. She was instrumental in bringing an educational electronic health record to Phoenix College for student training, one of the first community colleges in the country to do so, and led the team from MCCD that sought and ultimately was awarded one of the coveted federal HITECH HIT training grants. In 2010 the Arizona Health Information Management Association honored her with its special Lifetime Achievement Award.

Janelle Wapola is an assistant professor in the undergraduate and graduate programs in the Department of Healthcare Informatics and Information Management at the College of St. Scholastica in Duluth, Minnesota. Her instructional responsibilities are associated with health care information, specifically the electronic health record and project management. She is particularly interested in global HIM and the opportunities available to today's new HIM graduates. Wapola is the technology lead for the department and also serves as an HIT Consultant with the Regional HIT Extension Center serving Minnesota and North Dakota. She is a member of the American Health Information Management Association and currently serves as one of Minnesota's Delegates to the AHIMA House of Delegates.

How to Use the Text:
A Guided Walkthrough

CHAPTER 6 Problem, Medication, and Allergy Lists

CHAPTER OUTLINE

Workflow
Standards: Functional, Content, and Vocabulary
Functional and Content Standards
Vocabulary Standards

KEY TERMS

allergy and adverse reaction list
medication list
problem list
summary lists

OBJECTIVES

Upon completion of the chapter, the learner will be able to:

1. Describe the position of The Joint Commission and that of the Accreditation Association for Ambulatory Health Care (AAAHC) on summary lists in ambulatory patient records.
2. Explain why summary lists are included in the continuity of care record (CCR) and the continuity of care document (CCD) standard.
3. Identify specific capabilities an ONC-ATCB "certified" electronic health record (EHR) must have that support the creation and maintenance of (a) problem lists, (b) medication lists, and (c) allergy and adverse reaction lists.
4. Explain why a reference vocabulary (e.g., SNOMED-CT) is preferred over a classification system (e.g., ICD-9-CM or ICD-10-CM) as the basis for structuring the content of the problem list.
5. Describe an office workflow process that will assure that the summary lists in each patient's EHR are reviewed and updated routinely to maintain their accuracy, completeness, and currency.

Chapter Opener

Each chapter begins with an outline which lists an **overview of topics,** Key Terms to **highlight important concepts,** and Objectives to provide **focus for learning.**

Case Situations

Case Situations provide a **real-life point of view,** applying the concepts in the chapter to real workplace experiences.

Margin Glossary

Key terms are **defined two ways**: both in context in the text discussion, as well as in the margin of the page.

Case Situation continued

After 6 months of being fully involved with assessing, planning, and EHR product selection activities, the clinic providers and clerical staff were eager to implement their new electronic health record system. As they reviewed the many workflow changes that would be implemented to take full advantage of the EHR system, they also recognized that the types of computer workstations they installed would impact their ability to use the EHR system easily as a daily work tool.

This clinic has 11 exam rooms used by three family physicians, one physician assistant, and one nurse practitioner. The existing space and floor plan would not be changed because the clinic space had been renovated within the past three years. So the revised workflows took the existing space and floor plan into account. Therefore, the planning for new EHR workstations and related equipment (printers, scanners, etc.) would take these factors into consideration as well.

In order to retire the paper medical records completely, computer workstations were needed in every location where clinicians and clerical staff would need to view or enter data into the patient's record. Printers would be located in every location where clinicians and clerical staff needed to access printed materials to hand to patients. When the locations for the computer workstations and printers were identified, electrical and network wiring were installed to accommodate the equipment. The clinicians decided to use hardwired desktop computer workstations to avoid potential problems with mobile tablet devices—problems such as limited battery life, security issues with tablets that might be taken out of the clinic, potential damage from dropping, and additional technology required to support wireless connections. The clinicians established design principles for the exam-room workstations based on the recommendations given to them by their REC consultant:

- Position the workstation so the clinician can sit close enough to touch the patient and maintain easy eye contact with the patient while the clinician is seated at the workstation.
- Assure that each workstation is positioned at the ergonomically appropriate keyboard height, monitor-viewing height, and mouse position for clinicians.
- Have a readily available writing surface.

Quality Improvement Organization (QIO)
An organization that contracts with the federal government to perform tasks on its behalf under the Medicare program, focusing especially on quality and necessity of care issues.

eligible providers (EPs)
Health care providers that are qualified by regulations to participate in Medicare's or Medicaid's "meaningful use" incentive programs.

meaningful use
Relates to the actual ways that the EHR must be used to support patient care and specific ways that quality of care must be measured to receive incentive payments from Medicare and Medicaid Services as determined by the federal HITECH Act.

Summary

The Summary section concludes each chapter and **emphasizes major discussion points**.

Computer Exploration

These exercises ask you to **research topics** on the Internet or complete **practical, hands-on activities** using e-Medsys® Educational Edition 2.0 software.

Review Questions

These questions **assess the important concepts** of the chapter; they are printed on a separate page to be torn out and turned in.

SUMMARY

The workflow for the coding and billing process begins prior to the patient visit as part of the scheduling function and continues after the visit until payment for services is received. Using defined clinical vocabularies and established coding systems, patient-treatment documentation can be linked to diagnostic and procedural codes. In turn, codes can be applied to bills for submission to third-party payers. Standards for these processes are important for sharing and interpreting data accurately. HIPAA regulations identified standard code sets for submitting information for an ambulatory service bill, including the use of ICD, CPT, and HCPCS Level II codes. The ICD is an international classification system that is used in provider practices for recording diagnoses. Recording of procedures is done with the CPT nomenclature. CPT codes are actually Level I HCPCS codes. Level II HCPCS codes are used nationally for services and equipment that are not found in CPT. The SNOMED-CT® is the primary clinical vocabulary identified for use within an EHR. Both SNOMED-CT® and MEDCIN have been mapped to ICD, CPT, and other specialized vocabularies in order to permit standardization and consistency in the use of medical terms in an EHR. Once diagnoses and procedures are identified via a problem list or other means, an encoder can assist personnel with code assignment. If computer-assisted coding is applied, then no human intervention is required except for auditing purposes. CAC software programming facilitates code assignment either through natural-language processing or structured menu input. Audit trails can record the steps in each of those processes in the event that questions about assignment develop. Assigned codes then can be transferred to the billing component of the EHR system. Additional information is added to the bill from other data sources within the EHR, scrubbers are applied to edit codes and bills for errors, and then the bill is sent electronically to the primary payer. Communication with that payer or the patient continues electronically, if possible, until service payment has been received.

The billing function in the health care provider office has long included electronic procedures. In the EHR system, interoperability among the billing system and the medical record is key to increasing the accuracy and efficiency of this important business activity. Finally, the interaction of the two systems also supports gathering data to assist practice owners and managers in monitoring activities and performance and in making sound management decisions.

Computer Exploration

Significant amounts of information about Personal Health Records are available at this web site: http://www.myPHR.com/. Access the site and:

a. Click on "Start a PHR" at the top of the home page and then "Choose a PHR" on the drop-down menu that appears. Select "Web-based" under "Format" and "Free" under "Cost" (bottom of page) and then "Submit." Click links for at least two free products (e.g., MyMediConnect and IntuitHealthPHR—formerly iHealthRecord). Next return and select at least two products "For Purchase" under "Cost" (e.g., Mymedicalrecords.com and Lynxcare).

b. For each of the four products you select:

(1) Find the product demo, tour, or overview available via its web site and describe the product features that you find most appealing or useful as a potential customer.

(2) Review the FAQs (frequently asked questions) available via its web site or presented in videos and document at least four facts that you find most informative as a potential customer.

(3) Describe how the issue of "security" of personal health data is addressed within the content of this product's web site.

(4) Write a brief comparative analysis of the four PHR products: what was common among them, what was unique about one as compared to the others, etc.

REVIEW QUESTIONS

1. Plan, Select, and Implement are three of the four major steps associated with an EHR project. What is the other step, and what types of activities does it include?

2. Identify two major websites that provide free access to HIT Tools and sources for physician office practices to guide the organization through its EHR assess, plan, select and implementation activities.

3. How does an organization's EHR vision differ from its EHR goals?

4. What basic activities must be taken by the EHR selection task group when investigating the EHR product's appropriateness, reliability, and stability before making a final decision?

5. Who must be involved with defining the functional specifications for an EHR before a vendor is selected?

6. What are the differences between the CCHIT ambulatory EHR criteria and the Medicare/Medicaid "Meaningful Use" EHR criteria?

CHAPTER 1 Electronic Health Records: An Overview

CHAPTER OUTLINE

OBJECTIVES

Upon completion of the chapter, learners will be able to:

1. Define the terms *electronic medical record* (EMR) and *electronic health record* (EHR) and explain the difference between the two.
2. Describe the major components of an EHR.
3. Identify eight core functions/capabilities of an EHR.
4. Define terms and key concepts used to describe characteristics of an EHR.
5. Describe benefits of an EHR and provide an example of each for the healthcare practice setting.
6. List frequently identified challenges to implementation of EHRs.
7. Explain the roles of ONC, NHIN, RHIOs, HIEs, SNOs, RECs, ACOs, and organizations such as the CCHIT in electronic record initiatives.
8. Identify initiatives that are attempting to assist practices in adoption and funding of an EHR.
9. Describe the status of electronic record adoption in health care provider offices.
10. Describe a smart card and explain how it can be used to support patient care.

KEY TERMS

Accountable Care Organization (ACO)
alerts
Centers for Medicare and Medicaid Services (CMS)
Certification Commission for Healthcare Information Technology (CCHIT)
data repository
electronic health record (EHR)
electronic medical record (EMR)
eligible providers (EPs)
Health Information Exchange (HIE)
Health Information Technology for Economic and Clinical Health Act (HITECH)
interoperability
meaningful use
National Health Information Network (NHIN)
Office of the National Coordinator for Health Information Technology (ONC)
Quality Improvement Organization (QIO)

continues

KEY TERMS continued

Regional Health Information Technology Extension Centers (RECs)

Regional Health Information Organizations (RHIOs)

reminders

smart card

standards organizations

Sub-Network Organizations (SNOs)

telemonitoring

treatment protocols

VistA-Office EHR

INTRODUCTION

Computers have been used in health care provider offices for decades. As is true in most health care organizations, the introduction of computers in practices often was associated with payment for services or the billing and patient accounts functions. Next steps included practice management software designed to coordinate scheduling and patient registration with billing, accounting, and administrative features. Some practices also have established electronic linkage with a diagnostic testing laboratory system or a hospital information system that provides timely transfer of some diagnostic test results. Computers also may be used by health care providers to perform research on a disease or its treatment, to communicate with other providers, to track referrals, or to monitor practice productivity. Reports vary, but it is estimated that by 2010 less than half of practices had implemented components of an electronic health record (EHR) system, and far fewer had fully functional systems. Practice size is an important factor, with smaller practices generally having a lower adoption rate. Important efforts to use computers to record and access the full range of a patient's office experiences in a coordinated manner are receiving national attention, primarily due to some new programs and funding incentives.

This chapter will provide a definition of an EHR along with background information to explain the importance of the current national, regional, and state programs supporting the implementation of EHR systems in health care provider settings. The challenges ahead will become evident through a discussion of the status of EHR implementation in practice settings and the hurdles that still must be overcome before coordinated systems are common in the United States.

ELECTRONIC HEALTH RECORD DEFINITION AND DESCRIPTION

electronic health record (EHR) An electronic record of health-related information on an individual that conforms to nationally recognized interoperability standards and that can be created, managed, and consulted by authorized clinicians and staff across more than one health care organization.

electronic medical record (EMR) An electronic record of health-related information on an individual that can be created, gathered, managed, and consulted by authorized clinicians and staff within one health care organization.

The current understanding of what an electronic health record is has evolved as technology, system capabilities, and health care information needs have grown. The term **electronic health record (EHR)** does not describe only a computerized version of a medical record, but rather an entire system that documents health care services, the information gathered to make decisions about health care, and then can share that information with other health care providers. Some literature will use other terms such as **electronic medical record (EMR)** for the same or similar systems. To reduce confusion in the use of terms and provide a common foundation for further discussion in the United States, The National Alliance for Health Information Technology published a report in 2008 that provided the following definitions:

> Electronic Medical Record – An electronic record of health-related information on an individual that can be created, gathered, managed, and consulted by authorized clinicians and staff within one health organization.
>
> Electronic Health Record – An electronic record of health-related information on an individual that conforms to nationally recognized interoperability standards and that can be created, managed, and consulted by authorized clinicians and staff across more than one health care organization.

According to these definitions, **interoperability**, the ability of record systems to communicate and exchange information with each other across systems and multiple organizations, differentiates the EHR from the EMR. This text focuses on the capabilities of an EHR through its use in the practice setting.

Nationally, a number of government agencies, voluntary groups, and health-related associations are involved in providing guidelines to assist in making the EHR more uniform. These groups are referred to as **standards organizations**. Some standards organizations focus just on the EHR, while others develop standards in other areas as well. As a result of the work of one standards organization, more than 160 functions for an EHR have been identified and defined. These EHR functional criteria expanded upon a list of eight core functions originally identified by the Institute of Medicine (2003). These EHR core functions can be found in Table 1-1, including examples of each function.

What does this mean for the practice setting?

Most practice settings currently own or lease computer systems (hardware) that incorporate computer programs (software) for a variety of processes (health care and supporting tasks) that involve both people (practice employees and patients) and day-to-day office activities (policies and processes). In an EHR, each system would collect and send data to an electronic holding place known as a **data repository**. Data from one system would share with other systems, and all pertinent data would be available to providers whenever they see a patient. Data collected would include all patient and payment identifiers, patient

interoperability
The capacity of systems to communicate and exchange information with one another.

standards organizations
Government agencies, voluntary groups, and industry associations involved in establishing guidelines to assist in bringing uniformity to business processes or products.

data repository
Electronic holding place for data.

TABLE 1-1 Core Functions of an Electronic Health Record

EHR FUNCTION	EXAMPLES
Health information and data	Ability to record patient history and physical, other assessments, a problem list, visit notes, vital sign monitors.
Order entry and management	Ability to write orders that can be transmitted to pharmacies, laboratories, or providers electronically; alerts if drug orders show potential drug interactions.
Results management	Ability to receive diagnostic and treatment reports electronically; ability to receive alerts if abnormal findings occurred.
Decision support	Ability to obtain information electronically on drugs appropriate for prescribing or therapy research; ability to receive alerts if anything in the patient's history shows potential for adverse reactions.
Electronic communication and connectivity	Ability to share patient information electronically with another provider or a secure network of providers; ability to access medical and drug information electronically.
Administrative processes	Ability to record patient identification and payment information; ability to request and receive data on the diagnoses of the practice's patient population.
Patient support	Ability to provide patients with educational material; ability to communicate electronically with patients.
Reporting and population management	Ability to report the results of research drug responses electronically; ability to submit public health information directly to the state department of health.

reminders Automated notices to practitioners or patients regarding actions that need to be taken.

alerts Automated notices to practitioners of information that requires immediate or special attention.

visit history, problem lists, medications, and so forth. Based on this information, the EHR system could produce **reminders** to patients about, for example, the need to schedule an appointment; or it could supply the service and diagnostic information needed to submit a bill to a third party for payment without reentering information. All information that currently is considered to be part of a patient or client record also would be part of the data repository, including reports of all diagnostic and therapeutic procedures and results, images, orders, and treatment plans. Beyond that, the EHR could generate automated notices to health care providers of those aspects of patient care requiring urgent attention. These notices, called **alerts**, might be based on allergy or drug interaction lists or other patient information. Orders could be tracked, and adverse results from any diagnostic test would produce another type of physician alert so that patient care plans could be adjusted as necessary. Patient data also could be passed from the data repository to laboratories, pharmacies, and payers through communicating or interfacing software.

Four other major components provide added capabilities:

- Accessing research (best practices) information.
- Sharing of diagnostic and treatment information among providers.
- Reporting required information to public health agencies.
- Communicating with patients.

treatment protocols Established guidelines for treatment of specific diseases.

First, the EHR would permit access to current research on disease management and provide information to assist in care delivery, planning, and patient management. Current drug information, effective **treatment protocols** (established guidelines for treatment of specific diseases), and access to expert knowledge bases could provide valuable and timely information for clinical decisions.

telemonitoring Using telecommunications technology to gather physiologic or diagnostic data and transmit it to a health care provider who can evaluate patients who are located a distance from the care provider setting.

Second, the EHR would allow sharing of treatment information among care providers to the level that the patient and the system permits. As a result, duplication of diagnostic tests and adverse drug and treatment interactions would be decreased, and providers would have accurate information for care no matter where the patient might be seen. Record components or data elements shared across providers would be defined, and the shared information would have established confidentiality restrictions. One model for this type of data sharing across provider settings is the continuity of care record (CCR). The CCR consists of a standard set of patient data that can be sent from one health care provider to another in order to assist in a patient's transfer from one health care setting to another. The CCR will be described in greater detail in Chapter 13. Another type of sharing of patient information over distances is referred to as **telemonitoring**. Patients in their homes are connected to a vital signs device or other medical monitoring device. Text and/or image data collected by the device is transmitted via a telecommunications system to the EHR in the provider's office for interpretation and medical management.

Third, data required for public health reporting—for example, the diagnosis of some sexually transmitted diseases, or a disease incidence such as individuals diagnosed with influenza—could be transmitted electronically from the EHR system to the public health agencies that track them. Authorized data also could be reported directly from the EHR system to licensing or accrediting organizations.

Finally, ongoing communications between providers and patients, as well as transfer of information contributed by patients to support their own care, also would have a place in the EHR.

As this description indicates, a fully functional EHR is a robust product that can have a huge impact on both the care provided and the processes performed in the health care provider setting. An EHR also requires careful attention to confidentiality and security precautions as well as a large financial investment. Because adoption requires adjustments in almost every aspect of the practice's clinical and administrative work processes, it is important to understand what rewards and challenges are ahead.

IMPORTANCE OF ELECTRONIC RECORDS

Patients, health care providers, payment organizations, researchers, and public health services, among others, all benefit from an electronic health record system. Table 1-2 identifies some major benefits of an EHR as noted in a growing number of studies, and provides examples of each benefit.

In fact, a growing number of studies have found that miscommunications (including those responsible for adverse drug reactions), missing information, inaccurate information, inaccessible information through misfiles and inaccessible records, and mishandling of information are responsible for a significant portion of patient adverse events such as treatment complications or even death. As indicated in this chapter, the EHR responds to each of these problems. With benefits so obvious, what reasons are given for *not* adopting an electronic record?

Other studies have identified reasons that EHR adoption has not been more widespread. Among them are: lack of funding; lack of physician or staff support; insufficient time or knowledge on how to purchase, install, and implement a system; reluctance to make the changes in workflow required for success; costs overriding the benefits received from a system (return on investment); and difficulty in transferring a prior medical record into the new system. Other concerns often voiced involve: the complex security and confidentiality precautions that must be part of any comprehensive computer record system; technology barriers, including a lack of standards that would allow systems to share information; products and vendors that change frequently; patient fears, particularly in relation to confidentiality of information; and human resistance to change. Efforts must be spent to address all of these hurdles to successful implementation. The federal government is taking the lead in resolving several of these issues.

ELECTRONIC RECORD INITIATIVES

The movement toward electronic record systems in health care is evident throughout the United States. As a result of the studies previously noted, government groups as well as health care providers have become aware of the advantages of electronic systems. This will not be a quick or easy process. Electronic systems involve changes at every level of health care and by everyone that works or interacts with health care. The cost of new or updated systems is another challenge. However, the vision of a fully functioning system, with its potential for improving the quality of care and eventually reducing health care costs, provides the motivation to keep moving in that direction.

TABLE 1-2 Benefits of an Electronic Health Record

BENEFIT	EXAMPLES
Improves clinical decisions, supporting evidence-based medicine.	Access to medical, treatment, and medication research literature provides current information while care is under way. Imaging capabilities provide opportunities to exchange information among practitioners more quickly for expert interpretation.
Decreases errors.	System drug alerts highlight potential medication interactions or when diagnosis and gender do not agree. Documentation is legible.
Improves coordination of care.	Interoperability among clinical and administrative applications permits access to pertinent patient identification and clinical medical information among health care organizations and health care providers. No matter where the patient is located, important care information will be available. Pharmacy orders can be sent electronically.
Improves quality of care.	Timely diagnostic and therapy reports mean that treatment is more focused. Evaluation of treatment steps and outcomes against those of other providers helps to identify best practices and establish diagnosis-based treatment protocols.
Increases practice efficiency.	Information from a practice management system can be communicated to the care system and vice versa, eliminating duplicate data entry. More than one user can access a record at the same time. Provider documentation is recorded as it occurs, eliminating backlogs in charting. Bills are submitted and paid on a timely basis. Office workflow is streamlined.
Improves patient communication and satisfaction.	Accurate treatment decisions can contribute to a faster recovery. Patients can contribute medical information and gain access to information to help them better understand treatment and become true partners in their care. Patient appointment alerts can be generated automatically, supporting timely screening and follow-up care.
Easily provides data for research or disease monitors.	Data links easily can transfer information required for participation in approved research projects or state and federal government disease and biohazard reporting. Public health reporting and health data compiled about selected populations contribute to research on diagnosis and effective treatment of diseases, and the knowledge gained can be applied to individual cases. Earlier interventions and appropriate care result.
Decreases cost of care.	Efficiencies incorporated from the additional information available and from reduced duplication of testing can save money for the practice, the patient, and the entire health care system. The number of malpractice cases is reduced as a result of decreased risk of errors and greater patient satisfaction. Savings also are created from the elimination of paper record handling, photocopying, and storage and streamlined office processes.
Increases staff recruitment and productivity.	As more health profession students are exposed to electronic records and tools available in an EHR as part of their training, use in health care settings will be expected. Appropriate use of documentation templates and ease of data entry impacts productivity.

National, Regional, and State Efforts

Efforts are under way at national, regional, and state levels to encourage the adoption of EHRs. Many projects are sponsored by government groups, but others are private or cooperative efforts. For example, in 2004 President George W. Bush formed the **Office of the National Coordinator for Health Information Technology (ONC)** and made electronic health records a primary focus of that office. The stated goal was to have a national system, or **National Health Information Network (NHIN)**, in place by the year 2014 that permits sharing of health care data among those involved in health care provision. From the federal government's perspective, these efforts are aimed at reducing errors in medical treatment, decreasing costs, and increasing quality of health care in the United States. Educating consumers regarding EHRs is another focus; as an example of that effort, ONC launched a web site, HealthIT.gov (http://www.healthit.gov/), in 2011 to provide information for patients and providers on health information technology. For many of the same reasons, regional and local groups in many geographical areas within the United States have formed **Sub-Network Organizations (SNOs)**, also referred to generically as **Health Information Exchanges (HIEs)**. The network of Veterans Administration facilities that spans the entire nation is a prime example of an SNO. Exchanges that are specifically organized by geographic regions, such as a state or part of a state, may be referred to as **Regional Health Information Organizations (RHIOs)**. It is ONC's goal that state and regional efforts of this nature be aligned with national efforts.

Accountable Care Organizations (ACOs) are another type of network of health care providers that are tied together not only for the purpose of better serving a group of patients, but also for reducing costs for that selected patient population while focusing on maintaining quality of care. The proposed ACO integrated model begins with health care organizations and providers gathering data in a practice database and then sharing specific parts of their practice health data with defined groups, including other providers treating their patients who are part of an SNO, HIE, RHIO, or ACO network. In turn, the network provides information across the country to other providers or authorized individuals via an NHIN. These regional, distributed, and national networks share information regarding routine and emergency treatment, share information to monitor disease outbreaks and bioweapon attacks, share information to perform research, and share information to evaluate the quality of care (Mon, 2005).

In order to share information successfully within these types of regional, state, and national networks, data standards are required. Therefore, both federal government programs and voluntary cooperative efforts are under way to develop various types of standards for use within electronic health record systems. Discussion of these standards is included in each chapter of this textbook as they relate to the content of the chapter.

Standards being developed address everything from the clinical terminology that is used in the EHR systems to the functions that the EHR systems must perform. For example, in 2004, three national health care information management and technology associations came together to form the **Certification Commission for Healthcare Information Technology (CCHIT)**. This independent, nonprofit commission received a contract from the U.S. Department of Health and Human Services (HHS) to develop functional standards and a testing process to certify EHR products. The first efforts of the CCHIT focused on setting criteria and a certification process for ambulatory (physician office and clinic)

Office of the National Coordinator for Health Information Technology (ONC)
Federal government office introduced to lead and coordinate efforts toward a National Health Information Network.

National Health Information Network (NHIN)
National system under development that will permit electronic sharing of health care data among those involved in care provision across the United States.

Sub-Network Organizations (SNOs)
National, regional, or local efforts established for electronic sharing of patient health care data among care providers.

Health Information Exchange (HIE)
National, regional, or local efforts established for electronic sharing of patient health care data among care providers; subdivisions of the NHIN that also may be referred to as SNOs.

Regional Health Information Organizations (RHIOs)
Network of regional health care providers established for electronic sharing of patient health care data.

Accountable Care Organization (ACO)
A type of network of providers that are tied not only in serving a group of patients, but also in reducing costs for that selected population while focusing on quality of care.

EHR products. To gain certification, EHR products are inspected for their functionality (that is, what the EHR can do), interoperability (that is, can the EHR easily share information with another system), and security (that is, can the EHR adequately protect data from unauthorized access). The first "certified" ambulatory EHR vendor products were announced in July 2006. In 2007, the CCHIT began certifying inpatient care (acute hospital) products and has expanded to other types of health care settings since then.

Certification Commission for Healthcare Information Technology (CCHIT)
An independent, nonprofit organization formed to establish functional, interoperability, and security criteria and to certify EHR products as meeting those criteria.

Health Information Technology for Economic and Clinical Health Act (HITECH)
Legislation authorizing a process to certify organizations to perform product reviews on behalf of the government and to award grants for further adoption of EHRs.

Regional Health Information Technology Extension Centers (RECs)
Regional centers that offer technical assistance, guidance, and information on best practices to support and accelerate health care providers' efforts to become meaningful users of Electronic Health Records.

VistA-Office EHR
A component of the Veterans Administration's electronic health record system available for use in non-VA ambulatory care settings.

Centers for Medicare and Medicaid Services (CMS)
Federal government office that oversees the Medicare and Medicaid programs.

The next step in these EHR standard-setting efforts was part of the **Health Information Technology for Economic and Clinical Health Act (HITECH)** of 2009. Part of this legislation authorized ONC to set up a process to review and approve additional EHR certification organizations to perform EHR product reviews on behalf of the federal government. See Chapter 3 for further information about these ONC-Approved Certification and Testing Bodies.

The HITECH Act also includes several other efforts to encourage EHR adoption. For example, funding was provided to:

- [S]upport States to establish health information exchange (HIE) capability among health care providers and hospitals . . .
- [E]stablish **Regional Health Information Technology Extension Centers (RECs)** to offer technical assistance, guidance and information on best practices to support and accelerate health care providers' efforts to become meaningful users of EHRs . . .
- [F]und research focused on achieving breakthrough advances to address well-documented problems that have impeded adoption. . . . (United States Department of Health and Human Services, 2010)

Another barrier that has been addressed is funding assistance for health care provider practices. Effective October 2006, federal Stark regulations (regulations that greatly limit what type of assistance health care systems can provide to care providers) were loosened to permit some sharing of the costs of new systems between health care providers and health care organizations. Electronic prescribing and EHRs were both identified in Stark regulations. Several states also have provided low interest loan programs to support small physician practices with access to funds for EHR implementation projects. Some large health care systems are offering small clinics access to their EHR system through a technology-sharing arrangement. This shared arrangement greatly reduces EHR startup and maintenance costs while providing the practice with a state-of-the-art system and all the benefits of an EHR.

Four early national initiatives provided other funding examples. The federal government as well as health plans developed programs that rewarded practices incorporating EHRs, resulting in cost savings through efficiencies and improved patient management. Via contracted services, the federal government also encouraged further development of the Veterans Administration (VA) ambulatory record—**VistA-Office EHR**, a component of the VA's electronic health record—so that it could be used by those outside the VA at minimal cost. A third effort was headed by the **Centers for Medicare and Medicaid Services (CMS)**, the federal government office that oversees the Medicare and Medicaid programs. Through its contracted state **Quality Improvement Organizations (QIOs)**, CMS initiated programs that provided consultation to primary care practices with ten or fewer physicians regarding the choice and implementation of EHR systems. In return the QIOs received selected diagnostic and patient care information. An offshoot, an online interactive web training site, provided free education to small- and medium-sized physician practices on how to implement technology adoption.

The most recent effort to encourage adoption is funded by the federal HITECH Act of 2009. **Eligible providers (EPs)**, (see Table 1-3 for provider list) and eligible hospitals can qualify for Medicare or Medicaid incentive payments when they implement an EHR product that has been certified by one of the organizations approved by the federal government for that purpose, and use it in ways that meet the **"meaningful use"** objectives as defined by Medicare/Medicaid. "Meaningful use" relates to the actual ways that the EHR must be used to support efficient, quality, and coordinated patient care, which includes electronically exchanging information and being able to directly report quality measures information. "Meaningful use" incentive payments began in 2011 and are planned to continue through 2015 for those EPs who are able to continue to demonstrate they are using their EHR system in ways that meet the "meaningful use" criteria. "Meaningful use" criteria are to be released in three stages. Stage 1 criteria were released in February 2011, Stage 2 in August 2012, and Stage 3 criteria are expected to be released in a subsequent years. Pertinent "meaningful use" criteria from Stage 1 will be presented throughout the coming chapters as examples of these standards.

On the state level, legislation or special task force efforts encouraging EHR adoption through cooperative projects and funding support also are under way. For example, the HITECH Act is helping to fund Health Information Exchanges (HIEs) and Regional Health IT Extension Centers (RECs) at state or regional levels. In addition, some states such as Minnesota and Washington have passed legislation to provide grant funding to physician office practices to support steps toward implementation of an EHR. Due to the federal grants noted above, most states now also have initiatives in place to develop criteria for state health information networks, provide incentives for EHR implementation, and continue exploration of funding alternatives.

Quality Improvement Organization (QIO)
An organization that contracts with the federal government to perform tasks on its behalf under the Medicare program, focusing especially on quality and necessity of care issues.

eligible providers (EPs)
Health care providers that are qualified by regulations to participate in Medicare's or Medicaid's "meaningful use" incentive programs.

meaningful use
Relates to the actual ways that the EHR must be used to support patient care and specific ways that quality of care must be measured to receive incentive payments from Medicare and Medicaid Services as determined by the federal HITECH Act.

TABLE 1-3 Summary of the HITECH Act EHR Stage 1 Incentive Programs for EPs

	MEDICARE	MEDICAID
Eligible Providers (if a provider is eligible under both programs, a choice must be made between the two).	Doctors of medicine, osteopathy, dental surgery, dental medicine, podiatry, or optometry; chiropractors.	Physicians, nurse practitioners, certified nurse-midwives, dentists, some physician assistants.
EHR Functional Measures.	20 measures (15 core measures and 5/10 from choice menu).	Same, however states can require 4 from the choice menu.
Clinical Quality Measures.	6 measures (3 core and 3 from choice menu).	Same.
Administrative Authority.	Federal government.	State governments.
Maximum Incentive.	$44,000.	$63,750.
First Year to Begin the Program.	2011.	Depends on the state, 2011 in 21 states.
Last year to Begin the Program.	2014.	2016.

Health Care Provider Efforts

A fully functional EHR system cannot be implemented overnight in any setting. However, significant efforts are under way. Research has reported varying figures in relation to adoption. The 2009 National Ambulatory Care Study conducted by the National Center for Vital and Health Statistics (NCVHS) revealed that only 6.9% of the reporting physicians were using a fully functional EHR and 21.8% reported using a basic EHR system. Those figures can be compared to 4.5% and 16.9% respectively reported in 2008. A "basic" EHR system is defined as one that captures patient demographics, a patient problem list, clinical notes, orders for prescriptions, and that permits viewing of laboratory and imaging results. A "fully functional" EHR system is defined as one that includes all functions of the basic system, plus medical history and follow-up, orders for tests, prescription and test orders sent electronically, warnings of drug interactions or contraindications, highlighting of out-of-range test levels, and reminders for guideline-based interventions. Another national study from 2008, the National Ambulatory Medical Care Survey by the Centers for Disease Control and Prevention (CDC) had more positive findings. This survey questioned nonfederal, office-based physicians who primarily provided direct patient care. Resulting probability estimates indicated that 28.8% had all-electronic records and another 17.4% had part-paper and part-electronic records (CDC, 2010). Although progress is being made, universal use of EHRs is still a distant goal.

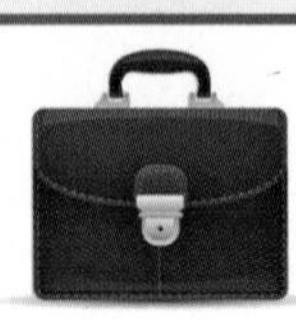

Case Situation

A group of five specialists from an existing multi-specialty clinic decided to leave the clinic and set up their own practice partnership. Because the new group practice must be organized from the ground up, the care providers decided to begin with an EHR system. They chose a vendor that provided both electronic medical record and practice management systems that interfaced with each other, although prior records brought to the practice were all paper-based. The chosen vendor was one that had received CCHIT certification for its products. The office administrator was the coordinator for the project. The practice used an information technology consultant for add-on design and implementation of the system, and it continues to use individuals outside the practice for technology support. Digital voice recording is used for dictation, and those who transcribe the recording have direct input to the medical record component of the EHR. Scheduling, billing, accounts management, and other business-related functions are performed with the practice management program, which permits data exchange with the medical record program. The group planned carefully for security, confidentiality, and remote backup of their system. In addition to the new software and hardware, the group updated telephone lines and other office equipment and also added laptop computers. All staff including care providers were trained prior to implementation and had ample opportunity to practice with the system before it went live. Problems discovered during training were "triaged" for either immediate attention or future resolution. As a result, the actual implementation, one provider at a time, went quite smoothly. Prior treatment paper records are being scanned into the system as time permits. This group has applied for incentives available under the HITECH "meaningful use" program.

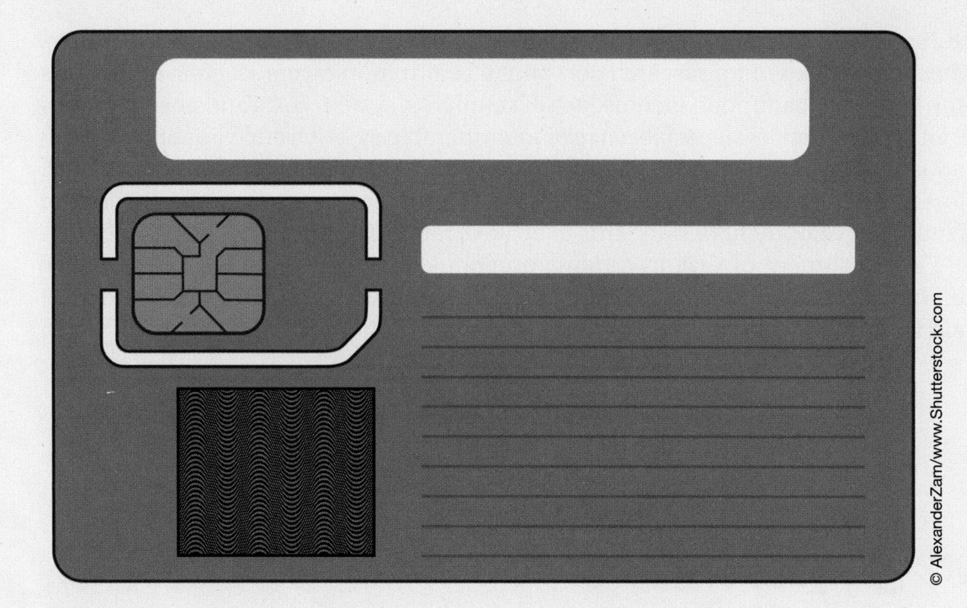

Figure 1–1 Smart Card example.

ELECTRONIC HEALTH RECORDS IN THE FUTURE

Imagine traveling anywhere in the world with the knowledge that, no matter what injury or sickness you encounter, health care providers will have access to your health care data. The information could be shared via an international network of secure health information or via data that you carry on a tamper-proof microprocessor, inserted into a **smart card** similar to a credit card (see Figure 1-1) or on a computer chip implanted in your body.

smart card
Patient-held portable summary of important health information digitized on a medium the size of a credit card.

Under this scenario, knowledge of life-threatening allergies and current medications can be considered immediately in treatment decisions. Information is then added to the source data so that follow-up care can be coordinated with the patient's primary physician once the individual returns home. Researchers using international databases are able to pinpoint locations of disease outbreaks as they occur, improving timely interventions. International research efforts via shared health care data-bases could find cures or effective treatments for some of the world's most devastating diseases. Quality and length of life might improve for millions. Certainly the EHR could not take full credit for these advances, but timely and accurate sharing of vital health care information is essential for them to occur.

SUMMARY

Electronic health records are defined as electronic medical records that are shared across multiple health care settings. Eight major EHR capability categories have been specified by the Institute of Medicine. These categories include health information and data, order entry and management, results management, decision support, electronic communication and connectivity, administrative processes, patient support, and reporting and population management. The benefits associated with use of EHRs include providing information for clinical decisions, improved continuity and quality of care, saving time and increasing efficiency, improving patient satisfaction and general quality of life, decreasing costs, contributing to information needed for research and public health monitoring, decreases in errors and increases in staff satisfaction. Hurdles to EHR adoption include lack of standards, system costs and need for funding support, lack of time to evaluate and implement systems, absence of interoperable systems and variability in vendors, security and privacy issues, and lack of confidence by providers and consumers as well as resistance to change. Each hurdle must be addressed. Efforts are under way from federal and state governments and geographic regions to deal with several of these issues, including development of standards to achieve interoperability of systems, adoption of clinical vocabulary standards, and establishment of various funding programs. Incentives for physician-practice adoption have taken a giant step forward with the passing and implementation of the federal HITECH Act in 2009 that established a Medicare/Medicaid Incentive Payment Program focused on achieving "meaningful use" of EHRs in health care practices by 2016.

Computer Exploration

1. The Centers for Medicare and Medicaid web site provides further information on the criteria for meaningful use of EHRs that will be used to provide practice incentive funding. Enter http://www.cms.gov/EHRIncentivePrograms/ in your browser and then click over "CMS EHR Meaningful Use Overview" found in a column of topics on the left side of the page. Describe the time frames used for the adoption phases.
2. The US Department of Health and Human Services web site provides descriptions of the eight HITECH Act Programs. Access the web site, http://healthit.hhs.gov then click over the topic "HITECH Programs" found in a list on the left side of the page. Read further about each of the programs. How does each program impact physician practices?
3. The list of organizations approved by ONC to certify EHR products as meeting "meaningful use" criteria can be found at the "Authorized Testing and Certification Bodies" (ACTB) link from the "Regulations and Guidelines" and then "Standards and Certification" sections of the Department of Health and Human Services home page at http://healthit.hhs.gov/. Access the list of approved organizations and then provide the following information:
   - **a.** How many organizations are currently approved by ONC as authorized testing and certifying bodies?
   - **b.** Of those organizations, how many certify complete EHRs and how many certify EHR modules?
4. Now choose the "Certified Health IT Product List" from the same standards subsection and respond to the following:
   - **a.** List the names of at least five companies that produce certified ambulatory care EHR software products.
   - **b.** Do these five companies offer modular or complete EHRs?
   - **c.** Which ONC certification organization approved their product?
5. Search the Internet and identify at least two companies that produce smart cards.
   - **a.** List the name of each company.
   - **b.** Compare the capabilities of the smart cards from the companies.
   - **c.** How are the smart cards of these two vendors currently being used?

REFERENCES

Centers for Disease Control and Prevention. (2010). National ambulatory medical care survey: 2008 summary tables. Retrieved from http://www.cdc.gov/nchs/ahed.htm

Institute of Medicine. (2003). *Key capabilities of an electronic health record system. Patient safety: Achieving a new standard of care*. Washington, DC: National Academies Press.

Mon, D. T. (2005). An update on the NHIN and RHIOs. *Journal of AHIMA, 76(6)*, 56–57, 59.

National Center for Health Statistics. (2009). National ambulatory care study. Retrieved from http://www.cdc.gov/nchs/data/hestat/emr_ehr_09/emr_ehr_09.pdf

The National Alliance for Health Information Technology. (2008). *Defining key health information technology terms*. Washington, DC: Office of the National Coordinator, Department of Health and Human Services.

US Department of Health and Human Services. (2010). HITECH programs. Retrieved from http://healthit.hhs.gov/

REVIEW QUESTIONS

1. In addition to hardware and software, the EHR includes other components. List three other components and describe their role in the EHR.

2. Define the following concepts:

   a. alerts

   b. interoperability

   c. data repository

   d. reminders

   e. treatment protocols

   f. telemonitoring

   g. smart card

3. The practice submits a complete bill to Blue Cross for services provided to patient Janet Smith. Which of the eight core EHR capabilities is being described?

4. The practice submits data electronically to the state's health department on a child who has evidence of abuse. Which of the eight core EHR capabilities is being described?

5. Provide a practice setting example for each of the following EHR benefits:

   a. clinical decision support

   b. coordination of care

   c. quality of care

   d. time savings and increased efficiency

   e. increased patient communication and satisfaction

   f. decreased errors or cost

   g. data for research and public health monitoring

   h. increased productivity and staff satisfaction

6. List at least five reasons given by practices for their reluctance to adopt an EHR.

7. Describe the role of the ONC, NHIN, SNO/HIE/RHIO/ACO, REC, and groups such as the CCHIT in relation to the electronic health record.

8. VistA-Office EHR and the HITECH Act are potential efforts to address the cost of an EHR.

   a. Which is an adaptation of the Veterans Administration electronic record?

   b. Which would provide incentives to physicians for meeting EHR-related "meaningful use" criteria?

9. According to the CDC, what percentage of office-based physician practices had a fully functional EHR in 2008?

CHAPTER 2 Taking Steps Toward a Successful EHR Implementation

CHAPTER OUTLINE

OBJECTIVES

Upon completion of the chapter, the learner will be able to:

1. List the four major phases of work associated with an electronic health record (EHR) project.
2. Locate credible and useful web-based resources to support health care provider practices through each phase of an EHR project.
3. Describe the role that Regional HIT Extension Centers are funded to play in support of EHR implementations in physician office practices.
4. Identify the basic activities that must be taken to investigate an EHR product before a final selection decision.
5. Use the Internet to access four nationally recognized sources for identifying and evaluating ambulatory EHR products, and compare the types of EHR product information provided by these sources.
6. List five major interrelated activities that are essential to complete during the implementation phase (before "go-live") of an EHR project.

KEY TERMS

CCHIT Functional Criteria for Ambulatory EHRs

Certified Health IT Product List (CHPL)

EHR goals

EHR project plan

EHR vision

functional requirements

Health IT Adoption Toolbox

Health Information Technology Toolkit for Physician Offices

implementation activities

Medicare/Medicaid EHR Certification Standards for "Meaningful Use"

readiness assessment

Regional HIT Extension Centers (RECs)

request for proposal (RFP)

vendor selection

INTRODUCTION

As discussed in Chapter 1, there are a significant number of activities underway at national, regional, and state levels to encourage the adoption of EHR systems; at the national level specifically they are the activities funded under the ARRA's HITECH Act and the Center for Medicare and Medicaid's "Meaningful Use" Incentive Payment Program. These efforts are focused on encouraging and supporting EHR implementations in the health care provider practice setting. Anyone preparing to work in a health care provider office must develop a clear understanding of how an EHR project and an EHR system will affect how that office functions. This chapter will provide an overview of the phases of work associated with bringing clinicians and office staff through a project that concludes with the successful implementation of an EHR in a health care provider practice setting.

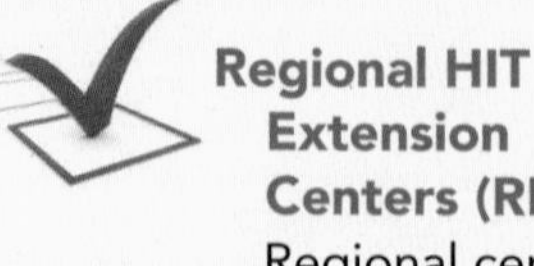

Regional HIT Extension Centers (RECs) Regional centers that offer technical assistance, guidance, and information on best practices to support and accelerate health care providers' efforts to become meaningful users of Electronic Health Records.

Health IT Adoption Toolbox Developed by HHS's Health Resources and Services Administration (HRSA), this toolkit is a compilation of planning, implementation, and evaluation resources to help community health centers, other safety net providers, and ambulatory care providers implement health IT applications in their facilities. Staff from community health centers and a variety of stakeholders in the health IT arena have reviewed and contributed to the toolbox to ensure the resources are accurate, relevant, and effective in supporting health IT in health centers.

Health Information Technology Toolkit for Physician Offices Developed by Stratis Health, this toolkit helps physician offices assess their readiness, plan, select, implement, make effective use of, and exchange important information about the clients they serve. The toolkit contains numerous resources, including tools for telehealth, health information exchange, and personal health records.

TAKING STEPS TOWARD THE EHR

Making the transition from a paper-based health record system to a computer-based one is a significant project for any health care organization, including the health care provider office practice. Suzanne Columbus (2006) advises that "the first things a practice needs are time, stamina and leadership" because the "average implementation for a solo practitioner can take anywhere from 12 to 18 months, including planning, design, implementation and training."

There are numerous resources available to health care provider practices to support them in their efforts to plan for and implement an EHR system. Three excellent resources are described here:

1. The HITECH Act 2009 called for the creation of over 60 **Regional HIT Extension Centers (RECs)** across the nation to provide health care providers with low-cost access to training, information, guidance and technical support in their efforts to select, implement, and effectively use an EHR system in their practice setting. A full listing of grant-funded Regional HIT Extension Centers is available at http://www.healthit.gov/rec#listing.
2. The U.S. Department of Health and Human Services' Health Research and Services Administration (HRSA) **Health IT Adoption Toolbox** located at http://www.hrsa.gov/healthit/toolbox/HealthITAdoptiontoolbox/index.html.
3. Stratis Health's **Health Information Technology Toolkit for Physician Offices** located at http://www.stratishealth.org/expertise/healthit/clinics/clinictoolkit.html.

The four common steps an organization must take when it makes a commitment to an EHR project are:

- Assessing
- Planning
- Selecting
- Implementing

A brief discussion of these basic steps and associated activities is presented here.

Step One: Assess

When a practice makes the strategic decision to adopt an EHR and commits financial resources to it, an important first step is a **readiness assessment** to gain a baseline understanding of the practice's long-term EHR vision. Commonly the readiness assessment focuses on several aspects of the practice's current status:

- Clinician and staff attitudes toward the EHR.
- Clinician and staff skills.
- Financial situation.
- IT systems and staffing.

Sample assessment tools are available for each. Figures 2-1 and 2-2 provide example content from the HIT attitudes assessment and IT staffing inventory tools from the Stratis Health Information Technology Toolkit for Physician Offices. The data collected through these tools helps the practice understand the issues, concerns, and training needs of its staff that must be addressed as the practice moves from a paper-based to a computer-based health record system.

Step Two: Plan

Using the information gained from the Step One "Assess" activities, the practice can define its EHR vision and the goals it wants to achieve by implementing an EHR system. Then an EHR project plan designed to achieve the practice's vision and goals can be developed. The **EHR project plan** documents the organization's vision, goals, and anticipated schedule and budget for selecting a vendor and for completing EHR implementation activities.

The **EHR vision** is the desired future state of the health care provider office practice once the EHR is fully implemented. A vision can be presented in words or in graphic form. Typically, EHR visions speak to the practice's desire to have real-time access "24/7" to each patient's past and current clinical information in order to improve the efficiency of the practice, to improve the quality of care provided to its patients, and to increase patient satisfaction with the services they receive.

The **EHR goals** set by health care provider office practices usually concern improvements in clinical and office work processes or improvements in the outcomes of patient care to be achieved as a result of implementing the EHR system. Reductions in the cost of providing care as well as increasing patient satisfaction with the practice's services and/or staff satisfaction with their work are also common goals established for EHR systems.

The remainder of the project plan usually outlines several phases of work. The project plan also provides an estimate of the staff time that must be dedicated to each phase. For example, preparing the physical space and hardware infrastructure involves purchasing equipment and installing communications lines. At the same time, the practice likely will review its workflows as well as its policies and procedures to identify where changes or a redesign might be needed. It may be necessary for the practice to hire extra staff to handle some parts of the project implementation effort and/or to provide temporary backup staff for regular practice staff when regular practice staff are needed for EHR project work.

Step Three: Select

With the project plan in hand, the practice is ready to step into EHR **vendor selection** activities. The group who leads the vendor selection effort must include representatives from the clinical, administrative, and office areas of the

readiness assessment
Evaluation of a practice's work, workflow, existing technologies, applications, hardware, etc., to determine its status in preparation for EHR implementation.

EHR project plan
Anticipated schedule and budget for selecting a vendor and completing EHR implementation.

EHR vision
A statement of the desired future state of a health care practice once the EHR is fully implemented.

EHR goals
Statements regarding desired improvements in clinical and/or office processes or in outcomes of patient care as a result of EHR implementation.

vendor selection
The process of developing a request for proposal, receiving vendor responses, and evaluating them against established criteria in order to determine a specific EHR product for implementation.

STRATIS HEALTH | HEALTH INFORMATION TECHNOLOGY TOOLKIT | PHYSICIAN OFFICES

Section 1.1 Adopt – Assess

HIT Attitudes Assessment

Use this assessment to help understand your organization's readiness for adopting an electronic health record (EHR) and other health information technology (HIT). Understanding early attitudes and beliefs can help with effectively planning and providing the right education.

Instructions for Use: Surveying and Determining Results

1. Distribute the survey below in paper and/or electronic form to all staff at your clinic. Indicate a relatively short response time; one or two weeks is plenty of time to respond.
2. Do not circulate the interpretation of results as part of the survey. You will use the interpretation information to help your HIT steering committee and organizational leadership understand the results. You may then share other forms of the results with the entire community of respondents.
3. Once you have received all of the completed surveys, tally the results for each of the three respondent position types (physicians, nurses and other clinicians, administrative/operations staff) and record results using the results form below (one form for each position type). If you have several different facilities, you may want to tally by facility as well. Record the number of respondents and the percent responding from all potential respondents in the category. For example, if you have 12 physicians on the medical staff at your clinic and receive seven responses—that is a 58 percent response rate. In addition to the actual responses, the response rate is a factor that may indicate level of interest.
4. The structure of the questions is designed to prevent someone from merely selecting answers in only one category (e.g., all Agree). Some statements are written in a manner that agreement might be considered a negative; other statements are written so agreement might be a positive. Agreement may be a risk factor (denoted by red), a cautionary area (denoted by yellow), or a strength (denoted by green).
5. Once you have tallied all responses, identify how many statements are in each of the risky (red), cautionary (yellow), and strength (green) areas. If many statements reflect risk, this obviously indicates a high overall risk. In this case, your challenge is considerable education and careful planning. A small number of statements with risk generally indicates overall interest and comfort with HIT—and the areas of risk can be relatively easily targeted in your educational activities.
6. Use the information in the Interpreting Results section to initiate discussion in your organization. Plan what you will do for each area of risk.

Section 1.1 Adopt – Assess – HIT Attitudes Assessment - 1

Figure 2-1 Example readiness assessment tool: HIT attitudes assessment.

HIT Attitudes Assessment

This assessment will help us understand the organization's readiness for adopting an electronic health record (EHR) and other health information technology (HIT). At this time, we are seeking your impressions about potentially adopting EHR or other HIT. This will help us with effectively planning and providing the right education for everyone.

Instructions

Please complete this survey and return to: ______________________ by: ____________.

Indicate your position by checking the appropriate box:

☐ Physician
☐ Nurse and other clinician (e.g., PA, RN, CMA, dietician, lab tech, pharmacist, PT, social worker)
☐ Administrative/operations staff (e.g., administrator, biller, coder, communications/customer services, finance, reception/front desk, scheduling, IT)

Note: If you are a physician/clinician with administrative responsibilities, please check only physician or other clinician.

Concerning HIT and EHR, check the column that most closely describes how you feel about each of the following statements:	Strongly Agree	Agree	Neutral	Disagree	Strongly Disagree
1. HIT, in general, increases overall efficiency.					
2. Computerized alerts and reminders can be annoying.					
3. Our patients and/or their families expect us to use a computer for their records.					
4. HIT and EHR will improve my personal productivity.					
5. HIT and EHR are difficult to learn how to use.					
6. Use of HIT and EHR in front of patients or their family members is depersonalizing.					
7. HIT is not as accurate or complete as paper records.					
8. HIT improves quality of care and patient safety.					
9. Once all documents are scanned into the system, we will have a complete EHR.					
10. A first step toward a successful EHR is addressing workflow and process improvements.					
11. We are in an age where we must exchange data electronically with others and HIT helps us do this.					
12. Health care is too complex anymore without access to clinical decision support provided by HIT.					
13. HIT is not as secure as paper records.					
14. We cannot afford an EHR.					
15. HIT can have unintended consequences if we don't apply professional judgment in its use.					

Section 1.1 Adopt – Assess – HIT Attitudes Assessment - 2

Figure 2-1 *(Continues)*

(Continued)

Results Form for (Select position type: Physicians, Other clinicians, or Administrative/operations staff)

Responses from facility ______________________ (insert number responding and percent response)

Concerning HIT and EHR, participants checked the column that most closely describes how they feel about each of the following statements:	Strongly Agree	Agree	Neutral	Disagree	Strongly Disagree
1. HIT, in general, increases overall efficiency.					
2. Computerized alerts and reminders can be annoying.					
3. Our patients and/or their families likely are expecting us to use a computer for their records.					
4. HIT will improve my personal productivity.					
5. HIT and EHR are difficult to learn how to use.					
6. Use of HIT in front of patients or their family members is depersonalizing.					
7. HIT is not as accurate or complete as paper records.					
8. HIT improves quality of care and patient safety.					
9. Once all documents are scanned into the system, we will have a complete EHR.					
10. A first step toward a successful EHR is addressing workflow and process improvements.					
11. We are in an age where we must exchange data electronically with others and HIT helps us do this.					
12. Health care is too complex anymore without access to clinical decision support provided by HIT.					
13. HIT is not as secure as paper records.					
14. We cannot afford an EHR.					
15. HIT can have unintended consequences if we don't apply professional judgment in its use.					
Date Completed:					
Total	**Strength:**		**Caution:**	**Risk:**	
Highlight or circle the statements above where responses indicate a risk factor for the organization.					

Interpreting Results

Use the following information to initiate discussion about your findings:

1. **HIT, in general, increases overall efficiency.** Physician offices have many ways to become more efficient through greater access to data, more complete and legible documentation, and reducing rework. Agreement with this statement is healthy, although interpretation must be coupled with an analysis of the response to statement #4. Many people believe in overall efficiency, but won't accept changes for personal productivity gains. Disagreement with this statement may require you to give more specific examples of HIT functionality and more thorough expectation setting.

Section 1.1 Adopt – Assess – HIT Attitudes Assessment - 3

Figure 2-1

2. **Computerized alerts and reminders can be annoying.** Provision of alerts and reminders is an inherent, but not the only, part of clinical decision support. Too many alerts can be annoying, but having none defeats the purpose of HIT. A balance of agreement and disagreement may reflect the appropriate skepticism for finding just the right level of alerting. Strong agreement with this statement may demonstrate resistance to change; strong disagreement may be unrealistic.
3. **Our patients and/or their families likely are expecting us to use a computer for their records.** Many more patients and their family members have used or use computers than health care delivery organizations realize. Increasingly more patients and their family members wonder about how well their clinicians are keeping up to date if they are not using computers. Agreement with this statement recognizes that patients and their families have an important role to play in health care. Disagreement with this statement identifies the need for managing change in staff and patients/their families.
4. **HIT will improve my personal productivity.** Setting realistic expectations about productivity is important. Some physicians and clinicians have heard that using a computer takes longer; others expect to see great time savings. Strong agreement with this statement may reflect unrealistic expectations. Agreement is the desired state. Disagreement with this statement may signal the need for education, especially in reassuring clinicians that typing proficiency is not required for their use of HIT.
5. **HIT and EHR are difficult to learn how to use.** Some skepticism about the difficulty of learning to use HIT and EHR is healthy; being overconfident (strong disagreement) of one's ability to learn to use HIT and EHR can actually work against its adoption. Even if some physicians or clinicians may have used HIT at another organization, they still will have a learning curve with any new HIT or EHR. Any of the middle-of-the-road answers to this question are generally considered a good sign of readiness. Strong agreement may be evidence of resistance to change.
6. **Use of EHR in front of patients is depersonalizing.** Use of EHR at the point of care is essential to gain quality, safety, and efficiency value. Studies demonstrate that the perception of depersonalization is a physician/clinician perception not shared by most individuals. Agreement with this statement signals that physicians/clinicians may not be confident in their computer skills or are generally resistant to change. New forms of communication with patients and their families may need to be introduced. Role playing with staff is a good strategy to overcome this concern.
7. **HIT is not as accurate or complete as paper records.** This concern has arisen because unintended consequences with HIT have occurred (see also statement #15) and of how different the output of HIT may be in relationship to the paper record. Agreement with this statement demonstrates potential resistance to change. It indicates a need for education about what is possible to accomplish with HIT and viewing HIT as a tool, not a substitute for the physician/clinician. Care also must be taken to ensure that all forms of documentation improvement and data quality auditing normally done with paper records is not eliminated in the electronic environment.
8. **EHR improves quality of care and patient safety.** A primary purpose of EHR is to improve safety and quality of care. These are essential goals and if not recognized could be an issue in gaining adoption of EHR. However, EHR alone does not improve safety and quality of care, so strong agreement could signal unrealistic expectations.

Section 1.1 Adopt – Assess – HIT Attitudes Assessment - 4

Figure 2-1 *(Continues)*

(*Continued*)

9. **Once all documents are scanned into the system, we will have a complete EHR.** This belief arises because many health care organizations have used document scanning to supplement various electronic applications to reduce the risks of a hybrid record environment. Unfortunately, while some risk is reduced, other potential new risks remain because scanned documents may be more difficult to retrieve than paper charts, and they do not generate clinical decision support. Agreement with this statement suggests a narrow view of what constitutes HIT, especially an EHR.
10. **A first step toward a successful EHR is addressing workflow and process improvements.** Agreement with this statement represents a strong understanding of EHR and willingness to change. The vast majority of EHR failures have come about because workflow and process changes were not attended to. Disagreement puts the organization at high risk and must be addressed through leadership commitment to the time and resources needed to address this.
11. **We are in an age where we must exchange data electronically with others and HIT helps us do this.** Cautious optimism might be the best response about exchanging data electronically, especially as systems are not fully interoperable and full-blown interfaces actually may not be necessary where access to summaries or ability to view data may be sufficient. Disagreement suggests resistance to change.
12. **Health care is too complex anymore without access to clinical decision support provided by HIT.** Improvement in quality of care is probably the primary long-term benefit of HIT. Disagreement with this statement may suggest that current quality issues are not recognized, or suggest a lack of appreciation for HIT functionality.
13. **HIT is not as secure as paper records.** HIT can be made more secure than paper records if policies about security access controls, audit trails, and proper workstation utilization measures are adopted. Disagreement with this statement suggests need for education about computer security and commitment to policy enforcement.
14. **We are not able to afford an EHR.** A healthy skepticism about cost is important. Strong disagreement suggests an unrealistic view of resource requirements; strong agreement may be used as an excuse not to acquire an EHR for other reasons.
15. **HIT can have unintended consequences if we don't apply professional judgment in its use.** A number of articles have recently described problems with unintended consequences of HIT. Virtually all of the articles, or at least responses to the articles, have recognized that in large measure the results have come about because of lack of attention to workflow and process design, or because of reliance solely on the computer rather than professional judgment.

For support using the toolkit

Stratis Health • Health Information Technology Services

952-854-3306 • info@stratishealth.org

www.stratishealth.org

StratisHealth

Section 1.1 Adopt – Assess – HIT Attitudes Assessment - 5

Figure 2-1

STRATIS HEALTH　HEALTH INFORMATION TECHNOLOGY TOOLKIT　PHYSICIAN OFFICES

Section 1.1 Adopt - Assess

IT Staffing Inventory

Use this IT Staffing Inventory to help you determine what IT staffing skills may be needed to implement specific health information technology (HIT).

Instructions for Use

1. Consider using different forms if you are planning multiple HIT projects. Otherwise, identify the specific project for which the first inventory is conducted and update the form for any subsequent projects as needed.
2. Review the column of IT Skills and check off the Skills Needed for the project under consideration. Where choices exist, be specific. For example, in Applications, do you need a person with Java or C++ programming skills? If you have not selected a product yet, you may need to put "?" in this column until you determine skills.
3. Identify the IT Staff, Clinicians, and Other Staff by name, who have the skills needed. For example, for implementing clinical messaging, in addition to IT staff to participate in hardware installation and network connectivity, clinicians should be involved in some of the workflow and implementation functions.
4. Identify in the Plan for Acquiring Skills column how you will go about getting the skills—hire additional staff, send existing staff to training, use a third party temporarily or permanently, etc.

HIT Project: (describe) Completed by: (names) Date inventory completed: (date)

IT Skills	Skills Needed	IT Staff (Names)	Clinicians (Names)	Other Staff (Names)	Third Party	Plan for Acquiring Skills
Strategy and Planning						
1. Maintain strategic IT plan (1.1 Visioning and Strategic Planning, and 1.1 Application Interface Inventory) consistent with financial/operational/clinical needs						
2. Keep abreast of technical, application, and industry progress and events						
3. Keep abreast of clinician needs to be sure current IT program is responsive						
4. Maintain good relations with vendors						
5. Develop and monitor IT budget: capital and operations (1.2 Total Cost of Ownership and Return on Investment)						

Section 1.1 Adopt – Assess – IT Staffing Inventory - 1

Figure 2-2 Example readiness assessment tool: IT staffing inventory. (*Continues*)

(Continued)

IT Skills	Skills Needed	IT Staff (Names)	Clinicians (Names)	Other Staff (Names)	Third Party	Plan for Acquiring Skills
6. Participate in vendor analysis, selection, and contracting (Adopt-Select section)						
Implementation						
1. Plan implementation details, including rollout strategy, consistent with contract (Utilize-Implement section)						
2. Manage implementation plan, including issues resolution (2.1 Issues Management)						
3. Assist in mapping current processes and identifying opportunities for improvement (1.2 Workflow and Process Redesign, and 2.1 Workflow and Process Improvement)						
4. Assist in recommending chart conversion and hybrid record risk management strategies (1.2 Chart Conversion Planning)						
5. Acquire vendor certification, if necessary						
6. Develop or manage development of interfaces (2.1 System Build)						
7. Perform system build to configure system for organizational needs (2.1 System Build)						
8. Conduct HIT system testing (2.1 Testing Plan)						
9. Maintain change control log as changes are made during implementation or ongoing use (2.1 Change Control)						
10. Recommend and perform appropriate file and data conversions						
11. Assist in training users (2.1 Training Plan)						
12. Support go-live preparation and actualization (2.1 Go-live Checklist)						
Operations						
1. Perform ongoing system utilization monitoring; use in overall capacity planning						

Section 1.1 Adopt – Assess – IT Staffing Inventory - 2

Figure 2-2

IT Skills	Skills Needed	IT Staff (Names)	Clinicians (Names)	Other Staff (Names)	Third Party	Plan for Acquiring Skills
2. Perform system backup; monitor fail-over server as applicable						
3. Perform daily/weekly/monthly/year end processing as required						
4. Assure good response time and little/no system downtime						
5. Assure network performance at optimal levels						
6. Order and maintain adequate stock of supplies (spare equipment, batteries, cables, storage media, etc.)						
7. Install vendor-provided updates, releases, patches; maintain version control						
Help Desk Functions						
1. Respond to routine questions and problems regarding software; appropriately escalate to vendor						
2. Knowledge of operating systems as applicable: (e.g., Windows, Linux, Oracle, SQL, Unix, Open VMS)						
3. Respond to routine questions and problems regarding hardware; appropriately escalate to vendor						
4. Respond to routine questions and problems regarding network and telecommunications; appropriately escalate to vendor						
5. Provide refresher training on applications to staff as needed; train new and temporary staff on applications						
6. Reset passwords as applicable						
Security (1.1 HIT Security Risk Analysis)						
1. Conduct security risk analysis to determine appropriate levels of security measures for environment; perform periodic security evaluation						

Section 1.1 Adopt – Assess – IT Staffing Inventory - 3

Figure 2-2 (*Continues*)

(Continued)

IT Skills	Skills Needed	IT Staff (Names)	Clinicians (Names)	Other Staff (Names)	Third Party	Plan for Acquiring Skills
2. Maintain access control lists and establish access (assign unique user ID and password or other authentication methods) as authorized and consistent with access control policy						
3. Maintain audit controls; review logs to identify potential confidentiality issues						
4. Develop and implement sound security procedures in relation to organizational policy, HIPAA, HITECH, and other regulatory requirements						
5. Provide periodic training and reminders about security						
6. Maintain disaster recovery and business continuity plans. Periodically perform tests/drills (1.1 HIT Security Risk Analysis)						
7. Protect information assets from external threats (e.g., malware protection, intrusion detection/prevention, firewalls)						
8. Respond to security incidents and maintain security incident reports; appropriately escalate to practice management and/or authorities						
9. Set up a virtual private network (VPN)						
10. Establish digital signature as applicable						
11. Manage device and media security, destruction and disposal						
Applications						
1. Ensure applications are kept current (e.g., clinical practice guidelines, clinical decision support rules, data sets, codes, vocabulary)						
2. Utilize vendor-supplied toolset to customize screens and templates as necessary (Examples: PowerBuilder, MS Visual Studio, Visual Basic, C++, Java, M, Delphi)						

Section 1.1 Adopt -- Assess – IT Staffing Inventory - 4

Figure 2-2

IT Skills	Skills Needed	IT Staff (Names)	Clinicians (Names)	Other Staff (Names)	Third Party	Plan for Acquiring Skills
3. Maintain intranet and internal Web site						
4. Maintain Web portals, personal health record, and other Internet-based applications						
5. Maintain interfaces as applications using HL7 and other standard protocols are upgraded						
6. Produce reports using various report writers (Examples: Crystal, Easytrieve, FoxFire, MS SQL)						
Database						
1. Develop and carry out plan to manage data storage						
2. Maintain data models and dictionaries						
3. Maintain master person index/record locator service						
4. Audit data entry quality						
5. Optimize database performance (DBMS examples: DB2, Informix, MS Access, Oracle, MS SQL, Sybase, MUMPS, Caché)						
Network						
1. Manage network servers						
2. Install and maintain wireless access points and other devices as applicable for wireless access						
3. Install and maintain routers, hubs, and other network devices and netware, as applicable for local area network						
4. Manage VoIP as applicable						
Hardware						
1. Install, inventory, and maintain workstations, printers, and other peripherals						
2. Install and maintain servers: main, fail-over, back up, email, Fax, others						
3. Manage storage devices; storage area network						

Section 1.1 Adopt – Assess – IT Staffing Inventory - 5

Figure 2-2 *(Continues)*

(Continued)

IT Skills	Skills Needed	IT Staff (Names)	Clinicians (Names)	Other Staff (Names)	Third Party	Plan for Acquiring Skills
4. Install and maintain Citrix, VMware as needed						
5. Construct and maintain data center in keeping with user system availability and disaster recovery requirements						
6. Develop hardware replacement/upgrade schedule						

For support using the toolkit

Stratis Health • Health Information Technology Services

952-854-3306 • info@stratishealth.org

www.stratishealth.org

StratisHealth

Section 1.1 Adopt – Assess – IT Staffing Inventory - 6

Figure 2-2

practice. This interdisciplinary task group will define the **functional requirements** for their EHR product. The EHR selection task group will obtain input from the future EHR users within the practice's staff (clinicians and office personnel) in order to finalize the EHR functional requirements. The functional requirements document clearly identifies and describes the expectations that clinicians and office staff have of the EHR so it can be a useful tool in their work. The functional requirements are used to develop a **request for proposal (RFP)**. An RFP is a document constructed by an organization and used by the organization to solicit bids from potential vendors for a product or service. The RFP will be sent to a small number of potential EHR product vendors.

As mentioned in Chapter 1, the Certification Commission on Health Information Technology's **CCHIT Functional Criteria for Ambulatory EHRs** standards are an excellent resource for identifying and describing the functions associated with state-of-the-art ambulatory EHR vendor products. The CCHIT criteria are based on broad-based health care industry expectations for EHR performance capabilities. Additionally, the ONC-ATCBs (see Chapter 3) utilize the **Medicare/Medicaid EHR Certification Standards for "Meaningful Use,"** published in 2010, to certify EHR products as being capable of supporting the Medicare/Medicaid "meaningful use" requirements. The health care practice can use the EHR functional criteria associated with either or both of these certifications as a starting point to identify its functional requirements.

Selecting the handful of EHR vendors who will receive the practice's RFP is also a challenge because the EHR vendor market is quite large. There are four excellent resources to help the EHR selection task group with this important task:

1. The EHR products that have been ONC-ATCB certified to support ambulatory practice sites are identified within the **Certified Health IT Product List (CHPL)** located at http://onc-chpl.force.com/ehrcert. It is free and open to the public.
2. CCHIT (http://www.cchit.org) provides a listing of "certified" ambulatory EHR products. The CCHIT site is also free and open to the public.
3. Center for Health Information Technology (http://www.centerforhit.org) provides a Physician Product Reviewer/EHR User Directory that is available only to individuals who are members of the American Academy of Family Practice (AAFP). It provides EHR product ratings that have been submitted voluntarily by AAFP members who currently are using an EHR in their practice. Reviewers use a five-point scale to rate products on quality, price, support, ease of use, and impact on productivity. The reviewers do not evaluate each product's functionality, but they do include information on practice sizes and locations.
4. The Medical Strategic Planning (MSP) EHR Selector™ product (http://www.ehrselector.com) is available to individual physician practices on a six-month or one-year subscription basis. A discounted subscription fee is available if the physician is a member of one of a group of "collaborator organizations". This online database provides comparisons of EHR products on important characteristics, including:
   - Practice size
   - Specialties using the product
   - Product features and functions
   - Standard codes and vocabularies
   - Training and support
   - Contract details

functional requirements Descriptions of the specific capabilities needed within an EHR to meet the goals of the practice.

request for proposal (RFP) An RFP is a document constructed by an organization and used by the organization to solicit bids from potential vendors for a product or service.

CCHIT Functional Criteria for Ambulatory EHRs Standards set by the CCHIT for the tasks an EHR must perform before it is approved as meeting the processing requirements in the ambulatory care environment.

Medicare/Medicaid EHR Certification Standards for "Meaningful Use" Standards set by the National Institute for Standards and Technology (NIST) for the tasks an EHR must perform before it is approved as meeting the Medicare/Medicaid "meaningful use" requirements in the ambulatory care environment.

Certified Health IT Product List (CHPL) Official listing of EHR vendor products certified to meet the Medicare/Medicaid "Meaningful Use" functional criteria.

This type of product comparison data can greatly assist the practice in selecting those EHR products and vendors that most closely meet their practice needs.

To meet the obligation to investigate fully the appropriateness, reliability, and stability of the EHR product and the EHR product vendor before a final decision is made, the practice's EHR selection task group must:

- Schedule on-site EHR-scripted product demonstrations that are focused on functions important to the practice's EHR users. Figure 2-3 provides excerpts from a demonstration script.
- Perform reference checks and site visits to other practice sites that have implemented comparable products from the vendor.
- Negotiate a contract that specifies precisely what is being acquired and also specifies the obligations of all parties regarding the implementation and ongoing support of the EHR system.

Users: a primary care physician, a nurse, a medical assistant
Script Patient: Jason Blue, birthdate 05/01/2007
Parent: Paula Blue
Address: 221 Jay Circle, Benton, OK

Activity	Expected Result	Pass with Comment	Fail with Comment
1. Log-in as medical assistant	Successful log-in		
2. Look up patient record for Jason Blue	Jason Blue (DOB 05/01/2007) is located		
3. Document reason for visit: "frequent headaches"	System accepts reasons for visit documentation		
4. Review allergy list and add "peanut" allergy	Updated allergy list		
5. Log-in as nurse	Successful log-in		
6. Use a template to enter vital signs: BP 90/55 Temp (oral) 98.6 F Pulse 80 Respirations 20	Template accepts the vital signs data and displays it		
7. Log-in as physician	Successful log-in		
8. Use a Pediatric "frequent headaches" template to document the assessment and plan of care	A pediatric template for "frequent headaches" exists and appropriately supports documentation of the assessment and plan of care		
9. Create a prescription for a medication	The prescription order is accepted by the system, the prescription prints and the medication list displays this newly prescribed medication		

Figure 2-3 Sample excerpt of an EHR demonstration script.

The Healthcare Information and Management System Society offers some excellent advice on Selecting the Right EMR Vendor in a brochure available free through its Web site: http://www.himss.org/content/files/SelectingEMR_Flyer2.pdf. In addition, excellent vendor evaluation, selection, and contracting guidance can be accessed through a Regional HIT Extension Center (REC).

Step Four: Implement

When the vendor contract is signed, **implementation activities** begin, setting in motion a complex set of interrelated activities that must be completed before the practice can "go live" with its EHR system. Specifically, these activities include:

- Establishing the technology setup (hardware, network, interface, and telecommunications).
- Customizing the EHR software (also known as doing "the build") so it will be tailored to the specific needs of the practice.
- Determining the processes and procedures for handling the paper documents associated with each patient's health record.
- Developing and/or revising policies and procedures that assure EHR system compliance with privacy, security, and legal requirements.
- Conducting the training sessions needed to assure that the practice's clinical and office staff are well prepared to "go live" with the EHR. Training must include lessons on navigating the EHR software and understanding the new workflows associated with using the EHR system in the patient care process and administrative processes of the practice.

implementation activities
A series of interrelated steps that must be completed before a practice can "go live" with a chosen EHR system.

The success of an EHR implementation is measured by the degree to which it effectively supports the day-to-day tasks and activities of each of its users within the practice setting. Each of these implementation steps must receive adequate attention in order to achieve that measure of success; failure to do so will limit the acceptance of the EHR and diminish its ability to contribute to improved efficiency and enhanced quality of care within the practice setting.

Once again, excellent implementation guidance can be accessed through a Regional HIT Extension Center (REC), the Stratis Health HIT Toolkit for Physician Offices, and the HRSA Health IT Adoption Toolbox described earlier in this chapter.

SUMMARY

When a health care practice begins an EHR project, it is best to follow an established series of steps and activities such as those outlined in the Stratis Health HIT Toolkit for Physician Offices or the HRSA Health IT Adoption Toolkit. The services provided through a Regional HIT Extension Center also should be explored to provide the practice with needed support in assessing, planning, selecting, or implementation activities. The practice must engage its executive and clinical leaders actively in order to establish a solid project management structure and plan. It also must involve the full range of future EHR users throughout the physician office practice in specifying functional requirements, selecting the vendor product, as well as planning the physical space and type(s) of computer workstations that will be most effective in meeting the EHR users' daily work needs. Successful EHR projects use established functional standards to guide the selection and development of the system; use best project management practices to organize and lead the project through the assessment, planning, vendor selection, and implementation phases; and assure compliance with security and legal requirements when establishing EHR system policies and procedures.

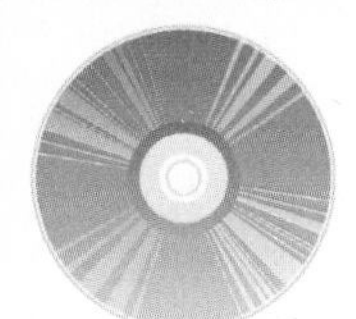

Computer Exploration

Using your e-Medsys® Educational Edition 2.0 access code provided with this text, complete the e-Medsys® Computer Exploration Exercises in Appendix B.

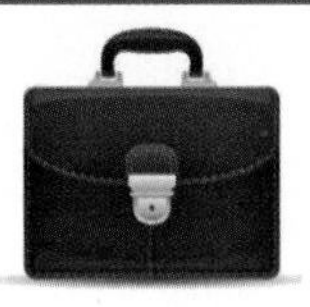

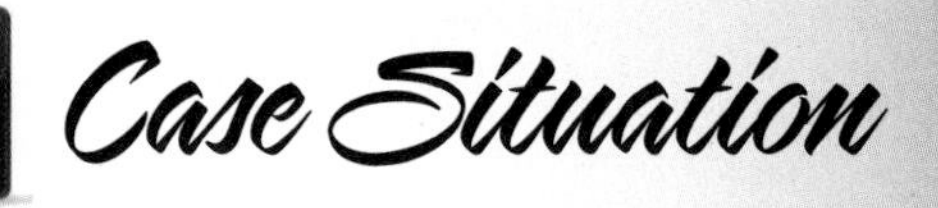

A group of five specialists from an existing multispecialty clinic decided to leave the clinic and set up their own practice partnership. Because the new group practice had to be organized from the ground up, the care providers decided to begin with an EHR system. They chose a vendor that provided both electronic medical record and practice management systems that interfaced with each other, although prior records brought to the practice were all paper based. The chosen vendor was one that had received CCHIT certification for its products. The office administrator was the coordinator for the project. The practice used an information technology consultant for add-on design and implementation of the system, and it continues to use individuals outside the practice for technology support. Digital voice recording is used for dictation, and those who transcribe the recording have direct input to the medical record component of the EHR. Scheduling, billing, accounts management, and other business-related functions are performed with the practice management program, which permits data exchange with the medical record program. The group planned carefully for security, confidentiality, and remote backup of their system. In addition to the new software and hardware, the group updated telephone lines and other office equipment and also added laptop computers. All staff including care providers were trained prior to implementation and had ample opportunity to practice with the system before it went live. Problems discovered during training were "triaged" for either immediate attention or future resolution. As a result, the actual implementation—one provider at a time—went quite smoothly. Paper records of prior treatment are being scanned into the system as time permits. This group has applied for incentives available under the HITECH "meaningful use" program.

REFERENCES

Amatayakul, Margret (January 2007). *Electronic Health Records: A Practical Guide for Professionals and Organizations*, 3rd Edition. Chicago, IL: American Health Information Management Association.

Ash, J. S., & Bates, D. W. (2005). Factors and forces affecting EHR system adoption: Report of a 2004 ACMI discussion. (1), 8–12.

Blumenthal, MD, MPP and Tavenner, Marilyn, RN, MHA (August 5, 2010). The "Meaningful Use" Regulation for Electronic Health Records. *New England Journal of Medicine*, 363, 501–504.

Center for Medicare & Medicaid Services. EHR Incentive Programs. CMS HER Meaningful Use Overview. Retrieved from https://www.cms.gov/EHRIncentivePrograms/30_Meaningful_Use.asp

Columbus, S. (2006, May). Small practice, big decision: Selecting an EHR system for small physician practices. (5), 42–46.

Fenton, S. H., Giannangelo, K., & Stanfil, M. (2006, June). Essential people skills for EHR implementation success. AHIMA Practice Brief. (6), 60A–D.

Healthcare Information and Management Systems Society. Selecting the right EHR vendor. Retrieved from http://www.himss.org/content/files/SelectingEMR_Flyer2.pdf

Healthcare Information and Management Systems Society. Making IT Happen: Strategies for Implementing the EMR/EHR. Retrieved from http://www.himss.org/content/files/davies/Davies_WP_Implementation.pdf

Health IT Standards and Testing. Meaningful Use Test Measures. Retrieved from http://healthcare.nist.gov/use_testing/finalized_requirements.html.

Health Resources and Services Administration HIT Adoption Toolbox. Retrieved from http://www.hrsa.gov/publichealth/business/healthit/toolbox/index.html

Office of the National Coordinator. Certified Health IT Product List. Retrieved from http://onc-chpl.force.com/ehrcert

Stratis Health. Health Information Technology Toolkit for Physician Offices. Resource Kit. Retrieved from http://www.stratishealth.org

REVIEW QUESTIONS

1. Plan, Select, and Implement are three of the four major steps associated with an EHR project. What is the other step, and what types of activities does it include?

2. Identify two major websites that provide free access to HIT Tools and sources for physician office practices to guide the organization through its EHR assess, plan, select and implementation activities.

3. How does an organization's EHR vision differ from its EHR goals?

4. What basic activities must be taken by the EHR selection task group when investigating the EHR product's appropriateness, reliability, and stability before making a final decision?

5. Who must be involved with defining the functional specifications for an EHR before a vendor is selected?

6. What are the differences between the CCHIT ambulatory EHR criteria and the Medicare/Medicaid "Meaningful Use" EHR criteria?

7. Name the organization that offers a subscription to an "EHR Selector" product, a resource for comparing ambulatory EHR products.

CHAPTER 3 The EHR Framework

CHAPTER OUTLINE

EHR Architecture, Hardware, Software, Networks, and Interfaces

EHR Architectures

Hardware, Software, Networks, and Interfaces

Human–Computer Interface (User) Devices

Functional, Data Content, and Vocabulary Standards

Functional Standards

Data Content Standards

Vocabulary Standards

Feature and Data Formats

Feature Formats

Structured and Unstructured Data

The Data Dictionary

Narrative Text Data

Imaged Data

Security Controls

Basic Technical Controls

Basic Physical Controls

Security Standards

Hybrid Records

OBJECTIVES

Upon completion of the chapter, the learner will be able to:

1. Explain the difference between a "client server" approach and a "software as a service" approach to implementing an electronic health record (EHR) system.
2. Identify three important decisions that clinicians, administrators, and staff must make concerning the human–computer interface (user) devices that they will be using to access the EHR system.

continues

KEY TERMS

administrative safeguards

audit trails

authentication protocols

client-server architecture or client-server model

Current Procedural Terminology—4th Revision (CPT-IV)

data dictionary

data-encryption protocols

data field

Diagnostic and Statistical Manual—Fourth Edition—Text Revision (DSM-IV-TR)

drop-down menu (pick list)

flow sheets

grids

Health Insurance Portability and Accountability Act (HIPAA)

HIPAA security standard

human–computer (user) interface devices

hybrid patient record

icons

imaged data

International Classification of Diseases—9th Revision—Clinical Modification (ICD-9-CM)

continues

KEY TERMS continued

International Classification of Diseases—10th Revision—Clinical Modification (ICD-10-CM)

legal source legend

Logical Observation Identifier Names and Codes (LOINC)

Meaningful Use (MU) EHR Certification Criteria

Meaningful Use (MU) Stage 1 Criteria—Risk Analysis

MEDCIN

menu (navigator) bar

narrative text data

National Drug Codes (NDC)

North American Nursing Diagnosis Association (NANDA)

Nursing Interventions Classification (NIC)

Nursing Outcomes Classification (NOC)

ONC-ATCB (Authorized Testing and Certification Body)

physical safeguards

risk analysis

RxNorm

software-as-a-service (SaaS) model

structured (discrete) data

Systematized Nomenclature of Medicine—Clinical Terminology (SNOMED-CT)

tabs

technical safeguards

toolbar

unstructured (text) data

user- and role-based access controls

OBJECTIVES continued

3. Describe the state of EHR product certification, the source of the functional standards for EHR certification, and the role of the ONC-ATCBs in EHR certification.
4. Explain what SNOMED-CT is and how it contributes to the quality of the data in an EHR.
5. Provide an example of structured data, unstructured data, narrative text data, and imaged data that would be found in an EHR.
6. Describe the purpose and content of a data dictionary.
7. Explain the purpose of tabs and icons within an EHR.
8. Explain the value that grids and flow sheets bring to an EHR.
9. List the three major safeguards that constitute a complete security program as specified in the HIPAA security regulations.
10. Explain the purpose of the risk analysis as required with the CMS MU Incentive Payment Program Stage 1 Criteria.
11. State how the American Health Information Management Association defines a "hybrid patient record."
12. Explain why the hybrid patient record creates a challenge to defining an organization's legal patient record.
13. Identify at least two reasons for a health care provider to use scanning as a component of their EHR system.

INTRODUCTION

Clinicians and staff who have a basic understanding of the components and features of an EHR system are much better prepared to support the practice in its efforts to integrate the EHR system into the practice's operations successfully. This chapter will provide:

- A brief description of the technologies required to support an ambulatory EHR system.
- An introduction to some important standards associated with an ambulatory EHR system: functional, data content, and vocabulary.
- A review of the basic user features of an ambulatory patient's EHR.
- An overview of key security policies and practices associated with an ambulatory EHR system.
- A discussion of the major issues involved with managing hybrid patient record systems as the health care provider practice transitions from a paper-based to a computer-based patient record system.

EHR ARCHITECTURE, HARDWARE, SOFTWARE, NETWORKS, AND INTERFACES

The EHR system implemented in a health care provider practice commonly is constructed in one of two ways: a **client-server model** (also called **client-server architecture**) or a **software-as-a-service (SaaS) model**. These two models will be compared in more detail later in this chapter. The specific model chosen by the practice will affect the hardware, software, and staff resources required to support the EHR system. However, no matter which model is chosen, the practice's clinicians and office staff will still need to adapt to using various types of computer hardware devices and learn how to use new computer software applications. A difficult part of the adjustment for the clinicians and office staff is likely to be learning how to locate, review, and document information in the EHR. Information in an EHR is organized quite differently than it is in the paper medical record and it also requires these individuals to document in more standardized ways than they have been documenting. At the same time, the EHR offers clinicians and office staff the benefit of more timely access to complete patient data to support their workflow and decision making.

client-server architecture or client-server model
One of two models for constructing a practice EHR; an annual licensing fee is paid to the EHR vendor for use of software, but all other components of the system are owned, operated, and maintained by the practice.

software-as-a-service (SaaS) model
The second model for constructing a practice EHR. With the SaaS approach, the practice purchases the hardware devices (computer terminals, laptops, etc.) and telecommunications system. The EHR product vendor continues to own, support, and maintain the servers, database software, and application software at the core of the EHR system.

EHR Architectures

A common approach taken by ambulatory practice settings to bring an EHR system into its daily operations is through a client-server model or client-server architecture. In this type of approach the practice pays the EHR product vendor an annual licensing fee, which allows the practice to use that vendor's EHR software application. The licensed EHR application software is then loaded on a dedicated computer (called a client server) that is fully owned, operated, and maintained by the practice. As a result, the practice must employ or contract with information technology (IT) experts of sufficient number and qualifications to manage the technical setup, perform routine maintenance, troubleshoot, and perform regular updates to the EHR system.

Increasingly, ambulatory EHR vendors offer access to their product through an "on-demand" application delivery process (initially called "application service provider" or "remote-hosted service") now commonly referred to as SaaS (software as a service). When using the SaaS option, the practice accesses the EHR application(s) and the data stored within the application(s) through a web browser and a secured Internet access point. The application(s) and the data are maintained in a remote-located data center that is maintained and managed by the EHR system vendor. SaaS benefits the practice by greatly reducing the hardware and personnel costs required to support the client server model. With the SaaS approach, the practice purchases the hardware devices (computer terminals, laptops, etc.) that clinicians and office staff will use to work within the EHR system. The practice also purchases the telecommunications system (e.g., a secured T1 line and Internet Provider Service) that supports secured web access from the practice environment into the remotely located EHR application. However, the EHR product vendor continues to own, support, and maintain the servers, database software, and application software at the core of the EHR system. The practice pays the vendor a monthly fee to maintain and support the system, to access the EHR system, and to store the practice's patient data on the system. The amount of the monthly fee usually is based on the number of clinicians and staff employed by the practice. Most important, the patient data documented by the clinicians and office staff in the remote-hosted EHR system remains the sole property of the practice.

Hardware, Software, Networks, and Interfaces

All EHR systems depend upon a sophisticated blend of equipment (hardware) and computer programs (software) to capture, store, display, and communicate data in ways that meet the varied needs of a wide range of users. Commonly, information technology (IT) products from many separate vendors will need to work together to create an EHR system for a practice. In some cases, the EHR vendor assumes the responsibility and cost for licensing and integrating any third-party products (e.g., a drug database, patient education materials, standard vocabularies, disease management protocols) into its EHR product. For example, Cerner's Millennium PowerOffice (an ambulatory EHR product) comes with an integrated third-party drug database (Multum), a third-party clinical alert/reminders protocol (Lynx), and several standard vocabularies (e.g., SNOMED CT, CPT-IV, ICD-9-CM, ICD-10-CM). In addition, the health care provider practice may wish to connect its EHR product (which it leases or has purchased from one vendor) with the practice's existing laboratory and/or practice management applications (which it leases or has purchased from another product vendor). In this case, the actual work of developing the electronic interface between the systems typically is done by the EHR vendor; however, the cost of creating the electronic interface between the practice's EHR product and these other types of third-party information system applications is always borne by the practice, and it can be quite expensive.

The bottom line is this: the technical setup of any EHR system requires the services of knowledgeable information technology specialists. In the client-server environment, the practice is responsible for acquiring the required IT staffing resources. In the SaaS (remote-hosted or on-demand) environment, the EHR vendor assumes the major portion of the IT responsibilities, with the practice responsible for the on-site setup of the user hardware and telecommunications devices required to connect to the remote-hosted EHR system and any electronic interfaces the practice requires from its other third-party applications. The larger the size of the practice, the more likely it will consider a client-server architecture for its EHR system. However, the SaaS model can be an appropriate choice for practices of any size.

HUMAN–COMPUTER INTERFACE (USER) DEVICES

Once the EHR is implemented, the best measure of its success is the extent to which clinicians and office staff use it to enhance their productivity and improve the quality of services they deliver to patients. Two key factors that impact the ease with which clinicians and office staff use the EHR in a practice setting are: (1) the types of **human–computer interface (user) devices** - i.e., hardware devices - selected for use by clinicians and office staff to interact with the EHR system; and (2) the actual location of those devices to support work activities and workflow.

human–computer interface (user) devices
The devices practice personnel use to interact with the EHR system; examples include wall-mounted or desktop computers, laptop computers, notebook or tablet personal computers, and personal digital assistants (PDAs).

The variety of user devices suitable for a practice's EHR system is expanding rapidly. Wall-mounted computer workstations commonly are used in examination rooms. Desktop personal computers (PCs) commonly are used in the patient registration area and other administrative office work spaces. Those user devices also often are complemented by laptop PCs on mobile carts, lightweight notebook or tablet PCs with point-and-click pen devices, and a variety of even smaller handheld mobile (wireless) communications devices, including personal digital assistants (PDAs), iPhones, iPads, and the like.

For each type of EHR system user (doctor, nurse practitioner, office clerk, medical assistant, lab technician, therapist, etc.), the usefulness of any specific type of user device can depend upon a variety of factors. Important considerations include where the device is located, what service or work process it will support, and whether the user usually is standing, sitting, or moving when using the device. The devices differ in other characteristics such as size and the resolution quality of the viewing screen. All these factors will affect the usefulness of any given device in various types of patient care situations. For example, a PDA may be suitable for reviewing lab results or writing a prescription order, but its small screen size and limited screen resolution make it unsuitable for viewing diagnostic images or lengthy narrative reports, and likewise make it unsuitable for entering a visit note or the results of an extensive physical examination.

Today, most user devices also can operate on a wireless network, which allows the user to review and input data from a single device while moving from one physical location to another within the practice setting. In that case, the specific locations of the wireless connection points within the practice setting, along with the size and weight of the user device, will determine how effectively a user can take advantage of the device's wireless capabilities. It is important to note that, when a practice attempts to determine appropriate locations for wireless access points, it also must consider the potential of the wireless system to interfere with electronic monitoring and medical devices.

The practice's clinicians and office staff must be involved to:

- Evaluate the types of user devices best suited for use in the practice.
- Determine how many of each type of device are needed so that there is an adequate number available when needed.
- Determine where the devices must be located to assure uninterrupted access where they are needed.

These decisions will play a major role in the ultimate success of the practice's EHR system because they will determine how much the EHR system actually is used to increase efficiency and the quality of care provided to patients.

FUNCTIONAL, DATA CONTENT, AND VOCABULARY STANDARDS

Standards are established within every type of business to assure basic and important uniformity of products, services, work processes, behavior, and so forth. Standards also guide those who develop and market products and services to customers, and provide assurances to consumers of the quality of the products and services they purchase. As EHRs have become more common in the marketplace, it is no surprise that the federal and state governments, along with the health care industry itself, now are recognizing the need for and developing standards focused on EHR products.

A brief discussion of three basic types of EHR standards is presented in this chapter: functional standards, data content standards, and vocabulary standards. All of these standard-setting efforts are important because they define the health care industry's expectations for the structure and function of the ambulatory electronic record, as well as defining the format(s) of the data captured within the electronic record. EHR systems that meet these standards make it possible to exchange patient data electronically between EHR systems and with other types of health information systems to support improved coordination, continuity and quality of patient care.

Functional Standards

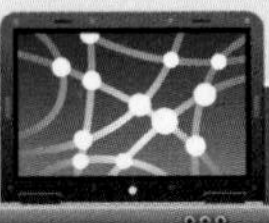

The functional criteria used by CCHIT to certify ambulatory EHRs can be viewed at the CCHIT website: http://www.cchit.org/.

As discussed in Chapter 1 and briefly mentioned in Chapter 2, the Certification Commission for Health Information Technology (CCHIT) began certifying ambulatory EHR vendor products in 2006.

Also introduced in Chapter 1 and briefly discussed in Chapter 2, the Center for Medicare and Medicaid's (CMS) Meaningful Use (MU) Incentive Payment Program incorporates another set of functional standards for ambulatory EHR systems. To be eligible for MU incentive payments, eligible providers must have implemented an EHR application that has been certified through an authorized testing process to have the capabilities required to allow the provider to use the practice's EHR system in ways that meet the Meaningful Use Criteria and thus qualify for incentive payments.

The CMS MU Incentive Payment Program is being implemented in three stages. The functional standards used to certify EHR products that can support provider practices in their efforts to meet the Stage 1 MU criteria were published in July, 2010. The actual process of testing EHR applications to certify them for this purpose began in December 2010. In September 2010 CCHIT was one of the two certification organizations to become an **ONC-ATCB (Authorized Testing and Certification Body)**, thus authorized to conduct the MU-related EHR certification testing process. As the U.S. Department of Health and Human Services Office of the National Coordinator (ONC) recognizes additional organizations as ONC-ATCBs, each is acknowledged on the ONC's Health IT website: http://healthit.hhs.gov/. See Table 3-1 for an overview of the EHR functional certification criteria established to support eligible providers (EPs) in their efforts to achieve the Stage 1 MU Criteria. The full list of the Stage 1 MU criteria is available at http://healthcare.nist.gov/use_testing/finalized_requirements.html.

ONC-ATCB (Authorized Testing and Certification Body) Organization authorized to perform Complete EHR and EHR Module testing in order to certify them as being able to support health care organizations in their efforts to achieve "meaningful use" of their EHR systems as defined in the CMS Meaningful Use Incentive Payment Program.

Throughout the subsequent chapters in this book, more details on these functional criteria will be presented as they relate to the chapter's topic.

Data Content Standards

State health care facility licensing regulations, Medicare's Conditions of Participation (including the CMS MU Criteria), and accreditation agencies are three sources of standards for the content in a patient's health or medical record. Standards specified by each of these sources generally have significant similarities, but do vary in details. These data content standards will be evaluated further in Chapter 4.

Vocabulary Standards

When health care providers record a specific medical symptom, treatment, or diagnosis in the patient's record, the medical term (vocabulary) used must be understood by others involved in the care of the patient so they can interpret it correctly. However, the vocabulary used by health care providers is a complex set of medical terms that have evolved over hundreds of years. Today, many medical conditions can be described accurately by several different terms or variations on a term. For example, the terms "heart attack," "myocardial infarction," "cardiac infarction," and "infarct of the heart" all reflect the same diagnosis, yet they might not be interpreted in the same manner by various health care providers. Moreover, an EHR system might not recognize all of these terms as the same concept. Inconsistencies in vocabulary terms can cause errors in

TABLE 3-1 Sample of Health Information Technology Stage 1 Set of MU EHR Certification Criteria

CRITERIA #	CERTIFICATION CRITERIA	TESTING CRITERIA
§170.302 (a)	Drug-drug, drug-allergy interaction checks	(1) Notifications. Automatically and electronically generate and indicate in real-time, notifications at the point of care for drug-drug and drug-allergy contraindications based on medication list, medication allergy list, and computerized provider order entry (CPOE). (2) Adjustments. Provide certain users with the ability to adjust notifications provided for drug-drug and drug-allergy interaction checks.
§170.302 (b)	Drug formulary checks	Enable a user to electronically check if drugs are in a formulary or preferred drug list.
§170.302 (c)	Maintain up-to-date problem list	Enable a user to electronically record, modify, and retrieve a patient's problem list for longitudinal care.
§170.302 (o)	Access control	Assign a unique name and/or number for identifying and tracking user identity and establish controls that permit only authorized users to access electronic health information.
§170.304 (b)	Electronic prescribing	Enable a user to electronically generate and transmit prescriptions and prescription-related information.
§170.304 (d)	Patient reminders	Patient Reminders. Enable a user to electronically generate a patient reminder list for preventive or follow-up care according to patient preferences based on, at a minimum, the data elements included in: Problem list; Medication list; Medication allergy list; Demographics; and Laboratory test results.
§170.304 (j)	Calculate and submit clinical quality measures	(j) Calculate and submit clinical quality measures. (1) Calculate. (i) Electronically calculate all of the core clinical measures specified by CMS for eligible professionals. (ii) Electronically calculate, at a minimum, three clinical quality measures specified by CMS for eligible professionals, in addition to those clinical quality measures specified in paragraph (1)(i). (2) Submission. Enable a user to electronically submit calculated clinical quality measures...

(continues)

TABLE 3-1 *(continued)*

CRITERIA #	CERTIFICATION CRITERIA	TESTING CRITERIA
§170.306 (a)	Computerized provider order entry	Enable a user to electronically record, store, retrieve, and modify, at a minimum, the following order types: (1) Medications; (2) Laboratory; and (3) Radiology/Imaging
§170.306 (e)	Electronic copy of discharge instructions	Enable a user to create an electronic copy of the discharge instructions for a patient, in human readable format, at the time of discharge on electronic media or through some other electronic means.

Source: National Institute of Standards and Testing (http://healthcare.nist.gov/use_testing/effective_requirements.html)

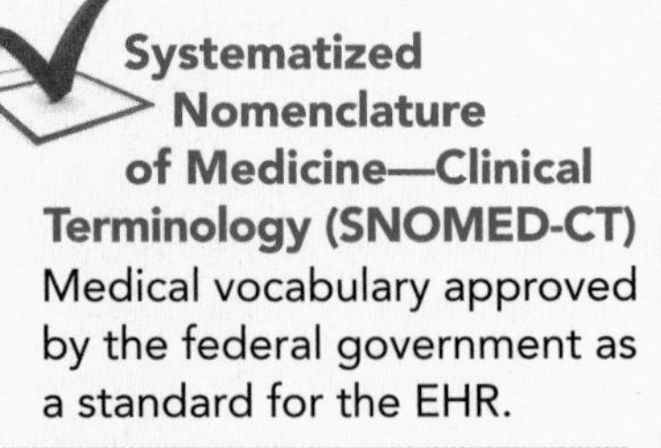

Systematized Nomenclature of Medicine—Clinical Terminology (SNOMED-CT)
Medical vocabulary approved by the federal government as a standard for the EHR.

MEDCIN
Point-of-care terminology that is fully mapped to the SNOMED-CT terminology.

Logical Observation Identifier Names and Codes (LOINC)
Terminology that supports electronic transmission of laboratory test orders and results.

RxNorm
Federally recognized standard for naming and identifying drugs; used by pharmacies for communicating prescriptions and assuring correct drug labeling.

National Drug Codes (NDC)
Federally recognized standard for naming and identifying drugs; used by pharmacies for communicating prescriptions and assuring correct drug labeling.

communication among health care providers and can lead to potential mistakes in patient care decisions. This is certainly also true in an EHR system when it is used to communicate among health care providers. Clearly, a common clinical vocabulary for use in electronic systems is needed to provide the foundation for accurate communications and data reporting.

In 2003, the federal government recognized the importance of standard vocabulary within an electronic health information system. To address this issue, in May 2004 the **Systematized Nomenclature of Medicine—Clinical Terminology (SNOMED-CT)** was adopted as a federal information vocabulary standard. SNOMED-CT is a product of the American College of Pathologists, with input from the United Kingdom's National Health Service. It is a vocabulary that is used internationally as well as in the United States. SNOMED-CT contains more than 300,000 unique clinical concepts, and it expresses these concepts by more than 900,000 descriptions. SNOMED-CT covers terms associated with diseases, procedures, body structures, organisms, findings, specimens, and so on. Under the federal SNOMED-CT license, this complex and detailed terminology was made available at no cost to software vendors and health care providers. As a result, today SNOMED-CT commonly is embedded in EHR systems as a standardized vocabulary. More detailed information about SNOMED-CT is available at http://ihtsdo.org/snomed-ct/.

Many other standard vocabularies exist to address specialized types of information in an EHR. Here we describe just a few of the most common ones encountered in ambulatory settings. **MEDCIN** is a proprietary standardized medical vocabulary developed by Medicomp Systems, Inc. MEDCIN terms have been linked to several other clinical terminology systems, including SNOMED-CT. This means that clinical findings captured in an EHR through MEDCIN terminology also can be translated into other terminologies, such as SNOMED-CT.

The following are examples of some vocabulary standards that are intended for more specific uses: laboratory tests and results, drugs and prescriptions, and nursing. The **Logical Observation Identifier Names and Codes (LOINC)** terminology is a federal health information standard that supports electronic transmission of laboratory test orders and results. **RxNorm** and **National Drug Codes (NDC)** are federally recognized standards for naming and identifying drugs used by pharmacies for accurately communicating prescriptions and assuring correct drug labeling. (See Chapter 9 for a more detailed explanation of RxNorm and NDCs.) The **Nursing Interventions Classification (NIC)**, **Nursing Outcomes Clarification (NOC)**, and **North American Nursing Diagnosis Association (NANDA)** are nursing terminology standards that are applied (respectively) to nursing interventions, nursing classification of patient/client outcomes, and nursing diagnoses.

Health care practices also may use the following coding/classification systems, which include clinical terms.

- The **International Classification of Disease, 9th Revision—Clinical Modification (ICD-9-CM)**. Note: ICD-9-CM will be replaced by **International Classification of Disease, 9th Revision—Clinical Modification (ICD-10-CM)** effective October 1, 2014.
- The **Current Procedural Terminology—4th Revision (CPT-IV)**
- The **Diagnostic and Statistical Manual—Fourth Edition—Text Revision (DSM-IV-TR)**, associated primarily with mental and personality disorders as well as life events or social problems that affect persons (see Green & Fenton, 2006).

See Chapter 11 for a more detailed discussion of these coding/classification schemes as they are used in EHR systems to support provider-office billing activities.

Although each of these terminology and classification systems can stand alone, most can be mapped from SNOMED-CT, making SNOMED-CT an especially robust standard vocabulary for use in EHR systems. Table 3-2 provides an example of several SNOMED-CT terms related to atrial fibrillation mapped to the ICD-9-CM and ICD-10-CM classification systems.

Nursing Interventions Classification (NIC)
Nursing terminology standard applied to nursing interventions.

Nursing Outcomes Classification (NOC)
Nursing terminology standard applied to patient outcomes.

North American Nursing Diagnosis Association (NANDA)
Nursing terminology standard applied to nursing diagnoses.

International Classification of Diseases—9th Revision—Clinical Modification (ICD-9-CM)
International coding classification system used for billing and public health reporting in all types of health care facilities.

TABLE 3-2 SNOMED-CT Terms Mapped to ICD-9-CM and ICD-10-CM

SNOMED TERM	TERMINOLOGY AXIS	SNOMED CODE	ICD-9-CM TERM	ICD-9-CM CODE	ICD-10 CM TERM	ICD-10-CM CODE
Atrial fibrillation	Finding	82343012	Atrial fibrillation	427.31	Atrial fibrillation	I48.0
Paroxysmal atrial fibrillation	Finding	421235014	Atrial flutter	427.32	Re-entry ventricular arrhythmia	I47.0
					Supraventricular tachycardia	I47.1
					Ventricular tachycardia	I47.2
					Paroxysmal tachycardia, unspecified	I47.9
Atrial fibrillation and flutter	Finding	300130013	Atrial fibrillation and flutter	427.3	Atrial fibrillation	I48.0
					Atrial flutter	I48.1

FEATURE AND DATA FORMATS

Menu bars and toolbars are common elements seen on computer screens that allow users to manipulate the applications run by the computer system. Tabs are typically used to move between one section (or view) within the patient's record and another section. Flow sheets, grids, templates, and "favorites" are features within EHR applications that help health care providers and office staff efficiently view large amounts of data in a patient's record and input data into the patient's record. Data in the EHR is formatted in a variety of ways—for example, structured data, narrative (text or unstructured) data, and imaged data. Health care providers and office staff who are familiar with these common feature and data formats in the EHR will find it easier to begin using the EHR in their daily work activities.

Feature Formats

When a user logs into an EHR system and enters into a patient chart, the screen format commonly includes a **menu (navigator) bar** (see Figure 3-1) located on the left side of the screen and a **toolbar** (see Figure 3-2) containing several **icons** across the top of the screen. Icons are an image, picture, symbol which represents a function or activity. Both features are designed to make navigating or moving through the patient chart easier for the user. For example, by clicking on a specific icon the health care provider or practice staff can *directly enter* data into that specific area of the patient record to enter data. Then, by clicking on a specific item within the menu (navigator) bar the health care provider or practice staff *can quickly access and review* that specific type of information as it currently is recorded in the patient's chart. It will take some training to gain a full understanding of how to use an EHR's specific menu (navigator) bar and toolbar most effectively.

Tabs, not unlike the tabs or dividers that separate sections of a paper-based patient record, are a common format feature on screens within a patient's chart in the EHR. Tabs also help the user to navigate the contents of the patient chart.

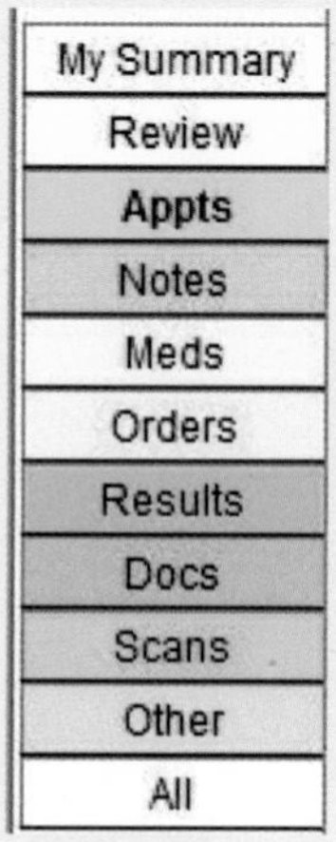
My Summary
Review
Appts
Notes
Meds
Orders
Results
Docs
Scans
Other
All

Reprinted with permission of TriMed Technologies, Corp.

Figure 3-1 EHR menu bar in e-Medsys®.

Reprinted with permission of TriMed Technologies, Corp.

Figure 3-2 EHR toolbar in e-Medsys®.

International Classification of Diseases—9th Revision—Clinical Modification (ICD-10-CM)
International coding classification system used for billing and public health reporting in all types of health care facilities, which will replace ICD-9-CM effective October 1, 2013.

Current Procedural Terminology—4th Revision (CPT-IV)
Coding nomenclature used for billing and public health reporting by ambulatory care service providers.

Diagnostic and Statistical Manual—Fourth Edition—Text Revision (DSM-IV-TR)
Coding classification system associated with mental disorders, personality disorders, and life events or social problems that affect people.

menu (navigator) bar
The first bar of icons across the top of a computer screen that (when chosen via a mouse click) allow standard functions of the software to be performed, making it easier to move through the system.

toolbar
The second bar of icons across the top of a computer screen that (when chosen via a mouse click) allow standard functions of the software to be performed, making moving through the system easier.

icons
An image, picture, or symbol used in a computer software program to represent a function or activity.

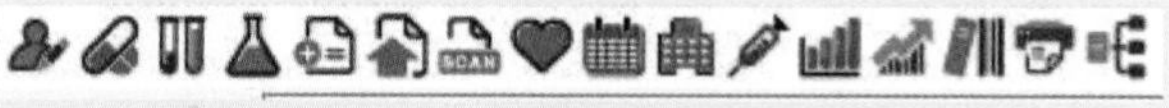

Demographics	Summary	Notes	CurMeds	Immun	CurChgs	UserDef	Flowsh	GrowthCh

Figure 3-3 EHR tabs in e-Medsys®.

The number and names of the tabs used within the EHR are generally customizable to the practice's needs at time of implementation. Each tab brings forward selected patient data from the EHR database. In e-Medsys® there are several tabs available to guide the health care provider to easily access different content in the patient's chart. (See Figure 3-3).

Grids in the EHR structure the data that is being entered into a format that resembles tables in Microsoft Word. However, each cell within the grid is associated with a data element and often contains a drop-down menu containing options from which to select. In addition, each of the cells in any one row on the grid contains a data element that is in some way associated with the data elements in each of the other cells on that row. For example, Table 3-3 shows a pain-evaluation grid with five data elements (i.e., five cells in the row) that all are related to describing a patient's pain: location, description, pain level, acceptable pain level, and pain alleviated by.

If the patient also had pain in other locations, the health care provider can add additional rows to the grid and similarly document a description of that problem. Data documented in a grid within the EHR is recorded efficiently and is read easily by all health care providers.

Flow sheets display data in a time sequence that allows healthcare providers to see trends more readily in the data they are monitoring; blood pressure, cholesterol levels, hemoglobin reading, blood sugar levels, and so forth." "(See also Chapter 7 discussion of graphics and charts.)

Structured and Unstructured Data

Most data documented in the EHR is associated with a specific data field. A **data field** is a defined area where a specific piece of information can be entered. Health care providers and others using the EHR enter visit, examination, and treatment data into the EHR through these data fields. Some data fields accept **structured (discrete) data** and others accept **unstructured (text) data**.

Structured data fields require that an individual either make selections from established lists of terms or enter data in a date or numerical form. For example, when a health care provider is documenting the "nature of pain" that a patient is experiencing, the provider could be asked to select—from a

tabs
Similar to dividers in a paper-based patient record, these markers highlight major sections of the EHR and so make navigation easier.

grids
Feature that enables the entry of structured data into an EHR in a format similar to a table.

flow sheet
A display of data in a time sequence, allowing care providers to see trends in areas (e.g., blood pressure, blood sugar level) they are monitoring.

data field
Defined area where a specific piece of information can be entered.

structured (discrete) data
Data fields where either numbers or dates must be entered or in which a selection from a defined list of options must be made.

TABLE 3-3 Pain Evaluation Grid

LOCATION	DESCRIPTION	PAIN LEVEL (1–10)	ACCEPTABLE PAIN LEVEL (1–10)	PAIN ALLEVIATED BY
Hip, left	Stabbing	8	5	Tylenol with codeine
Hip, right	Dull aching	2	5	Aspirin

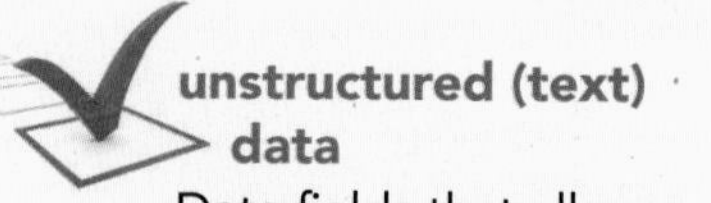

unstructured (text) data
Data fields that allow a user to enter data in free-text or narrative form.

drop-down menu (pick list)
Structured response choices presented within a data field.

drop-down menu (or pick list)—one or more of these six terms to describe the nature of a patient's pain: aching, acute, burning, chronic, dull, stabbing. The temperature data field may require the health care provider to document a number with a minimum of two whole digits and one decimal point (e.g., a number such as 98.2).

Unstructured data fields allow users to enter data in free-text (narrative) form. In some cases the unstructured data field in an EHR limits the length of the free-text entry to a predefined number of characters. In other cases the unstructured data field may be a rich text format that allows free-text entry with no character limit on the length of the entry. For example, a Chief Complaint data field may allow a free-text entry so the EHR system can capture the exact words the client uses to describe the reason for seeking an examination: "I have a raised reddish spot on my back between my shoulder blades. It seems to have gotten bigger over the past month. It doesn't itch or burn." Figures 3-4 and 3-5 are examples of structured and unstructured data fields commonly seen within examination or assessment documentation in an EHR.

Although structured data fields limit entries to only the choices provided, they are most efficient to use when there are a defined number of alternatives for expressing the data in a field. For example, when a State of Residence field exists in a form, it can be filled in efficiently when a person is presented with a structured listing of the 50 states and then asked to select the appropriate one. In that instance, State of Residence is a structured data field. Entering data into structured data fields can assure more consistency in the data, can save data entry time because far fewer keystrokes are required than when entering full text, and make it possible to produce lists and reports electronically based on data elements collected within the EHR system.

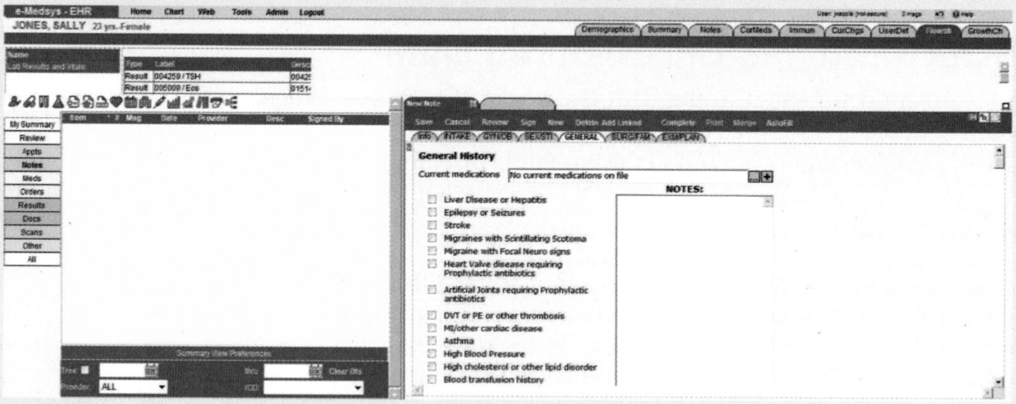

Figure 3-4 Structured data field in e-Medsys®.

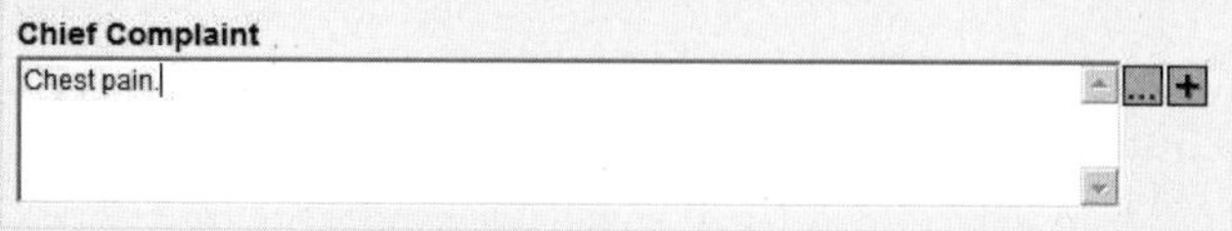

Figure 3-5 Unstructured data field in e-Medsys®.

The Data Dictionary

The total body of data fields that exist within the EHR is catalogued in the system's **data dictionary**. Within the data dictionary, each data field is, at a minimum, commonly "defined" by a unique title or label, an indication of its data type, a functional description, and a standard format. Each data element in the data dictionary represents a unique single data point. For example, oral temperature is a unique single data point and rectal temperature is a unique single data point; so are chief complaint, respiratory rate, blood sugar level—fasting, blood type, marital status, systolic blood pressure, diastolic blood pressure, and so on. An EHR system is capable of capturing such unique single data only when the data elements (or data fields) have been defined and built into the system via its data dictionary development software. Examples of the content of a data dictionary are shown in Table 3-4.

data dictionary A listing of each data field in a system; fields are defined by a unique title or label, an indication of the type of data, a functional description, and a standard format.

When an EHR system is implemented in an ambulatory practice, critical tasks are those of confirming the content of the product's existing data dictionary and, as needed, adding to it. The data dictionary of an EHR must be built or modified by an individual who is trained to use the specific software tool designed for that purpose. Such individuals will work closely with the practice's health care professional staff to assure that the data elements embedded in the EHR are sufficient to capture their examination findings, visit notes, and treatment documentation consistently.

TABLE 3-4 Examples of Data Dictionary Content for an EHR

FIELD NAME	DATA TYPE	FORMAT	EXAMPLE	DESCRIPTION
Oral temperature	Numeric	xxx.xx	100.36	Measure of body temperature in degrees Fahrenheit
Blood type	Alpha single select	A, A pos, A neg, B, B pos, B neg, O, O pos, O neg	A pos	One of nine possible blood types as determined by standard blood-typing techniques
Birth date	Date	mm/dd/yyyy	03/25/1956	Month/day/year of birth as stated by the patient being registered into the system or by their authorized representative; desirable to have confirmation based on a document with a picture ID
Patient last name	Text	Aaaaaaaaaa	Anderson	Surname as stated by the patient or client being registered into the system or by their authorized representative; preferable to have confirmation based on a document with a picture ID

Narrative Text Data

narrative text data A form of unstructured data not reflected in the EHR's data dictionary.

Patient health records historically have been filled with various types of reports that are presented as narrative text, referred to as **narrative text data**. Narrative text data is also a form of unstructured data; however, it is not reflected in the EHR's data dictionary. Narrative text is entered into the EHR through direct keystroke entry by the user or is transferred electronically into the EHR via a transcription system. Examples of narrative text include exam notes, pathology reports, and operation reports. When narrative text is entered into the EHR, it commonly is indexed or catalogued into the system by report type (e.g., History and Physical) so it can be linked to a standard location within the EHR and then easily located by an authorized user when needed.

Imaged Data

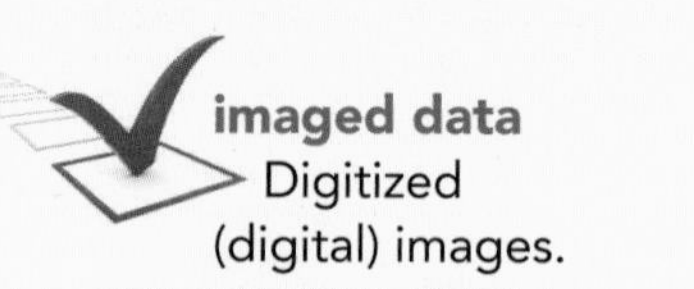

imaged data Digitized (digital) images.

Health Insurance Portability and Accountability Act (HIPAA) Federal legislation establishing regulations aimed at assuring the privacy and security of protected electronic health information.

HIPAA security standard Portion of the HIPAA regulations that identifies safeguards a health care organization must have in place to protect health care information.

administrative safeguards Assignment of security management, security training, and developing policies and procedures.

technical safeguards Automated processes that limit who is able to access the EHR and what they are able to do within the system.

physical safeguards Mechanisms that protect the equipment and the data associated with the EHR system.

Ambulatory EHRs also may contain digitized images, referred to as **imaged data**. Examples of this type of data include scanned signed consents, advance directives, or faxed reports received from other health care facilities. Digital images from diagnostic tests (e.g., CAT scans, MRIs, mammograms, EKG tracings) also can be incorporated into the ambulatory EHR. Like text (unstructured data), imaged data is catalogued, at a minimum, by report type when it is placed into the EHR so it can be linked to a standard location and easily accessed by authorized users.

SECURITY CONTROLS

Protecting patient data residing in EHRs from unauthorized access is identified routinely by health care providers and the consumer public as a leading concern. The **Health Insurance Portability and Accountability Act (HIPAA)** of 1996 established specific regulations at the national level aimed at assuring the privacy and security of protected health information that is collected, maintained, and transmitted in electronic form. The **HIPAA security standard** identifies three separate types of safeguards that a health care organization must have in place: administrative, technical, and physical controls to "safeguard protected health information from any intentional or unintentional use or disclosure that is a violation of the standards." (CMS, 2006):

- **Administrative safeguards** involve assigning responsibility for security management, establishing security training, and developing policies and procedures to guide the security-related behavior of the organization's human resources.
- **Technical safeguards** are the automated processes that limit who is able to access the EHR system and what they are able to do within the system. Encryption of data when it is stored or transmitted is also an aspect of technical control.
- **Physical safeguards** are mechanisms put into place that protect the equipment and the data associated with the EHR system.

Basic Technical Controls

Certainly EHR systems have the technical capacity to provide even better security controls on patient data than has been possible historically in paper-based health record systems. In particular, EHR systems commonly employ these types of technical security controls:

- **User- and role-based access controls**—limitations on what a user can view and do within a patient's EHR based on the user's job responsibilities.
- **Authentication protocols**—steps the EHR system requires users to take before it will accept their log-in and/or save the data they are entering into the patient's record.
- **Audit trails**—routine system tracking of all new log-in activity related to each patient's record in the EHR by user and role as well as continuous system tracking of each user's date/time pattern of logging in/out of the EHR system.
- **Data-encryption protocols**— system-generated manipulation (scrambling) of data during electronic transmission between two separate computer systems in order to prevent the data from being intercepted by an unauthorized party.

user- and role-based access controls
Limitations on what a user can view and do within a patient's EHR.

authentication protocols
Steps the EHR system requires users to take before it will accept their log-in and/or save the data they are entering.

audit trails
Routine system tracking of all activity related to each patient's record in the EHR by user and role.

data-encryption protocols
System-generated scrambling of data during electronic transmission to prevent the data from being intercepted.

These are the most basic technical control features of an ambulatory EHR system. They significantly protect the integrity and the privacy of patient data residing within the system.

However, in order to take full advantage of the technical security features built into EHR products, the practice will need to update its security policies and procedures to incorporate changes associated with the EHR implementation. For example, with respect to the use of the EHR system access controls, the practice must document policies and procedures related to:

- Who authorizes another individual to have access.
- Who determines the type of access rights assigned to an individual.
- Who is authorized to actually set up the access rights for an individual.
- Activating or deactivating user access in a timely manner.
- What penalties are in place for various types of violations of access privileges.

Basic Physical Controls

The practice must give special attention to assuring the security of the physical components of the EHR system—that is, preventing unauthorized access to computers, printers, faxes, and data storage media (USB devices, CDs, etc.). Paying close attention to where these devices are located and how they are secured when left unattended is a step in the right direction. An important but often-overlooked aspect of physical control concerns the methods used within the practice to store and dispose securely of hard-copy reports that have been scanned into the EHR or of hard-copy documents printed from the EHR that contain confidential patient information. Locked paper storage equipment along with well-placed printers and shredders are basic tools for handling the security of hard-copy documents.

Security Standards

One of the health outcome policies associated with the CMS "Meaningful Use" Incentive Payment System is to "ensure adequate privacy and security protections for personal health information." As a result, one of the Stage 1 MU Criteria

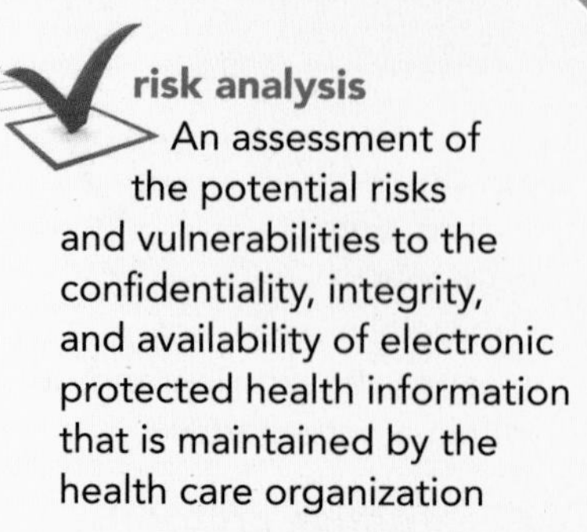

risk analysis An assessment of the potential risks and vulnerabilities to the confidentiality, integrity, and availability of electronic protected health information that is maintained by the health care organization

for Eligible Providers is to "[p]rotect electronic health information created or maintained by the certified EHR technology through the implementation of appropriate technical capabilities" and the requirement that the provider practice "[c]onduct or review a security risk analysis per 45 CFR 164.308(a)(1) and implement security updates as necessary." CFR 164.308 (a)(1) is a specific section of the HIPAA (1996) Security Rule that requires health care organizations to "[i]mplement policies and procedures to prevent, detect, contain, and correct security violations." A **risk analysis** involves an assessment of the potential risks and vulnerabilities to the confidentiality, integrity, and availability of electronic protected health information that is maintained by the health care organization.

The initial Stage 1 MU EHR certification criteria also include security-related standards that are tested during the ONC-ATCB certification process (see Table 3-5).

TABLE 3-5 Security Access Criteria in the Health Information Technology: Initial Set of MU EHR Certification Criteria

CRITERIA #	CERTIFICATION CRITERIA	TESTING CRITERIA
§170.302 (o)	Access Control	Assign a unique name and/or number for identifying and tracking user identity and establish controls that permit only authorized users to access electronic health information.
§170.302 (p)	Emergency Access	Permit authorized users (who are authorized for emergency situations) to access electronic health information during an emergency.
§170.302 (q)	Automatic Log-off	Terminate an electronic session after a predetermined time of inactivity.
§170.302 (r)	Audit log	(1) Record Actions. Record actions related to electronic health information. (2) Generate audit log. Enable a user to generate an audit log for a specific time period and to sort entries in the audit log.
§170.302 (s)	Integrity	(1) Create a message digest. (2) Verify upon receipt of electronically exchanged health information that such information has not been altered. (3) Detect the alteration of audit logs.
§170.302 (t)	Authentication	Verify that a person or entity seeking access to electronic health information is the one claimed and is authorized to access such information.
§170.302 (u)	General Encryption	Encrypt and decrypt electronic health information.
§170.302 (v)	Encryption when Exchanging Health Information	Encrypt and decrypt electronic health information when exchanged.

Source: National Institute of Standards and Testing (http://healthcare.nist.gov/use_testing/effective_requirements.html)

Ambulatory EHR products that apply for full certification by the CCHIT are evaluated against a set of security criteria in the same way that they are evaluated against the CCHIT's functional criteria.

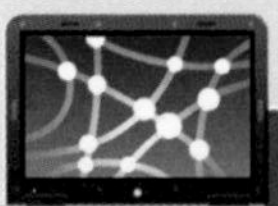

CCHIT security access criteria are available for review at the CCHIT website: http://www.cchit.org/.

HYBRID RECORDS

In its transition from a paper-based to a computer-based patient record system, it is likely that a practice will decide to maintain for some period of time a **hybrid patient record**: a patient record that has some electronic and some paper components. For example, a practice may have purchased a basic patient-documentation system to collect structured visit data, but text-based reports such as visit notes, transcribed examination reports, diagnostic imaging reports, and specialized laboratory reports that are not yet part of its initial EHR capabilities will be maintained in paper form. Later, the practice might add new capability to its EHR system, eliminating some of the paper components and increasing the types of data that are maintained electronically. Over the time that hybrid records exist, the ratio of record components maintained in the EHR to portions maintained in paper form might change from month to month or from year to year. Therefore, one of the special challenges in the hybrid record environment is making sure that the practice has a clear definition at all times of what constitutes the legal health record and where each piece of that legal health record can be found when needed, either within the EHR or on paper in a file folder. To assist with this process, the American Health Information Management Association (AHIMA) suggests that each health care organization develop and maintain a **legal source legend**, which is essentially a tracking instrument that "describes where and how to find specific documents that comprise the hybrid health record." (AHIMA eHIM Work Group, 2003). Table 3-6 shows a small

hybrid patient record
A patient record that has some electronic and some paper components.

legal source legend
A grid that describes where and how to find specific documents that constitute the hybrid health record.

TABLE 3-6 Excerpt from a Legal Source Legend for a Hybrid Patient Record System

REPORT/ DOCUMENT TYPE	MEDIA TYPE: P = PAPER E = ELECTRONIC	SOURCE SYSTEM APPLICATION (NONPAPER)	ELECTRONIC STORAGE START DATE	STOP PRINTING START DATE
Admission H & P	P/E	System 1	1/1/2005	1/1/2006
Physician Orders	E	System 1	1/1/2005	
Lab Results	E	System 2	1/1/2004	1/1/2004
Medication Record	E	System 1	1/1/2005	
Pathology Reports	E	System 2	1/1/2004	1/1/2004
Urgent Care and EMOR Records	P			

Source: AHIMA e-HIM Work Group (2003, appendix).

segment of a legal source legend that indicates what media type is the source for specific patient record documents. This legal source legend will be useful to those who must use the hybrid record to locate documents, and the tracking document easily can be easily updated to reflect exactly when various pieces of the legal record transition from paper-based to electronic form.

Document scanning is one way to eliminate some of the records-management challenges associated with a hybrid health record system. For example, scanning prior treatment records is one way to transition all or key pieces of existing patients' information into a new EHR. Scanning also can be used by a practice to incorporate documents coming from sources that do not have electronic transfer capabilities (e.g., lab results from an external laboratory, or transcribed Word documents). In addition, documents such as consents and authorizations that require paper in order to capture a legal signature can be scanned subsequently for integration into the EHR for safekeeping.

SUMMARY

When a health care practice is preparing clinicians and office staff for the transition to an EHR system, it is well advised to discuss openly the various issues associated with establishing a solid framework for an EHR system:

- Determining the human–computer interface (user) devices that will meet their needs most effectively.
- Incorporating established data content, vocabulary/terminology, and security standards.
- Defining the most appropriate data structure to link with the various types of documentation placed in the patient's record, recognizing that structured data is required to facilitate electronic data analysis and report generation.
- Managing the transitional hybrid health record from both a practical and legal perspective.

Computer Exploration

Using your e-Medsys® Educational Edition 2.0 access code provided with this text, complete the e-Medsys® Computer Exploration Exercises in Appendix B.

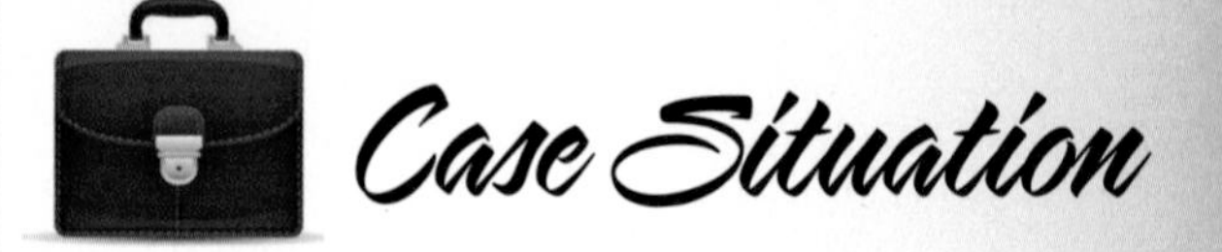

A small family-practice clinic made a decision to implement an electronic health record system. Because the clinician and clerical staff had no experience with using an EHR system and no expertise in project management, the clinic manager contacted the Regional HIT Extension Center serving their geographic area and contracted with the REC to guide her through the assessing, planning, selection and implementation activities.

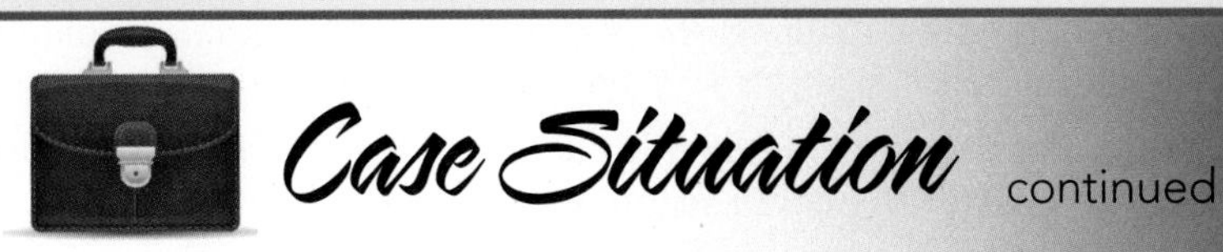

continued

After 6 months of being fully involved with assessing, planning, and EHR product selection activities, the clinic providers and clerical staff were eager to implement their new electronic health record system. As they reviewed the many workflow changes that would be implemented to take full advantage of the EHR system, they also recognized that the types of computer workstations they installed would impact their ability to use the EHR system easily as a daily work tool.

This clinic has 11 exam rooms used by three family physicians, one physician assistant, and one nurse practitioner. The existing space and floor plan would not be changed because the clinic space had been renovated within the past three years. So the revised workflows took the existing space and floor plan into account. Therefore, the planning for new EHR workstations and related equipment (printers, scanners, etc.) would take these factors into consideration as well.

In order to retire the paper medical records completely, computer workstations were needed in every location where clinicians and clerical staff would need to view or enter data into the patient's record. Printers would be located in every location where clinicians and clerical staff needed to access printed materials to hand to patients. When the locations for the computer workstations and printers were identified, electrical and network wiring were installed to accommodate the equipment. The clinicians decided to use hardwired desktop computer workstations to avoid potential problems with mobile tablet devices—problems such as limited battery life, security issues with tablets that might be taken out of the clinic, potential damage from dropping, and additional technology required to support wireless connections. The clinicians established design principles for the exam-room workstations based on the recommendations given to them by their REC consultant:

- Position the workstation so the clinician can sit close enough to touch the patient and maintain easy eye contact with the patient while the clinician is seated at the workstation.
- Assure that each workstation is positioned at the ergonomically appropriate keyboard height, monitor-viewing height, and mouse position for clinicians.
- Have a readily available writing surface.

REFERENCES

AHIMA e-HIM Work Group on Health Information in a Hybrid Environment. (October 2003). The complete medical record in a hybrid EHR environment. Part I: Managing the transition. AHIMA Practice Brief. Chicago: AHIMA.

ASTM [American Standards for Testing and Measurement]. (2007). Active standard: E2369-05 standard specification for continuity of care record (CCR). Retrieved from http://www.astm.org

CCHIT Certified 2011 Ambulatory EHR Certification Criteria. Retrieved from http://www.cchit.org

CMS [Centers for Medicare & Medicaid Services]. (2006). HIPAA security series: Security 101 for covered entities. Information. Retrieved from http://www.cms.hhs.gov/EducationMaterials/Downloads/Security101forCoveredEntities.pdf

CMS [Centers for Medicare & Medicaid Services]. Eligible Professional Meaningful Use Table of Contents Core and Menu Set Measures. Retrieved from https://www.cms.gov/EHRIncentivePrograms/Downloads/EP-MU-TOC.pdf

Corepoint Health. (2009). The Continuity of Care Document: Changing the Landscape of Health Information Exchange. Retrieved from http://www.corepointhealth.com/resource-center/white-papers

Federal Registry. (July 28, 2010). 45 CFR Part 170. Health Information Technology: Initial Set of Standards, Implementation Specifications, and Certification Criteria for Electronic Health Record Technology; Final Rule.

Fraser, G. (2005). Problem list coding in e-HIM. AHIMA Practice Brief. Chicago, IL: AHIMA.

Green, M. J., & Fenton, S. H. (2006). Clinical classifications and terminologies. In K. M. LaTour & S. Eichenwald Maki (Eds.), *Health information management: Concepts, principles and practices* (chap. 13). Chicago, IL: AHIMA.

National Center for Vital and Health Statistics. (2000). *Toward a national health information infrastructure.* Washington, DC.

National Institute of Standards and Testing (NIST). (July 2001). Special Publication 800-30. Risk Management Guide for Information Technology Systems. Retrieved from http://csrc.nist.gov/publications/nistpubs/800-30/sp800-30.pdf

National Institute of Standards and Testing (NIST). (February 7, 2011). Health IT Standards and Testing. Approved Test Procedures Version 1.0. Retrieved from http://healthcare.nist.gov/use_testing/finalized_requirements.html

Systematized Nomenclature of Medicine—Clinical Terms (SNOMED-CT). Retrieved from http://www.snomed.org

Wickham Lee, F. (2006). Data and information management. In K. M. LaTour & S. Eichenwald Maki (Eds.), *Health information management: Concepts, principles and practice* (chap. 5). Chicago, IL: AHIMA.

REVIEW QUESTIONS

1. How does a client-server model differ from a SaaS model as a method for accessing an EHR application?

2. What decisions should be made before the human–computer interface (user) devices (PCs, PDAs, notebooks, iPads, etc.) are purchased?

3. What standard vocabulary was adopted as a federal information technology standard in 2004 and can be mapped to other commonly used terminologies, such as ICD-9-CM, ICD-10-CM, MEDCIN and DSM-IV?

4. What standard medical terminology is associated with laboratory orders and results reporting?

5. What type of standard terminology systems are NIC, NOC, and NANDA?

6. A client's marital status is entered in the EHR system by selecting from a list of terms (single, married, divorced, widowed). Is this an example of structured data or unstructured data?

7. What is a data dictionary? How does it affect the EHR's ability to capture findings from an examination or assessment?

8. What purpose do icons serve within the EHR?

9. What do tabs reveal within the EHR?

10. How do grids differ from flow sheets in an EHR?

11. What are the three major types of safeguards specified in the HIPAA security regulations?

12. How do user- or role-based access control and data encryption serve to preserve the privacy of a patient's health record?

13. What is a "hybrid patient record"?

14. In what way does the hybrid patient record make it difficult to define the "legal patient record"?

15. For what purpose(s) would a health care provider practice use scanning as a component of its EHR system?

16. What does "ONC-ATCB" stand for and what service does an ONC-ATCB provide?

17. What is the nature and purpose of a HIPAA-required risk analysis?

CHAPTER 4 The EHR and Record Content

CHAPTER OUTLINE

OBJECTIVES

Upon completion of the chapter, the learner will be able to:

1. List the major purposes for a health care record.
2. Differentiate between source-oriented, integrated, and problem-oriented documentation.
3. Identify clinical and administrative record components and give examples of data recorded in each section.
4. Differentiate between the groups that develop licensure, certification, and accreditation standards.
5. Describe major sources for standards relating to content of health records.
6. Describe the basic content for an ambulatory care practice electronic health record.

continues

KEY TERMS

Accreditation Association for Ambulatory Health Care (AAAHC)

accreditation standards

administrative data

ambulatory care

American Association for Accreditation of Ambulatory Surgery Facilities (AAAASF)

American Health Information Management Association (AHIMA)

American Osteopathic Association (AOA)

certification standards

clinical data

Commission for the Accreditation of Birth Centers

Conditions of Participation (CoP), or Conditions of Coverage (CoC)

demographic information

Health Plan Employer Data and Information Set (HEDIS)

integrated record

licensure standards

Medicare

Medicaid

continues

KEY TERMS continued

National Committee for Vital and Health Statistics (NCVHS) Core Content of the Healthcare Provider Dimension

National Committee for Quality Assurance (NCQA)

problem-oriented record

source-oriented record

The Joint Commission (JC)

The Joint Commission's "Do Not Use" Abbreviation List

Uniform Ambulatory Care Data Set (UACDS)

OBJECTIVES continued

7. Describe general documentation guidelines used in an EHR.
8. Explain the difference between paper and electronic record systems for correcting documentation errors and adding signatures.
9. Describe the reasoning behind The Joint Commission's "Do Not Use" Abbreviation List and give examples of abbreviations that should not be used in health records.

INTRODUCTION

Most health care providers have established formats and content for their current practice records. It is likely this content has evolved over time based upon a variety of sources. Some content might have passed from one health care provider to another to meet established general or specialty medical documentation needs. Some may have been designed within the practice or obtained from medical organizations. Information found in the record must provide evidence of care delivered and communicate information to others both inside and outside the practice. Content must be sufficient to meet those needs. Standards set by outside regulatory or approval organizations also have an impact. When determining the content of electronic records, all of these sources are used in addition to standards for the functions expected of electronic health record (EHR) systems. Beyond that, there is also the possibility of some customization of record structure and content to meet individual provider or group preferences. This chapter provides an overview of the information needs, the guidelines, and the standards that help to define the content of the provider electronic health record.

RECORD PURPOSES

The primary purpose of a health record is to document care received, including the steps taken to identify a diagnosis or problem and to treat it. This evidence is important for the care of the patient both now and in the future. The health record is also a tool for communicating information to other care providers so that the entire health care team works together to provide quality services. In addition, information from the record may be used for other purposes such as billing and payment for services, research and public health reporting, quality of care evaluation, education and training of health care professionals, and planning for changes in the provider's practice. Patients, care providers, and organizations rely on the record for legal protection. All of those purposes need to be considered in determining record content. Table 4-1 summarizes the major purposes of ambulatory care health records and provides examples of uses for each purpose.

source-oriented record Patient record in which content is organized by the type of health professional entering data.

RECORD FORMATS AND TYPES OF DATA

Display of data in electronic health records may follow several established formats. A **source-oriented record** organizes content by the type of health professional entering data. For example, physician documentation would be

TABLE 4-1 Purposes of a Health Record

RECORD PURPOSES	EXAMPLE OF USES
Document care/services provided.	A physician records the results of a physical examination in a patient's health record.
Provide support for clinical decisions.	A physician uses the results of urinalysis and culture and sensitivity tests to prescribe an antibiotic for a patient's urinary tract infection.
Communicate with other care providers.	Results of a stress test consultation by a cardiologist are sent to the referring primary physician.
Evaluate quality of services.	Fifty health records of pediatric patients are reviewed by office staff to check if immunization policies are being followed.
Provide data for administrative decisions.	The governing board of a rural health clinic reviews a report of services provided to children to determine if there is sufficient need to hire a pediatrician.
Provide evidence for billing and payment of services.	A reimbursement specialist reviews a patient's health record to assign the correct evaluation and management (E&M) code.
Provide data for accreditation or licensure.	Surveyors from an accreditation association review health records of 30 patients currently being treated at a clinic to determine if care is being recorded accurately.
Provide data for research.	The records of 20 patients treated in an early intervention program for diabetes are compared to 20 who did not participate to evaluate whether the program made a difference in the progress of the disease.
Provide data for public health and health policy.	Positive results of tuberculosis testing are reported to the local health department for patient follow-up.
Educate health care professionals.	Medical assistant students receive part of their clinical training at a community health clinic where they review patient health records and assist in treating and educating patients.
Train office personnel.	A therapist new to a practice is oriented to the patient record system through an online tutorial and review of documentation completed by a therapist mentor.
Provide legal evidence of services rendered.	A practice responds to a subpoena for a patient record in response to a disputed claim for services.

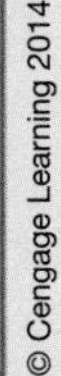

viewed in sections separate from recording done by a nurse or therapist. To read notes by all these individuals, one would need to move between several screens. In an **integrated record** material is organized by type of recording. Integrated progress notes, for example, would include notes made by a nurse, a physician, or any other provider on the same screen in date order (chronologically) or with the most recent documentation first (reverse chronologically). Computer systems have the capacity to integrate material that is entered by a variety of sources, adding flexibility to the visual presentation of data that cannot be found in paper-based records. In other words, depending on the need of the individual accessing a record, the documentation could be displayed in either of these sequences.

integrated record Patient record in which material is organized by type of recording.

problem-oriented record
Patient record organized by patient problems numbered in order as they are identified, where all recording refers back to the specific problem through documentation of its number.

clinical data
Components of a patient record that relate to the care and treatment provided to the patient.

administrative data
Documentation in a patient's record that is not related to care or treatment provided; includes demographic, financial, and consent information.

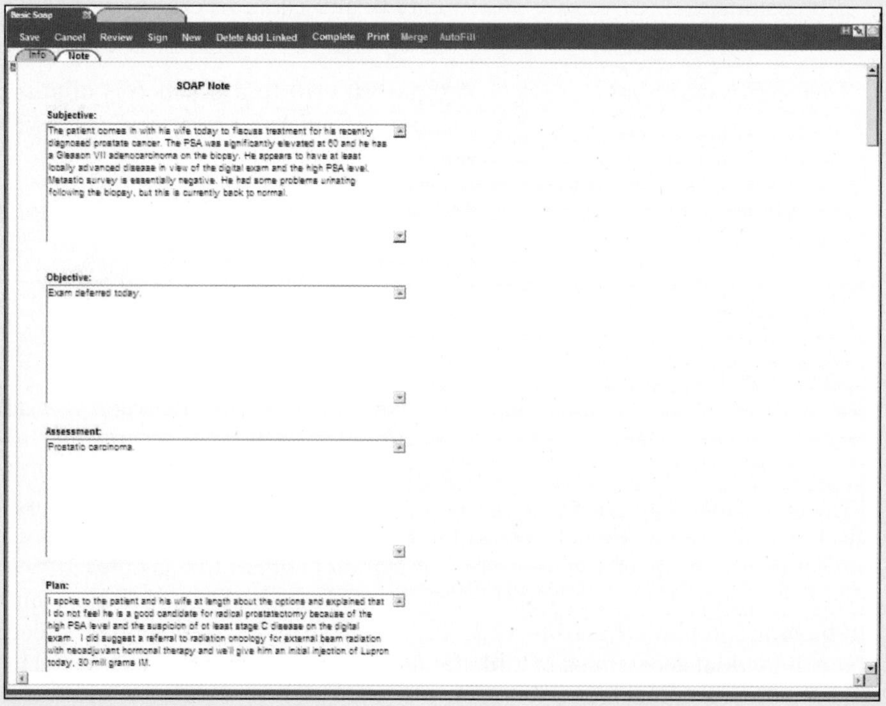

An electronic record also may be designed to reflect a **problem-oriented record** format. This format was designed in the 1960s by Dr. Lawrence L. Weed in response to his work with medical students. As the name suggests, this format organizes data by identified patient problem. Problems are recorded in a problem list and assigned a number. All recording relating to a specific problem is identified by that same problem number throughout the record. Problems sometimes are subdivided further into acute or short-term problems (e.g., an upper respiratory infection) and chronic or continuing problems (e.g., diabetes mellitus). A problem-oriented record also includes a database documenting information such as the patient's family, social, and medical histories; a physical examination; and initial diagnostic test results. A treatment plan or care plan then is developed for each problem. Progress notes recording the response to treatment also are identified by problem number and may be organized in what is called a SOAP format. The "S" in SOAP refers to subjective information that is supplied by the patient, family members, or others involved in care and often uses direct quotes from these individuals. Objective ("O") information includes observations of the care provider and significant findings from testing and evaluations. The "A" or assessment section of a SOAP note documents the conclusions of the care provider based on the previous subjective and objective information evaluated. The "P" or plan records the next steps determined by the provider for the patient's treatment. Notes may not always include all four SOAP components. If applied consistently, the problem-oriented record provides evidence of the thought processes used in health care decisions. Figure 4-1 shows an example of a SOAP note in an EHR.

Most records contain two major types of data: administrative and clinical. **Clinical data** includes all documentation that relates to the provision of care. This type of data begins with the patient history and physical examination and includes all diagnostic testing and procedural notes and recording by all health care professionals contributing to the patient's treatment. **Administrative data** identifies the patient, the patient's payment source, and pertinent patient contacts such as next of kin. It also includes patient rights statements and consents or acknowledgments

Basic Soap
Save Cancel Review Sign New Delete Add Linked Complete Print Merge AutoFill
Info Note

SOAP Note

Subjective:
The patient comes in with his wife today to discuss treatment for his recently diagnosed prostate cancer. The PSA was significantly elevated at 60 and he has a Gleason VII adenocarcinoma on the biopsy. He appears to have at least locally advanced disease in view of the digital exam and the high PSA level. Metastic survey is essentially negative. He had some problems urinating following the biopsy, but this is currently back to normal.

Objective:
Exam deferred today.

Assessment:
Prostatic carcinoma.

Plan:
I spoke to the patient and his wife at length about the options and explained that I do not feel he is a good candidate for radical prostatectomy because of the high PSA level and the suspicion of ot least stage C disease on the digital exam. I did suggest a referral to radiation oncology for external beam radiation with neoadjuvant hormonal therapy and we'll give him an initial injection of Lupron today, 30 milligrams IM.

Figure 4-1 Excerpt of a SOAP note in e-Medsys®.

concerning a practice's privacy policies and processes for maintaining the confidentiality of medical information. Patient identifiers, often referred to as **demographic information**, are gathered during the registration process when an individual presents himself or herself for health care services. The patient's name, address, gender, marital status, race or ethnicity, date of birth, and some type of unique patient identifier (such as the record number or account number) are all part of demographic information.

demographic information Patient identifying information gathered during initial contact and patient registration.

ambulatory care The health care category of patients who are not admitted to occupy a bed but rather seek health care services usually in the provider's office setting; the patient physically moves to the provider's location in order to receive care.

licensure standards Regulations established by each state for health care providers or facilities desiring to operate within the state's borders.

accreditation standards Guidelines developed by independent nonprofit groups that apply to health care facilities that voluntarily choose to comply.

certification standards Regulations, such as those developed by the Medicare program, that must be met in order to receive Medicare or Medicaid reimbursement; includes sections on patient records.

RECORD STANDARDS

When searching for standards that affect provider practice health records, **ambulatory care** is the terminology frequently used by regulatory bodies. Ambulatory care is a category of health care where patients are not admitted to occupy a bed to receive health care, instead seeking health care services usually in the provider's office setting. Health record standards occasionally may be found under other titles, such as clinics, or even more specifically under classifications such as rural clinics. There are also separate standards for ambulatory surgery centers and for urgent or emergency care providers. All potential sources need to be evaluated to ensure that a practice's health records include the documentation required to meet the standards that apply to its specific type of clinical practice.

Standards that can affect the content of a practice's electronic record include guidelines from internal organizational policies, provider or facility **licensure standards**, standards that apply to those providers who have earned specialty designations, **accreditation standards**, and **certification standards**. Addressing the need for interoperability between electronic record systems of health care providers across all health care settings has resulted in national standards for data in EHRs and for the functions that ambulatory electronic records should be able to perform. A more detailed discussion of each type of standard will be presented later in this chapter.

Organization Policies

Although not as complex as larger medical settings such as hospitals, many practices will have established office policies that include guidelines for clinical documentation. These policies are based on federal and state guidelines for practice, incorporate concepts from federal mandates, and establish restrictions to viewing medical information based on need and confidentiality. They might include identification of the types of health care professionals who actually may document in the record, the frequency of that documentation, the length of time that records need to be maintained (retention period), as well as guidelines for what actually must be documented. Because policies vary from practice to practice, it is important to check these formalized statements and ensure that the EHR can support the practice's guidelines.

Licensure Standards

The term *licensure* refers to standards established by each state for health care providers or facilities desiring to operate within the state's borders. Most states have facility licensure requirements for health care settings such as hospitals, long-term care facilities, and home health agencies, but do not have special licensure requirements for health care provider practices. However, pharmacies or laboratories located within practices may be required to obtain licenses to operate. The licenses often provide guidelines for recording of medications dispensed and laboratory test findings. These required elements must be part of the EHR.

More important for the practice setting, physicians, nurses, and some other allied health professionals must have individual professional licenses before they are allowed to provide services. Each state sets specific requirements for licensing of health care providers, including which categories of professionals must be licensed. These licensure standards usually will address the professional's responsibilities to document care provided in a timely fashion and to authenticate entries by signature; the standards also establish practice limits for the profession. Standards for health care professional's practice can include factors important to a record's content, such as whether or not a therapist can practice independently or must have medical supervision or physician orders for treatment. Knowledge of these professional practice standards and any record-related licensing requirements must be researched and incorporated into EHR documentation systems.

Specialty Designation Standards

Physicians who specialize in a particular area such as surgery often seek recognition of their skills and abilities by applying for a professional designation. Designation as a specialist indicates that the physician has advanced knowledge and experience within the specialty care area and meets the rigorous guidelines of the specialty group. Many times specific requirements about patient record documentation are among the items included in the specialty application when it is submitted for approval or included in the standards of the professional specialty once approval has been awarded. For example, the American College of Obstetricians and Gynecologists (ACOG) and the American Academy of Pediatrics (AAP) both publish guidelines that provide practices with care information that impacts the content of patient records. Other health professionals, such as nurse practitioners or physician assistants, also may have specialty designations and specific requirements for their documentation.

Accreditation Standards

Accrediting organizations are independent nonprofit groups that develop standards for health care facilities that voluntarily choose to comply. If the standards are met, the health care setting and its care providers are recognized as meeting challenging guidelines that support quality care. An on-site survey and supporting documents provided determine compliance. Once accreditation is received, monitoring continues as a requirement to maintain accreditation. Accreditation of independent ambulatory care settings is not as commonly found as it is in hospital-associated services such as outpatient clinics and surgery centers.

There are a number of organizations that accredit ambulatory care. The **Accreditation Association for Ambulatory Health Care (AAAHC)** focuses entirely on ambulatory settings and publishes its standards in its *Accreditation Handbook for Ambulatory Health Care*. The organization's web site lists the following types of facilities that, upon meeting eligibility guidelines, may apply for a survey to become accredited:

- Ambulatory health care clinics.
- Ambulatory surgery centers.

Accreditation Association for Ambulatory Health Care (AAAHC)
One of a number of voluntary organizations providing standards for and evaluating care in ambulatory care facilities; this organization focuses entirely on various types of ambulatory care settings.

- Birthing centers.
- College and university health centers.
- Community health centers.
- Dental group practices.
- Diagnostic imaging centers.
- Endoscopy centers.
- Federally Qualified Health Centers (FQHC).
- Health Maintenance Organizations (HMOs).
- Independent Physician Associations (IPAs).
- Indian health centers.
- Lithotripsy centers.
- Managed care organizations.
- Medical home organizations.
- Military health care facilities.
- Multi-specialty group practices.
- Occupational health centers.
- Office-based anesthesia organizations.
- Office-based surgery centers and practices.
- Oral and maxillofacial surgeons' offices.
- Pain management centers.
- Podiatry practices.
- Radiation oncology centers.
- Single specialty group practices.
- Surgical recovery centers.
- Urgent or immediate care centers.
- Women's health centers. (AAAHC, 2011b.)

Standards of this group are subdivided into core standards, which include a chapter on Clinical Records and Health Information, and adjunct standards, which address many of the specialty group requirements such as those for anesthesia services, pharmaceutical services, or radiation and oncology treatment services (AAAHC, 2011b).

The Joint Commission (JC) (formerly known as The Joint Commission for Accreditation of Healthcare Organizations, or JCAHO) provides standards for many types of health care settings, including ambulatory care practices. In addition to its *Standards for Ambulatory Care*, it publishes other ambulatory care-related accreditation guidelines for office-based practices, ambulatory surgery centers, imaging centers, sleep centers, urgent care centers, and laboratory and point-of-care testing services. Most of the standards in The Joint Commission's ambulatory care manual pertain to all ambulatory settings; this includes the Record of Care, Treatment and Services (RC) section that focuses on content of health records. Other standards sections, such as those for Medication Management (MM), Rights and Responsibilities of the Individual (RI), and Information Management (IM) include statements regarding documentation or with

The Joint Commission (JC)
One of a number of voluntary organizations providing standards for and evaluating care in ambulatory care facilities; this organization provides these services to a wide variety of types of health care settings in addition to ambulatory care facilities.

National Committee for Quality Assurance (NCQA)
One of a number of voluntary organizations providing standards for and evaluating care in managed care organizations.

American Osteopathic Association (AOA)
One of a number of voluntary organizations providing standards for and evaluating care in ambulatory care facilities, laboratories, and ambulatory surgery settings.

American Association for Accreditation of Ambulatory Surgery Facilities (AAAASF)
One of a number of voluntary organizations providing standards for and evaluating care in ambulatory surgery facilities.

Commission for the Accreditation of Birth Centers
A voluntary organization providing standards for and evaluating care in birthing centers.

Medicare
National program to provide federally funded health care assistance to the elderly in the United States.

Medicaid
A joint state- and federal-funded program providing health care benefits to populations below a defined income level.

Conditions of Participation (CoP), or Conditions of Coverage (CoC)
General name for the regulations that care providers must meet in order to participate in the Medicare/Medicaid programs.

indirect impact on documentation, so it is always a good practice to review all the standards for applicable guidelines. (JC, 2011.)

There are a number of other organizations that accredit specific types of ambulatory settings. For example: the **National Committee for Quality Assurance (NCQA)** accredits managed care organizations; the **American Osteopathic Association (AOA)** accredits laboratories, ambulatory care, and ambulatory surgery settings; and the **American Association for Accreditation of Ambulatory Surgery Facilities (AAAASF)**, and the **Commission for the Accreditation of Birth Centers** accredit those specific types of ambulatory settings. In addition, the accreditation standards for hospitals published by The Joint Commission include standards for hospital-associated outpatient, emergency, and surgical ambulatory sites. Whether or not a practice chooses to undergo accreditation review by any of these organizations, the standards of these groups provide excellent guidance on health record content.

Certification Standards

In relation to health record systems, certification refers to approval to receive reimbursement from the federal Medicare and/or Medicaid programs. **Medicare** programs provide federally funded health care assistance to the elderly. **Medicaid** is a joint federal/state funded program providing health care benefits to populations below a specific income level. Facilities that wish to become certified must meet either the **Conditions of Participation (CoP)** or **Conditions of Coverage (CoC)** that are published in the *Code of Federal Regulations*. Within ambulatory care, there are specific conditions pertinent to ambulatory surgery centers, rural health clinics, some behavioral care providers, and some rehabilitative care providers. All of these standards include guidelines for documentation practices and record content. Most practices, however, receive reimbursement based on the registration of individual health care providers as participating practitioners with the federal and state governments. Participating health care providers must follow these established guidelines in providing and documenting care and in billing practices.

Data Sets

Another action taken to further uniformity in data elements collected in ambulatory records was initiated by the U.S. Department of Health and Human Services. The end result of these efforts was the development of the **Uniform Ambulatory Care Data Set (UACDS)** approved by the National Committee on Vital and Health Statistics (NCVHS) in 1989 (Giannangelo, 2011). In 2001, as a result of their report, *Toward a National Health Information Infrastructure*, a new list of elements was published by the same group. The **NCVHS Core Content of the Healthcare Provider Dimension** was established for use by health care providers at or near the point of care. Its content is presented in Table 4-2. Core contents also were developed by the same organization for personal health records (see Chapter10) and for community health purposes.

In 2006, another type of data content standard was developed when the continuity of care record (CCR) core data set was approved by the American National Standards Institute (ANSI). This data set was established to identify record content that should be transmitted from one health care provider to another in order to assure good communication and efficient continuity of care for a patient seeing multiple providers or transferring care from one provider to another.

TABLE 4-2 NCVHS Core Health Data Elements for the Health Care Provider Dimension

PATIENT RECORD ELEMENTS
Personal identification information.
Socio-demographic identifiers (may include elements of longitudinal history such as family, social, and medical history, gender, birthday, age, race/ethnicity, marital status, living arrangements, education level, occupation).
Health insurance information (including covered benefits).
Legal consents or permissions.
Referral information.
Correspondence.
Patient history information (family history, immunizations, allergies, current medications).
Stated reason for visit.
External causes of injury/illness.
Symptoms.
Physical exams.
Assessment of patient signs and symptoms.
Diagnoses.
Laboratory, radiology, and pharmacy orders.
Laboratory results.
Radiological images and interpretations.
Record of alerts, warnings, and reminders.
Operative reports.
Vital signs.
Treatment plans and instructions.
Progress notes.
Functional status.
Discharge summaries.
Instructions about access.
Audit log of individuals who accessed patient record.
Patient amendments to patient record.
Provider notes, such as knowledge of patient, patient-provider interactions, patient's access to services.
OTHER ELEMENTS THAT SUPPORT CLINICAL PRACTICE
Protocols, practice guidelines.
Clinical decision support programs.
Referral history.

Source: National Center for Vital and Health Statistics. "Information for Health: A Strategy for Building the National Health Information Infrastructure." www.nchs.hhs.gov/nhiilayo.pdf (Retrieved)

Uniform Ambulatory Care Data Set (UACDS)
Basic list of information that should be found in ambulatory patient records, as initially approved in 1989 by the National Committee on Vital and Health Statistics.

National Committee for Vital and Health Statistics (NCVHS) Core Content of the Healthcare Provider Dimension
An update of the Uniform Ambulatory Care Data Set providing a list of elements to be found in health care provider patient records.

American Health Information Management Association (AHIMA)
A national member organization of health information management professionals that developed a core data set for ambulatory records; one of the Cooperating Party organizations that participate in recommendations regarding the content of ICD for use in the U.S.

Health Plan Employer Data and Information Set (HEDIS)
Defined set of information that is found in ambulatory records outlined by the National Committee for Quality Assurance as part of a system to measure and compare quality of care across physician providers.

The Standard Specification for the Continuity of Care Record states that the CCR includes "a summary of the patient's health status (for example, problems, medications, allergies) and basic information about insurance, advance directives, care documentation, and the patient's care plan" (ASTM 2007). The CCR core data set is an EHR content standard that applies to all types of health care provider organizations: ambulatory, inpatient, and long-term care (See Chapter 13 for a full discussion of the CCR).

Other data sets also have been proposed for some ambulatory record settings. For example, a work group formed by the **American Health Information Management Association (AHIMA)**, a national member organization of health information management professionals, developed "core data sets" for physician practice electronic health records. Specific data element lists were identified for new and established well-pediatric, well-adult, sick-pediatric, and sick-adult patient populations (AHIMA Work Group, 2003). A publication by another AHIMA Work Group provides a comprehensive list of organizations with core data sets affecting the EHR (AHIMA Work Group, 2004).

Although not designed to focus on documentation practices, the National Committee for Quality Assurance referred to previously has developed a **Health Plan Employer Data and Information Set (HEDIS)**. Intended to help employers compare managed care plans, the development of uniform data elements to be reported for participation in this program has a major impact on the content of a health care provider's records. Practitioners who participate in managed care plans may be required to supply this data as a condition for continued reimbursement, including participation in the Medicare or Medicaid programs. Data elements reported are seen as indicators of quality of services. Clinical measures included in HEDIS cover such diverse topics as diabetes care, immunization status for children and adolescents, monitoring of high blood pressure, and screening for breast and cervical cancer (see NCQA, 2007).

Finally, the federal HITECH Act referred to in Chapter 1 added clinical quality measures to "meaningful use" criteria. It requires practices to report on these clinical measures, in addition to initiation and use of an EHR, in order to receive incentive payments. For example, during years 2011 and 2012 quality measures include: computed tomography or magnetic resonance imaging reports for stroke patients; selection, ordering, and discontinuance of perioperative antibiotics; and treatment of children with upper respiratory infections without prescription or provision of antibiotics within three days of service. (U.S. Department of Health and Human Services, 2010.) Records must include the required report data to ensure all appropriate funding incentives are received.

The importance of using standardized data sets is also recognized by accrediting organizations. For example, The Joint Commission notes in its Elements of Performance for Standard IM.02.02.01, "The organization uses uniform data sets to standardize data collection throughout the organization." (2011, p. IM-8.) The rationale for this standard includes the following statements:

> Capturing data in standardized language can lead to greater data integrity and reliability, as well as an increased potential for ease of use by internal and external systems and users. The more consistent the organization's efforts are to capture accurate data in standardized language, the more likely the organization will be to rely on that data for patient-related purposes, including reimbursement, risk management, performance improvement, and infection surveillance. (2011, p. IM-8.)

More on standardized data and vocabularies can be found in Chapter 3.

A summary of the health record content standards referenced here can be found in Table 4-3.

TABLE 4-3 Examples of Standards that Affect Ambulatory Care Record Content

TYPE OF STANDARD	SAMPLE SPONSORING ORGANIZATIONS
Licensure (required to provide services in the state).	State specific standards; check state regulations to identify those that apply.
Specialty practice guidelines.	American College of Obstetricians and Gynecologists (ACOG), American Academy of Pediatrics (AAP).
Accreditation (voluntary).	Accreditation Association for Ambulatory Health Care (AAAHC), The Joint Commission (JC), National Committee for Quality Assurance (NCQA), American Osteopathic Association (AOA), American Association for Accreditation of Ambulatory Surgery Facilities (AAAASF), Commission for the Accreditation of Birth Centers.
Certification (required if receiving Medicare/ Medicaid reimbursement).	Conditions of Participation or Conditions of Coverage.
Data sets (voluntary; mandatory under some circumstances).	NCVHS Core Content of the Healthcare Provider Dimension, AHIMA Core Data Sets, Health Plan Employer Data and Information Set (HEDIS), "Meaningful Use" Quality Measures.

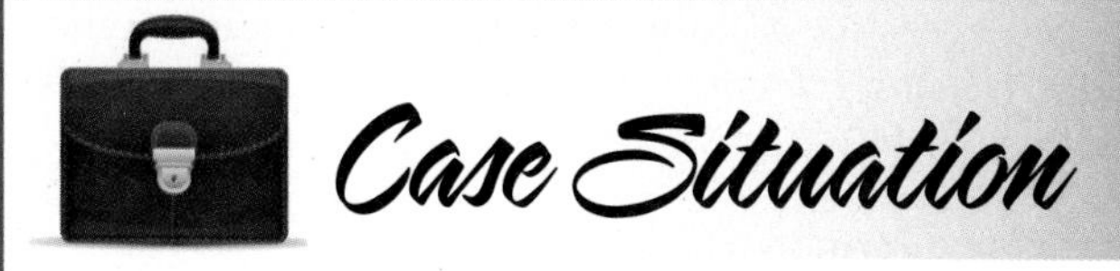

The corporate owners of a multi-specialty clinic have decided to add an on-site laboratory and pharmacy and an evening urgent care service. They understand that additional standards will apply to these services. State licensure is required for the laboratory and pharmacy, so these guidelines must be met prior to either department opening. State regulations are accessed to determine those requirements. The urgent care services are not licensed in this state. Since the group participates in the Medicare and Medicaid programs and is also a HEDIS participating managed care provider, the owners know that the pertinent Conditions of Participation, the NCQA standards (including HEDIS data elements), and "Meaningful Use" Quality Measures will need to be checked for compliance as far as services and service documentation are concerned. They are not sure what other recording might be needed, but elect to refer to the AAAHC and The Joint Commission standards to provide guidance. Anything learned can be used if the clinic decides to seek accreditation by one of those two groups in the future. By checking all of these reference sources and complying with the standards found in them, the owners believe that the new services will be approved and reimbursed and that financial incentives may be awarded as well.

RECORD CONTENT

Basic ambulatory record content can be determined by examining the standards and regulations that have been introduced in this chapter. Although this is not a comprehensive list, at a minimum ambulatory records should contain:

- Patient identification and demographic data.
- Patient consents and advance directives.
- Patient history (from patient and physician).
- Problem and allergy lists.
- Medication list.
- Physical examination findings and/or special assessments.
- Progress notes.
- Treatment plans and reports.
- Physician or other qualified health professional's orders.
- Diagnostic and laboratory test reports.
- Flow sheets and graphic charts.
- Immunization and injection records.
- Patient-disposition and patient-instruction information.
- Telephone contact information.

Each of these elements will be addressed in more detail in the following chapters.

DOCUMENTATION PRACTICES

In addition to the guidelines already described for record content, there are established principles for documentation practices that have been developed over time. They support both good practice and the legal defense of record content. As outlined by the American Health Information Management Association (see Smith, 2001), these guidelines include:

- Unity of the content and format of all records.
- Systematic organization of information in the record.
- Definition of those allowed to document in the record.
- Definition of who may receive and transcribe verbal orders.
- Timely documentation of services when they are provided.
- Clear identification of all authors of record entries.
- Use of only approved abbreviations and symbols.
- All entries become permanent.
- Errors in recording are identified as such; erroneous information is never deleted or obliterated.
- Patient corrections to records are inserted as addendums; original notes are not altered.
- Regular evaluation of record content both quantitatively (i.e., is the documentation complete? Are all required parts present?) and qualitatively (i.e., does the documentation meet established guidelines and policies?).

Fortunately, several of these practices are actually a part of an EHR system's design. For example, vendors include uniform content and systematic information organization as part of their software design. Guidelines for the use of abbreviations, timeliness of recording, and authorization for verbal order transcription come from the provider's practice policies. However, edit notices—alerts presented on screen to providers to assure compliance with documentation policies—can become part of the electronic record if desired. Still other documentation monitoring processes, such as quantitative and qualitative documentation reviews, may be adjusted for viewing electronically, but will remain similar to those processes performed on paper records. Other documentation guidelines do require significant adjustment for the EHR environment. They require further discussion, as follows.

Correcting Errors

The correction of errors in information recorded by a health care provider in an EHR requires a change in practices from paper-based recording. No information recorded at any time in a patient record should ever be totally deleted. However, errors in entries do need to be identified, and corrections must be made to the data or report within the EHR. Most EHR systems have the capability to delete or modify all types of data that may have been entered: orders, problems, assessment data, reports, and so on. When the "delete" or "modify" capability is selected, an "in error" or "modified" notation immediately is associated with the data in the record. In addition, the date/time/user identification is attached to the delete/modify action, and the date/time/user identification is attached to the new or modified data entered. The date, time, and user identification is added automatically by the system through system programs and the computer access code entered by the person making the record entry. This allows a reader of the documentation to follow the chronological sequence of recordings. Figure 4-2 displays an example of an audit trail history associated with a modification made in an entry.

Although the incorrect information no longer may appear on the screen after a correction has been made in an EHR, it is retained in a format so that it can be audited for legal purposes. Healthcare decisions may have been made based on content before the correction was inserted. A computer audit trail associated with the EHR will provide, if required, information about when specific entries were made, what information was available at what time, who made the correction, and so forth.

Chart History -- Patient Note -- JONES, SALLY

Review History

Review DateTime	Reviewed By
8/27/2012 12:51 PM	LAUREN WHALEN
7/6/2012 4:38 PM	JANELLE WAPOLA

Message History

Routed DateTime	To	From	Action	Priority	Message	Completed

Audit Trail

DateTime	Staff	Action	Module	Item Desc.	Misc.
8/27/2012 12:51 PM	lwhalen	VIEW	ChartViewerDetail		
8/27/2012 12:51 PM	lwhalen	VIEW	ChartViewerDetail		
8/27/2012 12:51 PM	lwhalen	UPDATE_SIGNED	DB	Updated Signed Item	

Figure 4-2 Example of an Audit Trail Notice for a modified EHR entry in e-Medsys®.

The Joint Commission's "Do Not Use" Abbreviation List
The Joint Commission's list of medical abbreviations that cause errors in interpretation and hence should not be found in the patient documentation of facilities that desire their accreditation.

Abbreviations

Abbreviations continue to create data quality problems in EHRs, just as they have in paper-based health records. Too often a single abbreviation can have multiple meanings, or one concept may have numerous abbreviations associated with it. For example, M can mean "myopia," "meter," "muscle," "thousand," or "male," and metastasis or metastases is often abbreviated "met," "metas," or "mets". The use of these types of abbreviations can lead to errors in communication between health care providers. Unfortunately, a comprehensive national abbreviations standard does not exist. **The Joint Commission's "Do Not Use" Abbreviations List** (see Table 4-4) is presented as a minimum national content standard that can and should be applied to documentation in EHR systems. It contains abbreviations that have been identified as having significant potential for causing errors in communication that could cause harm to a patient. Even though no comprehensive federal abbreviations standard exists, a good first step for a practice is to use credible sources (for example, Dorland or Stedman's Medical Dictionary and The Joint Commission's "Do Not Use" Abbreviations List) to develop a practice policy. The practice's abbreviations standard then can be used consistently by those who are building the EHR data dictionary and by those who are transcribing narrative reports for inclusion in the EHR.

Signatures

According to basic medical records standards, each health care provider entry in a health record must be signed by its author. The most important requirement related to a legal signature is that only the person making an entry should add the signature to that entry. A signature authenticates the entry; that is, it attests to the content of the entry and its accuracy. For this reason, authorization to sign documents done by one health care provider must not be given to others. This principle of authentication by signature also applies to consent and authorization forms that must be signed by the patient or the patient's representative.

TABLE 4-4 The Joint Commission's "Do Not Use" Abbreviations List

DO NOT USE	POTENTIAL PROBLEM	USE INSTEAD
U u (unit).	Mistaken for "0" (zero), the number "4" (four), or "cc."	Write "unit."
IU (International Unit).	Mistaken for IV (intravenous) or the number "10" (ten).	Write "International Unit."
Q.D., QD., q.d., qd (daily) Q.O.D., QOD, q.o.d., qod (every other day).	Mistaken for each other; period after the Q mistaken for "I" and the "O" mistaken for "I."	Write "daily" and write "every other day."
Trailing zero (X.0 mg) or lack of leading zero (.X mg).	Decimal point is missed.	Write "X mg" and write "0.X mg."
MS MSO_4 and $MgSO_4$.	Can mean morphine sulfate or magnesium sulfate; could be mistaken for each other.	Write "morphine sulfate" and write "magnesium sulfate."

Source: Reprinted with permission. © The Joint Commission, 2011, p. IM 8-9.

TABLE 4-5 The Joint Commission's Standard and Performance Elements for Signatures
STANDARD RC.01.02.01
ENTRIES IN THE CLINICAL RECORD ARE AUTHENTICATED.
ELEMENTS OF PERFORMANCE FOR RC.01.02.01
1. Only authorized individuals make entries in the clinical record.
2. The organization defines the types of entries in the clinical record made by nonindependent practitioners that require countersigning, in accordance with law and regulation.
3. The author of each clinical record entry is identified in the clinical record.
4. Entries in the clinical record are authenticated by the author. Information introduced into the clinical record through transcription or dictation is authenticated by the author. Note 1: Authentication can be verified through electronic signatures, written signatures or initials, rubber-stamp signatures, or computer key. Note 2:. . . For electronic records, electronic signatures will be date-stamped.
5. The individual identified by the signature stamp or method of electronic authentication is the only individual who uses it.

Source: Reprinted with permission. © The Joint Commission, 2011, pp. RC-4 and 5.

Status: **Saved:** jwapola 07/06/2012 04:21 PM **Signed:** jwapola 07/06/2012 04:21 PM

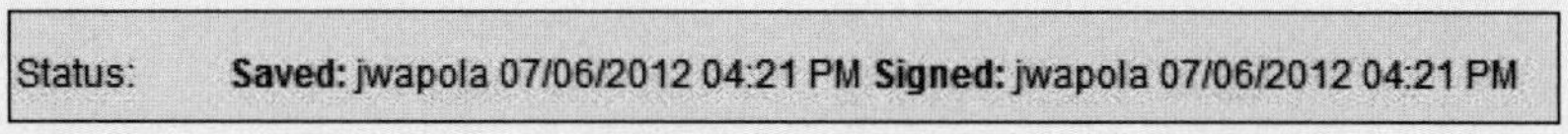

Figure 4-3 Example of an electronic signature in e-Medsys®.

Reprinted with permission of TriMed Technologies, Corp.

The importance of signing or authenticating records is recognized by most of the approval groups noted in the previous section on record-content standards. For example, the AAAHC notes simply that, in addition to clinical information, entries in a patient's record for each visit must include, "Authentication and verification of contents by health care professionals." (2011, p. 41.) On the other hand, The Joint Commission's ambulatory manual includes an entire Standard and Elements of Performance on the subject. That information can be found in Table 4-5.

Signatures in an electronic record system can be attached in several different manners. If the system has an electronic signature pad similar to those found in some retail stores, the patient or care provider can use the "pen" to sign on the pad's window in the designated box. This seems foreign to some individuals, and acceptance by the practice's patient population will need to be considered before this method is adopted. A more common method for health care provider use is to assign a computer key or keys that, when used, provides a signature. The key or keys must be used only by the assigned provider. An example of this type of electronic signature is shown in Figure 4-3.

A third method used more with patients is to continue using paper documents and then to scan the signed document into the electronic record for retention and viewing. A practice may use one or all three of these methods. If more than one method is adopted, practice policies should address which is to be used by whom and under what conditions. Before any specific type of electronic signature is adopted for use in a practice, state laws must be reviewed to make sure that it is legally acceptable for business and health care transactions.

SUMMARY

The format and content of ambulatory health records are essential to the successful application of electronic records in the practice setting. The record must be designed to fulfill its purposes, meet pertinent standards, record items needed for data sets, and follow established documentation guidelines, including appropriate correction of errors, use of abbreviations, and attachment of signature authentications. Uniformity in content will permit sharing of health care information across providers, benefiting the patient as well as care providers. If these guidelines are followed, more informed decisions that support continuity of care will result. An electronic health record not only documents patient treatment but also supports other functions that contribute to efficiency and quality of services and to management of the health care practice as a business.

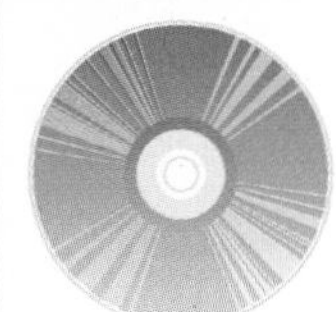

Computer Exploration

1. Many of the organizations introduced in this chapter have web sites that provide more information. Use the web sites listed below to explore an organization or organizations and gather the following information. (*Note:* Complete information may not be available from all web sites.)
   - **a.** How long has the organization been in existence?
   - **b.** What is the organization's purpose?
   - **c.** Who are the members of the organization?
   - **d.** What types of health care settings are serviced by the organization?
   - **e.** Does the organization provide standards for ambulatory care practices? If so, what is the name of the standards publication? How can it be obtained, and is there a cost associated with obtaining the standards? If the organization does not provide standards, what is its role with regard to EHR systems?
   - **f.** What are the steps in the organization's review/approval process?

Accreditation Association for Ambulatory Health Care (AAAHC)

http://www.aaahc.org

American Association for Accreditation of Ambulatory Surgery Facilities (AAAASF)

http://www.aaaasf.org

American Osteopathic Association (AOA)

http://www.osteopathic.org

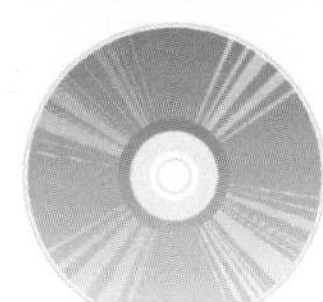

Computer Exploration continued

Commission for the Accreditation of Birth Centers

http://www.birthcenters.org

The Joint Commission (JC)

http://www.jointcommission.org

National Committee for Quality Assurance (NCQA)

http://www.ncqa.org

National Committee on Vital and Health Statistics (NCVHS)

http://www.ncvhs.hhs.gov

2. Search The Joint Commission's web site for the most current "Do Not Use" Abbreviation List. Are there additional abbreviations being considered for future inclusion in the list? If so, what changes are anticipated?

REFERENCES

AAAHC [Accreditation Association for Ambulatory Health care]. (2011a). *Accreditation handbook for ambulatory health care.* Wilmette, IL: AAAHC.

AAAHC. (2011b). Types of organizations accredited and AAAHC Accreditation Standards. Wilmette, IL: AAAHC. Retrieved from http://aaahc.org/

AHIMA e-HIM Work Group on Core Data Sets for the Physician Practice Electronic Health Record. (2003, October). Core data sets for the physician practice electronic health record (AHIMA Practice Brief). Chicago, IL: AHIMA. Retrieved from http://library.ahima.org

AHIMA Work Group on Core Data Sets as Standards for the EHR. (2004, September). E-HIM strategic initiative: Core data sets. Appendix A: Core data sets as standards for the EHR (pt. 1). Chicago, IL: AHIMA. Retrieved from http://library.ahima.org/

ASTM [American Standards for Testing and measurement]. (2007). Active standard: E2369-05 standard specification for continuity of care record (CCR). Retrieved from http://www.astm.org/Standards/E2369.htm

Giannangelo, K. (2011). Healthcare data sets and standards. In M. L. Johns (Ed.) *Health information management technology, An applied approach* (3rd ed., pp. 205–207). Chicago, IL: AHIMA.

The Joint Commission. (2011). *Standards for ambulatory care.* Oakbrook Terrace, IL: JC.

NCQA [National Committee for Quality Assurance]. (2007). HEDIS. Retrieved from http://www.ncqa.org/

National Committee on Vital and Health Statistics. (2001). *Information for health: A strategy for building the national health information infrastructure.* Retrieved from http://www.ncvhs.hhs.gov/nhiilayo.pdf

Smith, C. M. (2001). Documentation requirements for the acute care inpatient record. (AHIMA Practice Brief.) *Journal of AHIMA 72(3),* 56A–G.

U.S. Department of Health and Human Services. (2010, July 10). *Federal register 42 CFR parts 412, 413, 422 et al. Medicare and Medicaid programs; Electronic health record incentive program; Final rule, 75(144).* Washington, DC: National Archives and Records Administration.

REVIEW QUESTIONS

1. What is the primary purpose of a practice's health record?

2. What record purpose is associated with each of the following?
   a. Medical assistant records the height, weight, and vital signs of a patient?

   b. The results of the effectiveness of a new drug involved in a clinical research trial are reported to the study coordinator?

   c. Penicillin is not prescribed for a patient because the allergy list indicates the patient will have a reaction to it?

   d. The results of an annual mammogram are reported to the primary physician?

3. In which record format would documentation of a nurse, physician, and therapist be found in chronological (date) sequence?

4. Of the two major types of record data, which type includes the patient's name, address, payment source, next of kin, and treatment consents?

5. Which type of health record standard varies depending on the state in which the practice is located?

6. What type of health record standard is met when the practice is recognized as voluntarily meeting national indicators of quality care?

7. Which organization was specifically formed to accredit only ambulatory care settings?

8. What nationally recognized ambulatory care data sets have an effect on record content?

9. What are five guidelines outlined by AHIMA for good documentation practices that support legal defense of a record?

10. How does practitioner correction of errors in health records differ between a paper and an electronic health record?

11. Give two examples of abbreviations on The Joint Commission "Do Not Use" list and explain why each should not be used.

12. What are three alternatives for recording signatures in an electronic record?

CHAPTER 5 Patient Visit Management

CHAPTER OUTLINE

OBJECTIVES

Upon completion of the chapter, the learner will be able to:

1. Describe the general workflow that is part of patient visit management in an EHR environment.
2. Differentiate between a master patient/person index (MPI) and an enterprise master patient/person index (EMPI), and state the purpose of each to an EHR.
3. Provide examples of patient demographic information.
4. Describe the content of an MPI and explain how the content is used in a patient record search.
5. Describe processes used to gather billing information and to schedule patients in an electronic environment.
6. Indicate how consents, notices, authorizations for release of information, and advance directives are incorporated into an EHR.
7. Describe two methods for applying patient signatures to documents in an EHR.
8. Provide examples of Certification Committee for Healthcare Information Technology (CCHIT) criteria and accreditation guidelines for patient visit management functions.

KEY TERMS

Advance Beneficiary Notice (ABN)

advance directive

Assignment of Benefits

authorization for release (disclosure) of information

consent for treatment

durable power of attorney for health care

enterprise master patient/person index (EMPI)

living will

master patient/person index (MPI)

Notice of Exclusions from Medicare Benefits

Notice of Privacy Practices

practice management system (PMS)

unit record

INTRODUCTION

The functions of an electronic health record (EHR) in a health care provider practice go beyond the content of the health record itself. There are a number of office processes that tie into the health record and are necessary for the appropriate care of patients and for the success of a practice. Each of these associated functions uses data elements that connect it to the correct patient within the EHR system, and each contributes new information not found elsewhere. Some of these associated functions also require changes or adjustments in traditional practice processes in order to achieve a fully electronic health record environment.

Visit management processes begin when information is gathered during appointment scheduling prior to a patient actually seeing a health care provider. This information will determine when the patient can be seen, whether prior treatment records exist from within the practice and from other health care providers, and whether a bill for services can be initiated. Some tasks accomplished prior to treatment are required by law. The visit management functions described here are performed primarily by practice office staff or managers using practice management software. In the EHR environment the practice management and medical record components communicate directly with each other to facilitate the transfer of information and the use of both. Gathering quality (accurate, relevant, and complete) information when initiating a patient's visit means that the health care provider has a strong information foundation for all related processes. It also means that necessary information will be available for current treatment as well as any continuing care that might be required. Scheduling, registration functions, and patient identity management are the topics of this chapter.

WORKFLOW

The patient management process in an EHR environment begins in a similar manner as a paper environment, with a contact by a patient for an appointment with a health care provider. This contact usually is made via telephone by the patient, but could also be made in person, by e-mail, via the practice's secure Internet patient portal (see Chapter 10), or even by the office staff of a referring physician. Unless an appointment is made by the patient using a practice portal, the request usually is received by health care provider office personnel. The staff member first verifies the patient identification by accessing the practice's master patient index, or adding information to it if a new patient. Generally appointment options are presented beginning with the first available time and date that fits the visit parameters. Alternatives continue until a mutually acceptable choice has been made. The choice then is entered into the scheduling system along with the patient's basic identifiers. Questions also may be asked regarding a physician referral if one is needed and has not yet been received. The contact ends once a satisfactory appointment has been made and all required previsit information has been gathered.

Between the scheduling contact and the actual patient office visit, two additional processes may take place and be recorded in the practice management system. The need for these processes is determined as a result of information provided during scheduling. Using payment information, the office staff may need to contact the expected payer about the patient's health care benefits and receive prior approval for the visit. In addition, using the patient identifying information provided, a query can be made to a referring physician, a health system network, a SNO/HIE/RHIO/ACO, or the National Health Information Network (NHIN) regarding the existence of a patient's prior health care treatment record. The link for access to any previous care records found then can be shared with the provider who will treat the patient for review prior to the visit. If this is not done as a step before the visit, the health care provider or a staff member can do this on the day of the visit for access while the patient is being seen.

Once the patient arrives at the care provider's office, other steps in the registration process must take place. Obviously the patient must identify himself or herself so that the front office staff can check the appointment schedule and verify the patient's identification and payment information. That information will be checked and any changes will be reported and entered into the practice management system. If appropriate, a co-pay, deductible, or treatment payment will be requested. Depending on office policies, a general consent for treatment may be required. A notice of privacy practices must be reviewed and acknowledged by the patient or patient's representative. Consents and privacy notices each require the patient's or his/her representative's signature. If the individual is a new patient, and as policy indicates for continuing patients, the patient also may be asked to complete an assignment of benefits and a personal medical history, including the reason for the visit. Other information required usually includes an indication of whether the patient has executed an advance directive, and provision of additional payment or identifying information. In a practice with an EHR, these tasks all can be done via the patient portal prior to the visit (see Chapter 10) or on a computer in a designated private area to maintain confidentiality. If in the office, depending on the patient's comfort level with computers, data can be entered directly by the patient or the patient's representative, or a member of the office staff can interview the patient and enter the data. After the care provider has seen the patient, another set of visit management functions are performed. A follow-up appointment is scheduled if necessary either by the patient online or with the assistance of office staff. Referrals may be sent to other providers and drug prescriptions sent to the patient's pharmacy. In an EHR, these tasks can be done electronically. Coding, billing, and account processes must be completed (coding and billing are discussed in Chapter 11). Finally, follow-up appointment reminders can be sent via automatic generation of letters for mailing, lists for calling, or e-mails if patients have indicated approval for receiving them (see Chapter 10). At the next visit, the process begins again.

practice management system (PMS)
System that supports the financial and administrative functions of a practice; usually includes patient demographics, appointment scheduling, charge capture and billing, and report generation.

master patient/person index (MPI)
The key to locating a patient record, this listing includes patient identifying information and the assigned record number for all individuals ever receiving care by an organization.

MASTER PATIENT INDEX

A computer-based system designed to support many of the business process activities of health care provider office practices is called a **practice management system (PMS)**. PMS software has been around for some time, so most practice personnel are familiar with its functions. PMS applications either can be embedded within or be separate from and simply linked to the EHR. One application in an office practice management system is the **master patient/person index (MPI)**. The MPI is key to correctly identifying the patient and connecting different parts of an electronic record system. The master patient/person index includes patient identification information and assigned record numbers, if numbers are used. The goal is for the EHR to have only one longitudinal

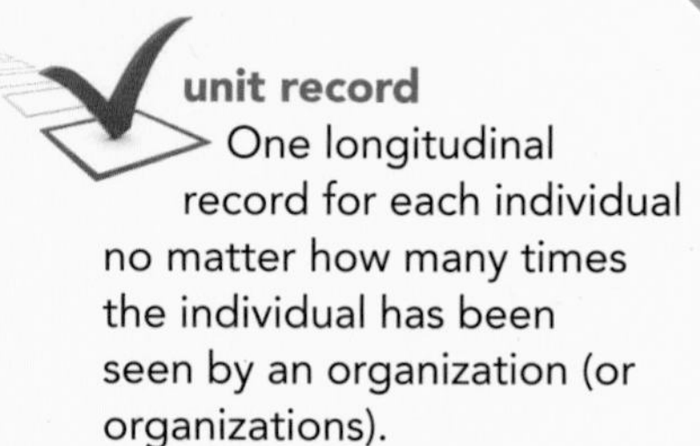

unit record One longitudinal record for each individual no matter how many times the individual has been seen by an organization (or organizations).

enterprise master patient/person index (EMPI) The key to locating a patient record in a health care organization with many component facilities, this listing includes patient identifying information and the assigned record number for all individuals ever receiving care by the entire organization.

record for each individual. In health information practice this is referred to as a **unit record**. A unit record means that no matter how many times a patient is treated at a particular setting, the information compiled during the visit can be retrieved as a single unit. Many health care regulations or accreditation standards require a unit record for quality of care purposes.

If the practice is part of a larger network of providers, then an additional goal is to support continuity of care for each patient by connecting the records of this practice with those of the same patient seen by others in the network. In a large health care organization made up of many levels of health care services (e.g., medical practices, hospitals, long-term care settings, home health services), the patient index may be known as an **enterprise master patient/person index (EMPI)** and will be shared across all the service components. Many benefits of EHRs will become evident only if information sharing can occur among all of a patient's health care providers. This requires that care providers identify their patients in the same manner so that the patient's records can be linked. Regional, national, and (someday) international networks of care providers will be able to share medical information because of defined patient index data.

Similar to an index in a book that identifies its contents, the master patient/person index lists the contents of the practice record database by identifying the patients who have medical information in the system. One of the first questions asked of patients desiring appointments is whether they have been seen by the practice in the past. This is done to determine if the practice already has an established relationship with a care provider and records for the patient. No matter what the response might be, the patient index should be queried. Patients may have forgotten prior visits or, in the case of an EHR, other provider treatment information may be available via a provider network or the NHIN. A patient index is a historical listing, which means that it must include all patients ever seen by the practice no matter how long ago those visits might have occurred. Thus the definition of a new patient is not the same as the definition used by some third-party payers for billing purposes, for whom the absence of visits for three years makes the patient automatically "new." Even if a patient's record eventually is transferred from an active EHR database to backup files, the entry in the index must remain to show that a record exists and to indicate its status and location.

The MPI itself consists of a listing of names of all individuals ever seen by the care providers in the health care practice. It is accompanied by certain other pieces of patient-identifying information and record numbers that help to identify each individual. Computers are programmed to compare names, dates of birth, and selected other pieces of information to identify possible "matches" via complicated algorithms. The importance of being precise in this process cannot be emphasized too strongly. It is the data in the MPI that links many components of the EHR and also allows data captured in other parts of the PMS to be fed directly into the correct patient's EHR. If errors are made in MPI entries, the result may be that vital health information about a patient is not brought to the care provider's attention or that precious treatment time is lost—with potentially serious implications. If the practice contributes data to an SNO (subnetwork organization) or NHIN, then the guidelines for identifying patients must be consistent across all health care providers who contribute to the network. It is therefore critical that standards addressing MPI data content and formatting be a part of MPI software. Although the purpose of the patient/person index is connecting the records of a patient seen in multiple visits or by multiple care providers, some of the demographic information gathered and stored also will be used to initiate the service payment record. Once entered in one screen, the same information can be transferred automatically from one location to another within the system through established database links.

MPI Content

Office personnel gather basic identification information required for querying the index during the first contact with the patient or the patient's representative. On the day of the appointment, other patient demographic data may be added as the registration process continues for new patients. The information's accuracy then must be verified at every visit thereafter. To assist in the process, it is important that the practice's policies for recording identifying information are used consistently by all personnel. For example, a practice policy should indicate if a full middle name is recorded or only a middle initial, or if titles such as "Dr." or credentials such as "M.D." are entered. Such a policy should be consistent with those of other care providers in the practice network, with the capabilities of the EHR system being used, and with any pertinent standards.

The most basic standards regarding demographic information are found in the AAAHC Handbook (see Chapter 4) and in the federal government Stage 1 Meaningful Use Objectives. The AAAHC criteria from the Clinical Records and Health Information section, part B notes:

> An individual clinical record is established for each person receiving care. Each record includes, but is not limited to:
>
> 1. Name
> 2. Identification number (if appropriate)
> 3. Date of birth
> 4. Gender
> 5. Responsible party, if applicable (2011, p. 40)

Demographic requirements from the Federal government Stage 1 Meaningful Use Objectives indicate that the record should include a patient's preferred language, gender, race, ethnicity, and date of birth. (Federal Register, p. 44370.) Accreditation standards of The Joint Commission (see Chapter 4) regarding patient identity expand on these basic examples. The standards are found in the section entitled "Record of Care, Treatment, and Services" (2011, RC.02.01.01):

> 1. The clinical record contains the following demographic information:
>   - The patient's name, address, phone number, and date of birth and the name of any legally authorized representative.
>   - The patient's sex, height, and weight.
>   - The legal status of any patient receiving behavioral health services.
>   - The patient's language and communication needs.

Usually much more demographic information will be gathered to identify and describe the patient fully. Demographic information in an EHR could include:

- Full name.
- Prior names, maiden name, and "also known as" (AKA) names.

- Address.
- Telephone numbers (home, work, cell, etc.).
- Date of birth.
- Age.
- Record number.
- Marital status.
- Gender.
- Race/ethnicity.
- Place of birth.
- Name and address of next of kin (e.g., spouse or parent).
- Name and address of guardian or custodial parent.
- Name, address, and relationship of an emergency contact.
- Social security number.
- E-mail address.
- Occupation.
- Name and address of employer.
- Dates of treatment.
- Name and address of third-party payer.
- Name of primary subscriber to the payment plan.
- Relationship of primary subscriber to the patient.
- Name of company or organization sponsoring the plan.
- Plan and group identification.
- Subscriber plan number.

Minors—unless emancipated or authorized by law to consent for treatment independently—will supply the following: names, addresses, and telephone numbers of parents and (if the parents are divorced or legally separated) an indication of which parent has custody. If a legal guardian has been appointed, then that individual's name and contact information also must be recorded. The patient's preferred pharmacy also can be noted, including its name, address, and telephone number. Examples of this type of data screen are shown in Figure 5-1.

MPI Searches

The patient's record number is usually the starting point for an EHR patient index search. However, if the patient is new or uncertain of the number, or if an alphabetical system is used, the patient's name will be the starting point. Because transposition of digits in a record number or letters in a name can occur and because names can be misspelled, other demographic information may be needed for the search. For example, the patient's date of birth and gender are often secondary data items chosen. An example of an initial patient index query is shown in Figure 5-2.

As you can see, no match was found for the patient with the information provided. If a direct match cannot be made with this data, the patient may need to be questioned further or the computer may search against other demographic data. As more demographic information is entered, the search will become more exact, but this also can limit greatly the number of matches. An

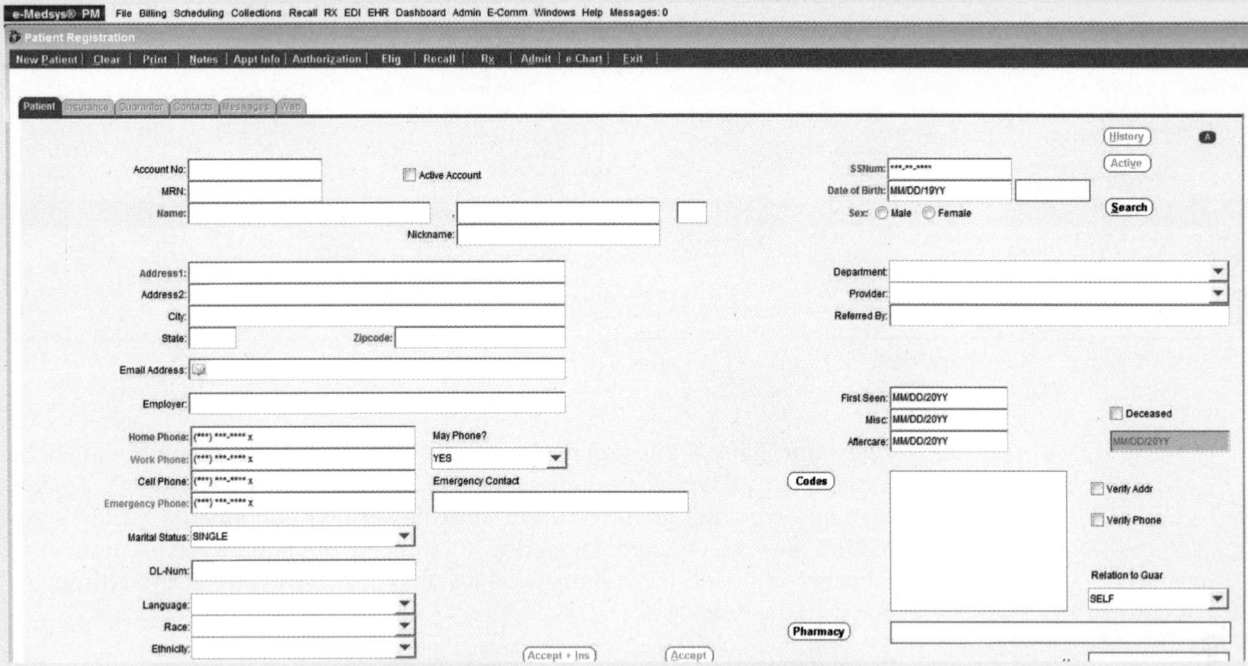

Reprinted with permission of TriMed Technologies, Corp.

Figure 5-1 Patient registration in e-Medsys®.

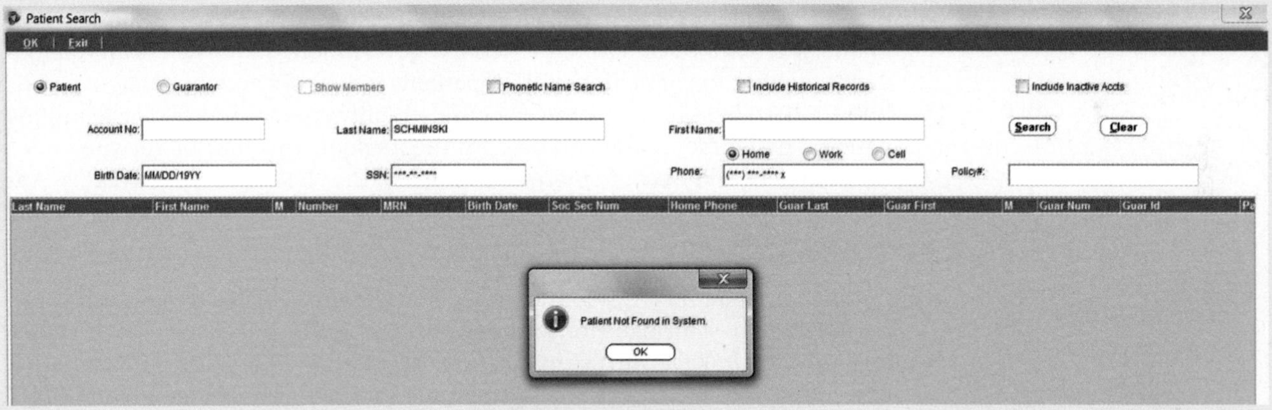

Reprinted with permission of TriMed Technologies, Corp.

Figure 5-2 Initial patient index query—no match found.

alternative to this type of search is for the computer system to identify close matches to the basic demographic information entered. These close matches are displayed as a listing of alternative individuals on the screen. Close matches may include patients with slight differences in spelling of a name (Peterson, Petersen, Pederson, Paterson, Patterson), with the same name but a different date of birth, with the same name and birth date but a different address, and so forth. An example of a screen with a patient entry and possible close matches is shown in Figure 5-3.

Additional information such as a maiden or former name, name of a spouse or parent, or treatment dates could be added for complete verification. If an exact match cannot be made, office personnel must ask the patient questions to

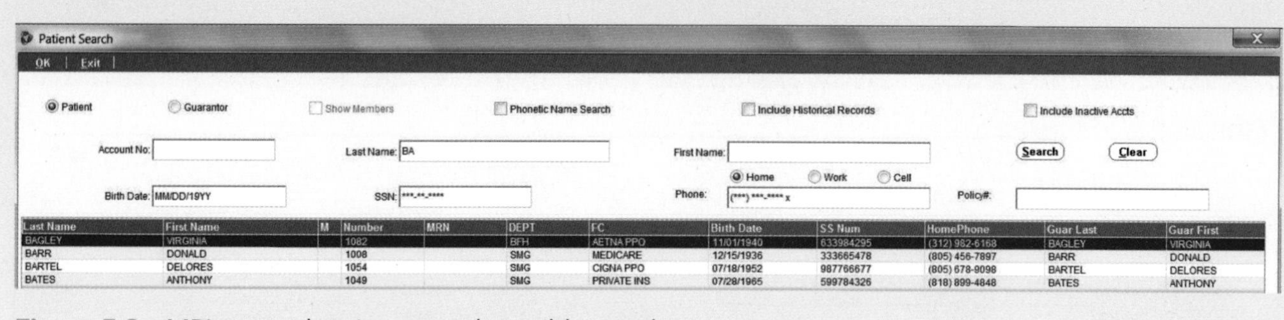

Figure 5-3 MPI query showing several possible matches to a name.

determine if any of the patient alternatives presented by the computer might be a match (e.g., "Have you ever lived at 1530 North Lincoln?"). If a match is made, then all demographic information must be verified and any inaccurate information must be updated. The index will indicate the patient record number or other record identifier, and the patient's record then can be retrieved through a link with the database.

If a match cannot be made, then a new index entry and patient record is initiated. The practice management system, via an automatic computer process, can assign a new health record number. If assigned, it also will appear in the index. In fact, the record number then becomes the key to accessing the EHR from the practice database, and the MPI becomes the source for identifying the number. The record number then becomes another identifier that can be used in a patient index query on any following visits. It also can be a link to the patient's financial record. At one time the federal government supported a unique patient identifier to connect records of patients nationally and included this in its initial HIPAA legislation. However, confidentiality concerns have placed unique national patient identifiers on hold for the present. This may be revisited once regional networks become more common or if the NHIN becomes a reality. Another possibility is that advances in computer algorithms may make a national identifier unnecessary.

If more than one record is found for a patient in the practice database, it is important that they be linked for continuity of care. Again, policies must be in place regarding the linkage, the use or deletion of record numbers, and the combining of records discovered. This is a critical function which is included in the CCHIT EHR criteria for an MPI.

In the future, the possible linking of data between care providers in a geographic region (or nationally) means that an additional step may be needed when registering a patient in an EHR system. An electronic request or query would be sent to the practitioner's SNO or the NHIN in order to locate and access any prior treatment information that might be useful to the current care provider. This could be done during the registration process or during the actual patient visit. It is clear that obtaining correct patient identification at the source of its collection is the key to an interoperable EHR system.

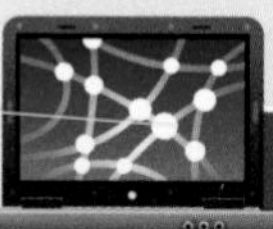

View the functional criteria used by CCHIT to certify ambulatory EHRs at the CCHIT website: http://www.cchit.org/.

SERVICE PAYMENT INFORMATION

Part of the initial registration information gathered by the practice relates to payment for services. Follow-up questions by the practice staff will depend on whether the patient is new to the practice or is a continuing patient. Some specialty practices only see patients who have been referred by another practitioner. If this is the case, staff will check that a referral has been received and may ask the patient for the referral number if the patient holds the referral document. The referral number then is entered into the EHR along with the referring practitioner's name and contact information for visit follow-up reports.

Correct information must be gathered regarding the name of the payment plan, the name of the person who is the primary subscriber to the plan, the subscriber's identification number in the plan, the relationship of the plan subscriber to the patient, the name of the company or organization sponsoring the plan, and plan and group numbers. If a patient has more than one payment plan, information needs to be gathered for all possible payment sources. This information is used by the office staff to determine in advance if prior approval for a visit is required from the payment plan, if the patient is authorized by a health plan for the visit, what payment parameters have been established, if there are any restrictions on services provided, and the amount of co-payments and deductibles to be requested from the patient. Because the federal government has begun issuing operating rules for simplifying health care payment transactions covered in the HIPAA legislation, eligibility and benefit information soon will easily be electronically obtained. An **Assignment of Benefits** form also may need to be completed to permit the third-party payer to send payment directly to the care provider instead of to the patient. However, fund transfers and claim statement production will occur electronically, if not already completed in that manner. Secondary payers may be contacted if the primary payer does not cover needed services.

If the patient is a Medicare patient and the provider knows that a particular service will not be covered by Medicare, a **Notice of Exclusions from Medicare Benefits** must be completed. This allows the provider to bill the patient for the services. If the provider believes that Medicare will not cover the type of care to be received because it could be considered unnecessary, an **Advance Beneficiary Notice (ABN)** must be initiated and presented to the patient prior to treatment by the care provider. This form informs the patient of this situation and allows the patient to choose whether to receive or not receive the service. A sample ABN as updated by CMS for use after September 1, 2011 is shown in Figure 5-4.

As with demographic information, the patient should be questioned about changes in plans or coverage at the beginning of every visit. It is also common practice to add a copy of the patient's actual insurance card to the record. The card contains plan contact information and an address for submitting claims. This information can be added to the EHR in two manners. The first is to photocopy the card and scan the photocopy into the record. This requires two time-consuming steps. A second alternative is to scan the card directly into the record using a business card reader. This type of scanner also can be used to scan driver's licenses or other cards that may have information needed by the practice.

Most of the billing process occurs after the patient visit, when diagnostic and procedural codes and service charges are added to the claim form to accompany the patient, payer, and care provider data already gathered. Coding and billing are described in more detail in Chapter 11. Because CCHIT functional criteria focus on electronic record functions versus those of a practice management or billing system, there are no specific standards in this area.

Assignment of Benefits Authorization by the patient for a third-party payer to reimburse the practice directly (instead of the patient) for services provided.

Notice of Exclusions from Medicare Benefits Document provided to a Medicare patient if the provider knows that a particular service will not be covered by Medicare; allows the provider to bill the patient for the services.

Advance Beneficiary Notice (ABN) Document given to Medicare patients if it is believed that a treatment or a portion of a treatment will be considered unnecessary by Medicare and consequently will not be reimbursed.

Patient's Name: Medicare # (HICN):

ADVANCE BENEFICIARY NOTICE (ABN)

NOTE: You need to make a choice about receiving these health care items or services.

We expect that Medicare will not pay for the item(s) or service(s) that are described below. Medicare does not pay for all of your health care costs. Medicare only pays for covered items and services when Medicare rules are met. The fact that Medicare may not pay for a particular item or service does not mean that you should not receive it. There may be a good reason your doctor recommended it. Right now, in your case, **Medicare probably will not pay for –**

Items or Services:

Because:

The purpose of this form is to help you make an informed choice about whether or not you want to receive these items or services, knowing that you might have to pay for them yourself. Before you make a decision about your options, you should **read this entire notice carefully.**

- Ask us to explain, if you don't understand why Medicare probably won't pay.
- Ask us how much these items or services will cost you (**Estimated Cost: $**________), in case you have to pay for them yourself or through other insurance.

PLEASE CHOOSE **ONE** OPTION. CHECK **ONE** BOX. **SIGN & DATE** YOUR CHOICE.

☐ **Option 1. YES. I want to receive these items or services.**
I understand that Medicare will not decide whether to pay unless I receive these items or services. Please submit my claim to Medicare. I understand that you may bill me for items or services and that I may have to pay the bill while Medicare is making its decision. If Medicare does pay, you will refund to me any payments I made to you that are due to me. If Medicare denies payment, I agree to be personally and fully responsible for payment. That is, I will pay personally, either out of pocket or through any other insurance that I have. I understand I can appeal Medicare's decision.

☐ **Option 2. NO. I have decided not to receive these items or services.**
I will not receive these items or services. I understand that you will not be able to submit a claim to Medicare and that I will not be able to appeal your opinion that Medicare won't pay.

Date **Signature of patient or person acting on patient's behalf**

NOTE: Your health information will be kept confidential. Any information that we collect about you on this form will be kept confidential in our offices. If a claim is submitted to Medicare, your health information on this form may be shared with Medicare. Your health information which Medicare sees will be kept confidential by Medicare.

OMB Approval No. 0938-0566 Form No. CMS-R-131-G (June 2002)

Figure 5-4 Advance beneficiary notice (ABN).

Source: Centers for Medicare and Medicaid Services. www.cms.hhs.gov/BNI/Downloads/cmsr131G.pdf (Retrieved 11/2/2011)

SCHEDULING

Scheduling a patient for an office visit is another PMS function that is done in conjunction with gathering patient demographic and financial information and accessing the MPI. For the scheduling software to operate efficiently, some key information must be stored in it for use each time a scheduling activity is initiated. For example, the names of all health care providers available to see patients must be stored in the system along with the days and office hours available for appointments for each of them. Care providers may block out times when they are at meetings, performing hospital visits, on vacation, and so forth. Another key factor is whether this is a new or established patient. Here the definition of "new" concerns payment, so a "new" patient is one who has not been seen in the past three years. Longer appointment time allotments generally are made for a first visit versus follow-up sessions, because patient assessment and evaluations must take place. For example, a first-time patient may require 45 minutes or an hour, whereas a patient returning for a medication check or therapy requires less time—perhaps only 15 to 30 minutes. Once all provider and visit parameters are entered in the system, choices of available dates and times will appear on the screen when the system is queried. Alternative open times will continue to be presented by the scheduling software until the patient can be scheduled satisfactorily. Figure 5-5 provides an example of a scheduling screen in a practice management system.

At the time the visit is scheduled, identification of the patient's payment source will be requested. To accommodate this aspect of the scheduling process, information on the common provider/payer relationships—in addition to payer pre-authorization requirements—can be embedded into the scheduling software. As a result, when scheduling staff enter the name of the payer, the patient's payer identification number, and the group and plan identification numbers, the scheduling system will alert the staff of special circumstances. The system will highlight cases where a provider/payer relationship does not exist or any situation when the patient may be required to obtain a referral from an attending physician or a preauthorization from a payer as part of the scheduling process.

Another scheduling alternative in a fully functioning EHR with an online practice patient portal (see Chapter 10) is using the portal request system for the patient to request a visit, or for a referring provider's office to request a visit for the patient. Patient portal scheduling options usually are given only to continuing patients with access codes, and referral scheduling may depend on the identity of the referral source. Once appropriate visit criteria are entered and a visit is

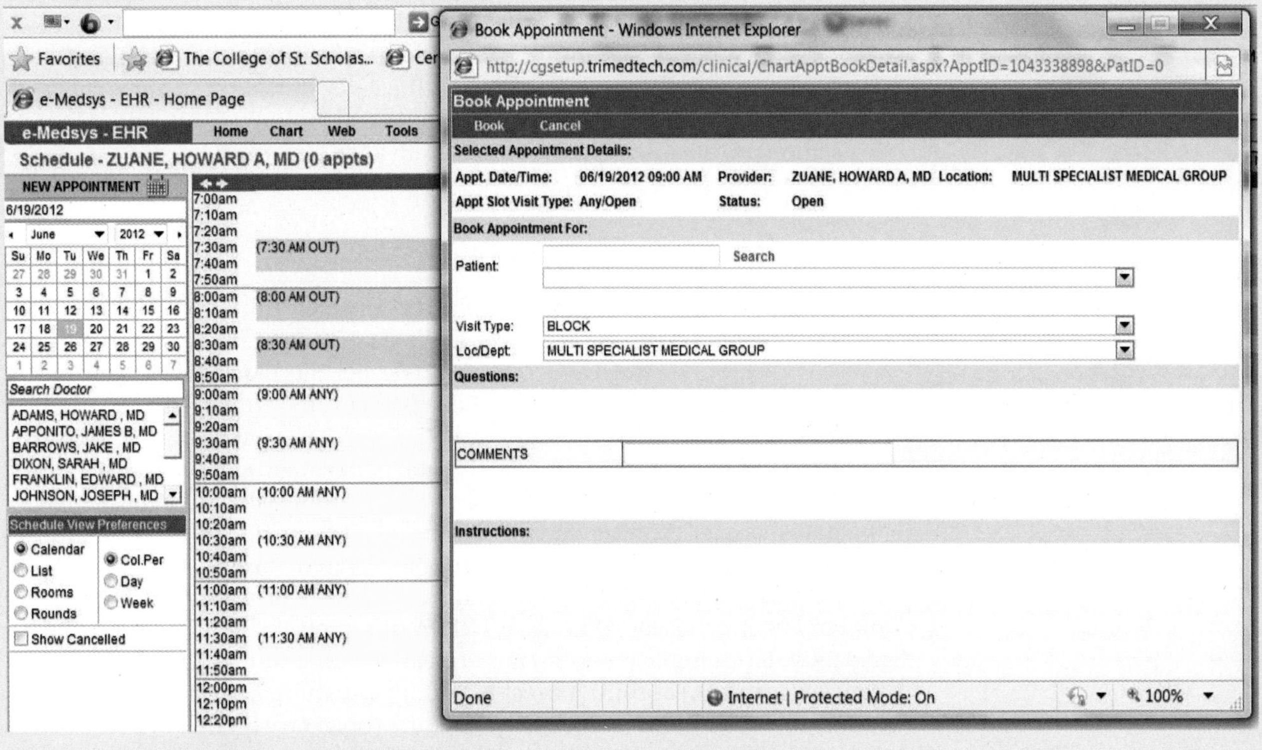

Figure 5-5 Example of scheduling building screen in e-Medsys®.

authorized, choices of dates and times are presented for selection. This option allows the patient or referral source to have more control over visit planning.

Patient e-mail or letter reminders, or lists for telephone calls regarding appointments, can be generated automatically by the scheduling system according to a timeline set by the practice. The EHR also can display each care provider's work schedule by day, week, or month. In addition, the schedule information can interact with the claims system to add the appointment date to the basic billing data already collected.

Patient cancellations, appointment mix-ups, and no-shows also must be documented in the EHR. On occasion these may have medical implications such as providing evidence of a patient's growing confusion. Some practices may have a policy that charges a fee for no-shows, and therefore a bill can be generated. Patterns of consistent missed appointments may mean that staff will need to counsel the patient.

There are few external standards or regulations for the scheduling function. The CCHIT functional criteria for ambulatory EHRs includes only one entry relating to scheduling. That criteria essentially requires that the EHR be able to display the patient appointment schedule.

CONSENTS, ACKNOWLEDGMENTS, ADVANCE DIRECTIVES, AND AUTHORIZATIONS

As a result of the federal Health Insurance Portability and Accountability Act (HIPAA) of 1996 and revised in the HITECH Act of 2009, the Department of Health and Human Services published rules relating to the privacy and security of confidential patient information. The rules apply to health care providers and health related entities that exchange personally identifiable information electronically. Of course these guidelines apply to an EHR environment, but they are already applicable to most health care provider offices as a result of their electronic submission of bills to payers. The rules provide guidelines for practices related to consents, acknowledgments, and authorizations. Other federal legislation provides guidelines regarding advance directives.

Consents and Notices

consent for treatment Documentation signed by the patient giving approval to the provision of routine care.

Historically it has been the common practice for at least all new office patients to sign a **consent for treatment** prior to anyone providing care. However, the final HIPAA privacy rule, effective October 15, 2002, permits those who are covered by the regulations (referred to in the standards as covered entities) to "use and disclose patients' protected health information for their own treatment, payment or healthcare operations and for the treatment, payment, and certain healthcare operations of other parties without prior written permission from the patient or the patient's legal representatives." (Petterson, 2011, p. 87.) Health care providers in the office practice using the EHR are covered entities. This final HIPAA privacy rule means that it is optional for a practice to have a patient sign a general treatment consent. Otherwise, HIPAA interprets the patient's contact with the provider as implied permission to treat and consequently a formal written consent (express consent) to treat is no longer required. Special consents still are required, however, for invasive procedures or when experimental research is involved. Whenever a signed consent is obtained from a patient, it must become part of the patient's record.

The HIPAA privacy rule does require that practitioners in a direct care relationship with a patient provide each patient a **Notice of Privacy Practices**. Usually this document is one that is printed and can be handed to the patient. It also can be included on the practice patient portal (if one exists) so that patients can print a copy as desired. An additional requirement of the HIPAA regulations is that the patient or the patient's legal representative acknowledge receipt of the notice via a signed statement. The acknowledgment signature can be obtained via an electronic pad if that technology is available in the practice. If the document is completed on paper, it can be signed and scanned into the EHR. At a minimum, the acknowledgment portion of the notice (the signature section) must become part of the patient's record. Figures 5-6A and 5-6B provide an example of a privacy notice and an acknowledgment of receipt of a privacy notice.

Notice of Privacy Practices
Information that HIPAA requires be provided to patients about the use and disclosure of information by the practice, patient rights and responsibilities in relation to the record, and contact information if questions arise.

If a patient is to undergo surgery, an invasive or surgical procedure with risk of complications, administration of anesthesia, or treatment with experimental drugs or procedures, then consents must be obtained from the patient or the patient's representative prior to the event. As with other consents and authorizations, consent for a procedure or special drug may be available online or on paper. If online, a signature pad is used for signatures and dates. Paper consents are completed manually and scanned into the record. Special consents also may be required for any type of audio or visual recording that is not for care purposes. Generally the same signature requirements will apply.

Advance Directives

An **advance directive** is a document that provides guidance to care providers about the wishes of a patient should he or she become incapacitated or no longer able to make decisions as a result of medical or psychiatric impairment. A directive also can name an individual who has been selected by the patient to make health care decisions in the event of incapacitation. Practices that accept Medicare or Medicaid funding are required by the federal Patient Self-Determination Act (effective 1991) to provide information to patients on their right to refuse or accept treatment and to express their health care wishes via advance directives. This information often becomes part of a patient's rights statement that may be printed with the notice of privacy practices. Two examples of advance directives are a **durable power of attorney for health care**, which gives another person the right to make health care decisions for the patient, and a **living will**. A living will outlines the wishes of the patient in relation to medical care in life-threatening situations and also can name a representative. Physician orders such as "do not resuscitate" must follow the patient's advance directive stipulations.

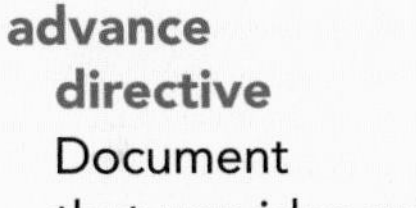

advance directive
Document that provides guidance to practitioners about the wishes of a patient should he or she become incapacitated or no longer able to make decisions because of medical or psychiatric impairment.

durable power of attorney for health care
Type of advance directive giving another person the right to make health care decisions for the patient.

living will
Type of advance directive that outlines the wishes of the patient in relation to medical care in life threatening situations; it also can name a representative.

Practices must make a notation in the patient EHR that an advance directive exists, but they are not required to make the actual document(s) part of the record. Often this information will be highlighted in some way to draw attention to it. An EHR is particularly effective in producing this type of special alert, because the software can be programmed so that information about an advance directive's existence appears on multiple screens within the EHR where treatment information is recorded or viewed. Figures 5-7A and 5-7B provide an example of an advance directive entry into a patient's EHR and the advance directive notation resulting from that entry to inform the care provider.

If the practice desires to include a copy of the actual advance directive in the EHR, the documents should be scanned and located in a section of the EHR intended for legal communications. Patients need to make sure that care providers

NOTICE OF PRIVACY PRACTICES

SAY SAN DIEGO, INC.

Effective Date: **April 14, 2003**

THIS NOTICE DESCRIBES HOW MEDICAL INFORMATION ABOUT YOU MAY BE USED AND DISCLOSED AND HOW YOU CAN GET ACCESS TO THIS INFORMATION. PLEASE REVIEW IT CAREFULLY.

WHO WILL FOLLOW THIS NOTICE

This Notice describes SAY San Diego, Inc.'s practices and that of:

- All employees, staff and other SAY personnel.
- Any member of a volunteer group we allow to help you while you are at SAY.

OUR PLEDGE REGARDING MEDICAL INFORMATION

We understand that medical information about you and your health is personal. We are committed to protecting medical information about you. We create a record of the care and services you receive at SAY. We need this record to provide you with quality care and to comply with certain legal requirements. This Notice applies to all of the records of your care generated by the facility. As required and when appropriate, we will ensure that only the minimum necessary information is released in the course of our duties.

This Notice will tell you about the ways in which we may use and disclose medical information about you. We also describe your rights and certain obligations regarding the use and disclosure of medical information.

We are required by law to:

- Keep your medical information, also known as "protected health information" or "PHI," private;
- Give you this Notice of our legal duties and privacy practices with respect to your PHI; and
- Follow the terms of the Notice that is currently in effect.

HOW WE MAY USE AND DISCLOSE YOUR PROTECTED HEALTH INFORMATION

The following categories describe different ways that we use and disclose protected health information. For each category of uses or disclosures we will explain what we mean and try to give some examples. Not every use or disclosure in a category will be listed. However, all of the ways we are permitted to use and disclose information will fall within one of the categories.

For Treatment

We create a record of the treatment and services you receive at SAY. We may use your PHI to provide you with medical treatment or services. We may disclose your PHI to doctors, nurses, technicians, or other facility personnel who are involved in taking care of you at SAY. For example, a doctor treating you for a chemical imbalance may need to know if you have problems with your heart because some medications affect your blood pressure. We may share your PHI in order to coordinate the different things you need, such as prescriptions, blood pressure checks and lab tests, and to determine a correct diagnosis. We also may disclose your PHI to people outside the facility who may be involved in your treatment, such as your case manager, or other persons for coordination and management of your health care. Your mental health information may only be released to health care professionals outside this facility without your authorization if they are responsible for your physical or mental health care.

For Payment

We may use and disclose your PHI in order to get paid for the treatment and services we have provided you. For example, we may need to give your health plan information about a medication, visit, or treatment session you received at SAY so your health plan will pay us. We may also tell your health plan about a treatment you are going to receive to obtain prior approval or to determine whether your plan will cover the treatment.

Figure 5-6a Sample of notice of privacy practices.

For Health Care Operations

We may use and disclose your PHI to carry out activities that are necessary to run our facilities and to make sure that all of our patients receive quality care. For example, we may use medical information to review our treatment and services and to evaluate the performance of our staff in caring for you.

Appointment Reminders

We may use and disclose your PHI to contact you as a reminder that you have an appointment for treatment or medical care at SAY.

Treatment Alternatives and Health-Related Products and Services

We may use and disclose your PHI to recommend possible treatment options or alternatives that may be of interest to you. Additionally, we may use and disclose PHI to tell you about health-related benefits or services that may be of interest to you.

Fundraising Activities

We may use your PHI to contact you in an effort to raise money for SAY and its operations. If you do not want SAY to contact you for fundraising efforts, you must notify, *the Director of Development; 3615 Kearny Villa Rd. Ste 101; 858-565-4148* and state that you do not want to receive further fundraising communications.

Individuals Involved in Your Care or Payment for Your Care

We may disclose your PHI to a friend or family member who is involved in your medical care or payment related to your health care, provided that you agree to this disclosure, or we give you an opportunity to object to this disclosure. However, if you are not available or are unable to agree or object, we will use our judgment to decide whether this disclosure is in your best interests.

Disaster Relief Purposes

We may disclose your PHI to an entity assisting in a disaster relief effort so that your family can be notified about your condition, status and location. We will give you the opportunity to agree to this disclosure or object to this disclosure, unless we decide that we need to disclose your PHI in order to respond to the emergency circumstances.

As Required By Law

We will disclose your PHI when required to do so by federal, state or local law.

To Avert a Serious Threat to Health and Safety

We may use and disclose your PHI when necessary to prevent a serious threat to your health and safety or the health and safety of the public or another person. Any disclosure, however, would be to someone able to help prevent the threat.

Workers' Compensation

We may release your PHI for workers' compensation or similar programs. These programs provide benefits for work-related injuries or illness.

Public Health Risks

We may disclose medical information about you for public health activities, such as those aimed at preventing or controlling disease, preventing injury or disability, and reporting the abuse or neglect of children, elders and dependent adults.

Military and Veterans

If you are a member of the armed forces, we may release your PHI as required by military command authorities. We may also release medical information about foreign military personnel to the appropriate foreign military authority.

Health Oversight Activities

We may disclose your PHI to a health oversight agency for activities authorized by law. These oversight activities include, for example, audits, investigations, inspections, and licensure. These activities are necessary for the government to monitor the health care system, government programs, and compliance with civil rights laws.

Figure 5-6a *(Continues)*

(Continued)

Lawsuits and Disputes

If you are involved in a lawsuit or a dispute, we may disclose your PHI in response to a court or administrative order. We may also disclose your PHI in response to a subpoena, discovery request, or other lawful process by someone else involved in the dispute, but only if efforts have been made to tell you about the request (which may include written notice to you) or to obtain an order protecting the information requested.

Law Enforcement

We may disclose PHI to government law enforcement agencies in response to a court order, warrant, subpoena, summons or similar process issued by a court.

Coroners, Medical Examiners and Funeral Directors

We may release PHI to a coroner or medical examiner. This may be necessary, for example, to identify a deceased person or determine the cause of death. We may also release medical information about patients of the facility to funeral directors as necessary to carry out their duties.

Specialized Government Functions

We may your PHI to authorized federal officials for intelligence, counterintelligence, and other national security activities authorized by law.
We may disclose your PHI to authorized federal officials so they may provide protection to the President, other authorized persons or foreign heads of state or conduct special investigations.

Inmates

If you are an inmate of a correctional institution, you lose the rights outlined in this Notice. Furthermore, if you are an inmate or under the custody of a law enforcement official, we may release your PHI to the correctional institution or law enforcement official. This release would be necessary (1) for the institution to provide you with health care; (2) to protect your health and safety or the health and safety of others; or (3) for the safety and security of the correctional institution.

Other Uses of Your Medical Information

Other uses and disclosures of your PHI not covered by this Notice or the laws that apply to us will be made only with your written authorization. If you provide us authorization to use or disclose your PHI, you may revoke that authorization, in writing, at any time. If you revoke your authorization, we will no longer use or disclose your PHI for the reasons covered by the authorization, except that, we are unable to take back any disclosures we have already made when the authorization was in effect, and we are required to retain our records of the care that we provided to you.

YOUR RIGHTS REGARDING YOUR PHI

You have the following rights regarding your PHI in our records:

Right to Inspect and Copy

With certain exceptions, you have the right to inspect and copy your PHI from our records. Usually, this includes medical and billing records.
To inspect and copy PHI that may be used to make decisions about you, you must submit your request in writing. A form will be provided to you for this request. If you request a copy of the information, we may charge a fee for the costs of copying, mailing or other supplies associated with your request.
We may deny your request to inspect and copy in certain circumstances. If you are denied the right to inspect and copy your PHI in our records, you may request that the denial be reviewed. With the exception of a few circumstances that are not subject to review, another licensed health care professional within SAY, who was not involved in the denial, will review the decision to deny access. We will comply with the outcome of the review.

Figure 5-6a

Right to Request Amendment

If you feel that your PHI in our records is incorrect or incomplete, you may ask us to amend the information. You have the right to request an amendment for as long as we keep the PHI. To request an amendment, you must submit your request in writing. A form will be provided to you for this request. We may deny your request for an amendment if it is not in writing or does not include a reason to support the request. In addition, we may deny your request if you ask us to amend PHI that:

- Was not created by us, unless you can provide us with a reasonable basis to believe that the person or entity that created the PHI is no longer available to make the amendment;
- Is not part of the PHI kept by or for the facility;
- Is not part of the PHI which you would be permitted to inspect and copy; or
- Is accurate and complete.

Even if we deny your request for amendment, you have the right to submit a Statement of Disagreement, with respect to any item or statement in your record you believe is incomplete or incorrect. If you clearly indicate in writing that you want this form to be made part of your medical record, we will attach it to your records and include it whenever we make a disclosure of the item or statement you believe to be incomplete or incorrect.

Right to an Accounting of Disclosures

You have the right to request an "accounting of disclosures." This is a list of the disclosures we made of your PHI other than our own uses for treatment, payment and health care operations, (as those functions are described above) and with other exceptions pursuant to the law.
To request this list or accounting of disclosures, you must submit your request in writing. A form will be provided to you for this request. Your request must state a time period that may not be longer than six years and may not include dates before April 14, 2003. The first list you request within a 12-month period will be free. For additional lists, we may charge you for the costs of providing the list. We will notify you of the cost involved and you may choose to withdraw or modify your request at that time before any costs are incurred.

Right to Request Restrictions

You have the right to request that we follow additional, special restrictions when using or disclosing your PHI for treatment, payment or health care operations. You also have the right to request that we follow additional, special restrictions when using or disclosing your PHI to someone who is involved in your care or the payment for your health care, like a family member or friend. For example, you could ask that we not use or disclose that you are receiving services at SAY.
We are not required to agree to your request. If we do agree, we will comply with your request unless the information is needed to provide you emergency treatment.
To request restrictions, you must submit your request in writing. A form will be provided to you for this request. In your request, you must tell us (1) what information you want to limit; (2) whether you want to limit our use, disclosure or both; and (3) to whom you want the limits to apply, for example, disclosures to your spouse.

Right to Request Confidential Communications

You have the right to request that we communicate with you about your appointments or other matters related to your treatment in a specific way or at a specific location. For example, you can ask that we only contact you at work or by mail.
To request confidential communications, , you must submit your request in writing. A form will be provided to you for this request. Your request must specify how or where you wish to be contacted. We will not ask you the reason for your request. We will accommodate all reasonable requests.

Right to a Paper Copy of This Notice

You have the right to a paper copy of this Notice. You may ask us to give you a copy of this Notice at any time. Even if you have agreed to receive this Notice electronically, you are still entitled to a paper copy of this Notice.
You may obtain a copy of this Notice at our website: http://www.saysandiego.org
To obtain a paper copy of this Notice, please contact your health care team.

Figure 5-6a *(Continues)*

(Continued)

CHANGES TO THIS NOTICE

We reserve the right to change the terms of this Notice. We reserve the right to make the revised or changed Notice effective for medical information we already have about you as well as any information we receive in the future. We will post a copy of the current Notice in the facility. The Notice will contain on the first page, in the top right-hand corner, the effective date. In addition, each time you register at or are admitted to the facility for treatment or health care services as an inpatient or outpatient, we will offer you a copy of the current Notice in effect.

COMPLAINTS

If you believe your privacy rights have been violated, you may file a complaint with SAY or the Federal Government. All complaints must be submitted in writing. **You will not be penalized or retaliated against for filing a complaint.** To file a complaint with us, or if you have comments or questions regarding our privacy practices, contact:

SAY San Diego, Inc.

SAY Privacy Officer

To file a complaint with the Federal Government, contact:

Office of Civil Rights (Room 515 F)

US Department of Health and Human Services

200 Independence Avenue, S.W.

Washington, D.C. 20201

(202) 619-0805

(202) 619-0553

Figure 5-6a

Say San Diego, Inc. http://www.saysandiego.org/documents/SAYprivacypractices.pdf (Retrieved 11/2/2011)

are aware of the existence of their advance directive or of any changes made to an existing directive. The CCHIT functional criteria include several that relate to advance directives. Among accrediting groups, the AAAHC indicates: "Discussions with the patient concerning . . . treatment alternatives and advance directives, as applicable, are incorporated into the patient's clinical record." (2011, p. 42.) AAAHC also adds that the patient has a responsibility to care providers to inform them "about any living will, medical power of attorney, or other directive that could affect his/her care." (2011, p. 19.)

Authorizations for Release of Information

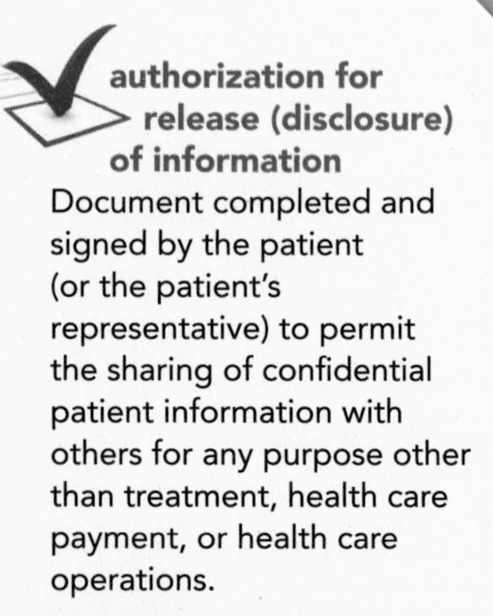

authorization for release (disclosure) of information
Document completed and signed by the patient (or the patient's representative) to permit the sharing of confidential patient information with others for any purpose other than treatment, health care payment, or health care operations.

Because the health care information contained in EHRs belongs to patients, patients have the legal right to control access to that information unless laws indicate otherwise. When patients request that protected, confidential information be shared for any purpose other than treatment, payment, or health care operations, the HIPAA privacy rule requires that the patient or the patient's representative sign an **authorization for release (disclosure) of information**. Both oral and written communications are covered by the regulations, which also provide guidelines covering their content, use, signatures, duration, and (if necessary) revocation. An example of an authorization to release information was provided in the Federal Register in 2000 and is shown in Figure 5-8.

State laws may specifically protect certain populations (e.g., psychiatric or AIDS patients) with special consent or process requirements. In this case, the laws or regulations that are the most restrictive are the ones that must be followed. If the authorization is a paper document, then it should be scanned and placed in the

NOTICE OF PRIVACY PRACTICES:
Acknowledgement of Receipt

ACKNOWLEDGEMENT OF RECEIPT

By signing this form, you acknowledge receipt of the *Notice of Privacy Practices* of SAY San Diego, Inc. ("SAY"). Our *Notice of Privacy Practices* provides information about how we may use and disclose your protected health information. We encourage you to review it carefully. Our *Notice of Privacy Practices* is subject to change. If we change our Notice, you may obtain a copy of the revised Notice by visiting our website at http://www.saysandiego.org or on request from your health care team.

I acknowledge receipt of the *Notice of Privacy Practices* of SAY.

Signature: ______________________________ Date:______________
(patient/parent/conservator/guardian)

INABILITY TO OBTAIN ACKNOWLEDGEMENT

To be completed only if no signature is obtained. If it is not possible to obtain the individual's acknowledgement, describe the good faith efforts made to obtain the individual's acknowledgement, and the reasons why the acknowledgement was not obtained:

Signature of provider representative:______________________________ Date:__________

Reasons why the acknowledgement was not obtained:

? Patient refused to sign.

? Other or Comments:

____

____

____

____

____

____

Figure 5-6b Acknowledgment of receipt of privacy practice notice.

Say San Diego, Inc. http://www.saysandiego.org/documents/SAYprivacypractices.pdf (Retrieved 11/2/2011)

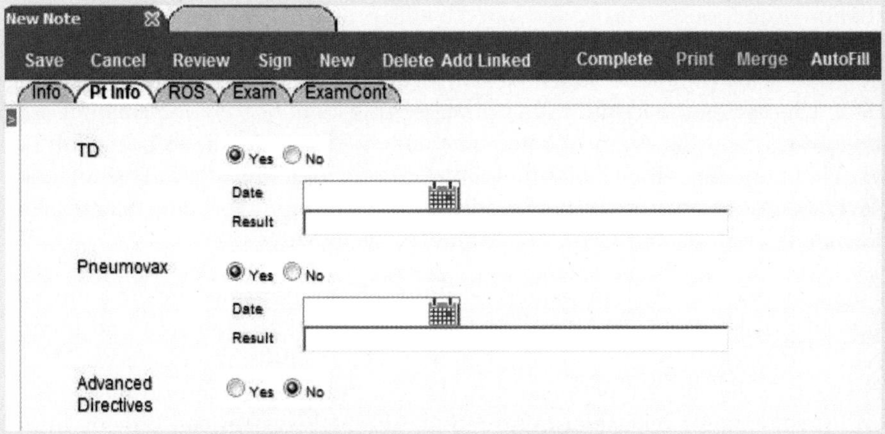

New Note

Save Cancel Review Sign New Delete Add Linked Complete Print Merge AutoFill

Info | Pt Info | ROS | Exam | ExamCont

TD — (•) Yes ( ) No
Date
Result

Pneumovax — (•) Yes ( ) No
Date
Result

Advanced Directives — ( ) Yes (•) No

Figure 5-7a Advance directive entry in e-Medsys®.

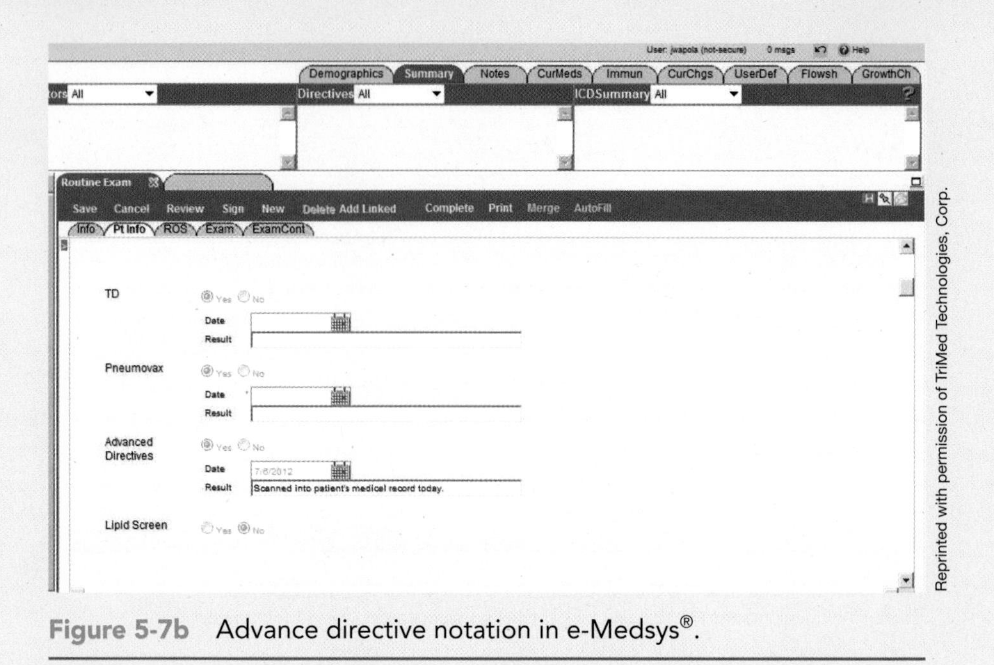

Figure 5-7b Advance directive notation in e-Medsys®.

legal communications area of the EHR. If electronic versions of an authorization are available and if electronic documents are accepted in the state where the practice is located, then the patient can sign via a signature pad. The EHR also must be programmed to provide a listing of all documents that are sent elsewhere for reasons other than treatment, payment, or health care operations, along with the date and time of each transmittal and to whom the information was provided. This listing becomes the "release of information" log required by the HIPAA privacy rule.

Although information requested and received from another health care provider does not require an authorization for information release, it is important to establish some method of identification of the source of the data and its timing. If the information is shared on paper, then the documents are scanned and placed in the communication section of the patient's record. However, if the information is shared electronically, the data may appear at multiple locations in the EHR. For example, test results may appear in the laboratory reports section and a history and physical in the history and physical section. For legal purposes the shared data must be identified as coming from another source, and the date and time of its receipt should be noted. Current health care decisions may rely on that information even though it is not generated by the practice. If questions ever arise regarding the shared information, it must be traceable to the correct source. Again, computers are capable of attaching source, date, and time notations to incoming data, which aids the identification process. This identification information may not always be visible on the computer screen, but it should always be retrievable via EHR audit files. The CCHIT functional criteria for ambulatory EHRs includes several entries concerning scanning, displaying, storing and printing release of information authorizations, consents, and privacy notices.

Finally, some information requests do not require protected health information. If this is the case, patient "de-identification" (i.e., removal of all identifying indicators) can be performed to meet the needs of the requester. These circumstances also are defined in the HIPAA privacy rule and do not require authorizations for release of information. The EHR system can provide information without identifiers through adjusting request criteria, a process much easier than blocking out this information by hand.

IHS-810 (4/09)
FRONT

DEPARTMENT OF HEALTH AND HUMAN SERVICES
Indian Health Service

FORM APPROVED: OMB NO. 0917-0030
Expiration Date: 1/31/2013
See OMB Statement on Reverse.

AUTHORIZATION FOR USE OR DISCLOSURE OF PROTECTED HEALTH INFORMATION

COMPLETE ALL SECTIONS, DATE, AND SIGN

I. I, ______________________________ , hereby voluntarily authorize the disclosure of information from my health record. *(Name of Patient)*

II. The information is to be disclosed by:	**And is to be provided to:**
NAME OF FACILITY	NAME OF PERSON/ORGANIZATION/FACILITY
ADDRESS	ADDRESS
CITY/STATE	CITY/STATE

III. The purpose or need for this disclosure is:

☐ Further Medical Care ☐ Attorney ☐ School ☐ Research
☐ Personal Use ☐ Insurance ☐ Disability ☐ Other *(Specify)* ________

IV. The information to be disclosed from my health record: *(check appropriate box(es))*

☐ Only information related to *(specify)* ________

☐ Only the period of events from ________ to ________

☐ Other *(specify) (CHS, Billing, etc.)* ________

☐ Entire Record

If you would like any of the following sensitive information disclosed, check the applicable box(es) below:

☐ Alcohol/Drug Abuse Treatment/Referral ☐ HIV/AIDS-related Treatment
☐ Sexually Transmitted Diseases ☐ Mental Health *(Other than Psychotherapy Notes)*
☐ Psychotherapy Notes ONLY (by checking this box, I am waiving any psychotherapist-patient privilege)

V. I understand that I may revoke this authorization in writing submitted at any time to the Health Information Management Department, except to the extent that action has been taken in reliance on this authorization. If this authorization was obtained as a condition of obtaining insurance coverage or a policy of insurance, other law may provide the insurer with the right to contest a claim under the policy. If this authorization has not been revoked, it will terminate one year from the date of my signature unless a different expiration date or *expiration event* is stated.

________________________ *(Specify new date)*

I understand that IHS will not condition treatment or eligibility for care on my providing this authorization except if such care is: (1) research related or (2) provided solely for the purpose of creating Protected Health Information for disclosure to a third party.

I understand that information disclosed by this authorization, except for Alcohol and Drug Abuse as defined in 42 CFR Part 2, may be subject to redisclosure by the recipient and may no longer be protected by the Health Insurance Portability and Accountability Act Privacy Rule [45 CFR Part 164] , and the Privacy Act of 1974 [5 USC 552a].

SIGNATURE OF PATIENT OR PERSONAL REPRESENTATIVE *(State relationship to patient)*	DATE
SIGNATURE OF WITNESS *(If signature of patient is a thumbprint or mark)*	DATE

This information is to be released for the purpose stated above and may not be used by the recipient for any other purpose. Any person who knowingly and willfully requests or obtains any record concerning an individual from a Federal agency under false pretenses shall be guilty of a misdemeanor (5 USC 552a(i)(3)).

PATIENT IDENTIFICATION	NAME *(Last, First, MI)*	RECORD NUMBER
	ADDRESS	
	CITY/STATE	DATE OF BIRTH

PSC Graphics (301) 443-1090 EF

Figure 5-8 HIPAA compliant authorization to release information. *(Continues)*

(Continued)

IHS-810 (4/09)
BACK

Instructions for Completing IHS Form 810 --

AUTHORIZATION FOR USE OR DISCLOSURE OF PROTECTED HEALTH INFORMATION

1. Print legibly in all fields using dark permanent ink.

2. Section I, print your name or the name of patient whose information is to be released.

3. Section II, print the name and address of the facility releasing the information. Also, provide the name of the person, facility, and address that will receive the information.

4. Section III, state the reason why the information is needed, e.g., disability claim, continuing medical care, legal, research-related projects, etc.

5. Section IV, check the appropriate box as applicable.

   a. **Only information related to** -- specify diagnosis, injury, operations, special therapies, etc.

   b. **Only the period of events from** -- specify date range, e.g., Jan. 1, 2002, to Feb. 1, 2002.

   c. **Other *(specify)*** -- e.g., CHS, Billing, Employee Health.

   d. **Entire Record** -- complete record including, if authorized, the sensitive information (alcohol and drug abuse treatment/referral, sexually transmitted diseases, HIV/AIDS-related treatment, and mental health other than psychotherapy notes).

   e. **IN ORDER TO RELEASE SENSITIVE INFORMATION REGARDING ALCOHOL/DRUG ABUSE TREATMENT/REFERRAL, HIV/AIDS-RELATED TREATMENT, SEXUALLY TRANSMITTED DISEASES, MENTAL HEALTH (OTHER THAN PSYCHOTHERAPY NOTES), THE APPROPRIATE BOX OR BOXES MUST BE CHECKED BY THE PATIENT.**

   f. **Psychotherapy Notes ONLY -- IN ORDER TO AUTHORIZE THE USE OR DISCLOSURE OF PSYCHOTHERAPY NOTES, ONLY THIS BOX SHOULD BE CHECKED ON THIS FORM. AUTHORIZATIONS FOR THE USE OR DISCLOSURE OF OTHER HEALTH RECORD INFORMATION MAY NOT BE MADE IN CONJUNCTION WITH AUTHORIZATIONS PERTAINING TO PSYCHOTHERAPY NOTES.**

   IF THIS BOX IS CHECKED WITH OTHER BOXES, ANOTHER AUTHORIZATION WILL BE REQUIRED TO AUTHORIZE THE USE OR DISCLOSURE OF PSYCHOTHERAPY NOTES ONLY.

   Psychotherapy notes are often referred to as process notes, distinguishable from progress notes in the medical record. These notes capture the therapist's impressions about the patient, contain details of the psychotherapy conversation considered to be inappropriate for the medical record, and are used by the provider for future sessions. These notes are often kept separate to limit access because they contain sensitive information relevant to no one other than the treating provider.

6. Section V, if a different *expiration* date is desired, specify a new date.

7. Section V, Please sign (or mark) and date.

8. A copy of the completed IHS-810 form will be given to you.

OMB STATEMENT

Public reporting burden for this collection of information is estimated to average 20 minutes per response including time for reviewing instructions, searching existing data sources, gathering and maintaining the data needed, and completing and reviewing the collection of information. An agency may not conduct or sponsor, and a person is not required to respond to, a collection of information unless it displays a currently valid OMB control number. Send comments regarding this burden estimate or any other aspect of this collection of information, including suggestions for reducing this burden to: Indian Health Service, 801 Thompson Ave., TMP Suite 450, Rockville, MD 20852, RE: PRA 0917-0030. Please DO NOT SEND this form to this address.

Figure 5-8

Source: U.S. Department of Health and Human Services, www.hhs.gov/forms/IHS-810_508.pdf (Retrieved 11/2/2011)

SUMMARY

The patient visit management concepts described in this chapter include the master patient/person index, service payment information, scheduling, consents, notices of privacy practices, advance directives, and authorizations for release of information. The master patient index is the key to locating the patient's EHR, often using a number assigned to each record, but always using patient demographic information. Information for initiating a bill and scheduling a patient is provided during the first contacts with the patient. These functions may be part of the EHR product itself or may be part of separate software programs—known as practice management systems—that interface with the EHR. The benefit of linkage of systems is that common information/data elements must only to be entered once and then can be transferred automatically to another system or systems.

General consents for treatment are optional according to the HIPAA privacy rule, but certain special procedures that are invasive or have risks associated with them still require informed consent. HIPAA does require a notice of privacy practices with a patient's (or patient's representative's) signature acknowledging receipt. Advance directives provide guidance to health care workers about the patient's wishes for treatment. A living will and a durable power of attorney for health care are two examples of advance directives. Authorizations to request or release information also must meet HIPAA guidelines. In the EHR environment, patient or patient representative signatures can be obtained in two ways. If the practice has the capability, the documents can be presented online and signatures applied via a connected signature pad. If that is not possible, the documents can be completed on paper and then scanned into the EHR. All documents noted above must become part of the EHR.

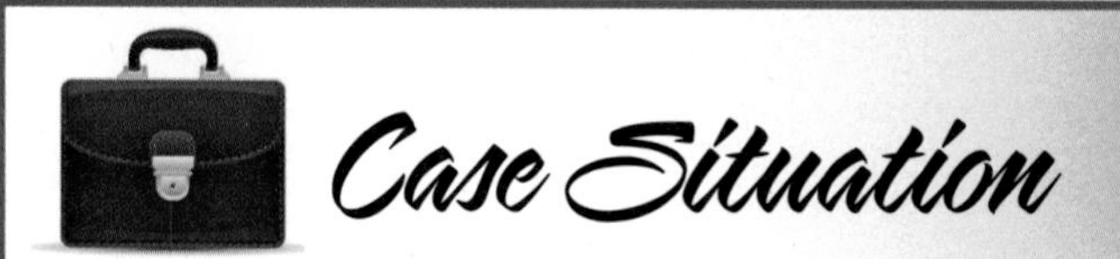

A patient calls a therapy practice, remarking that his primary physician is referring him for a series of sessions after surgery for replacement of an anterior cruciate ligament. A member of the front office staff obtains the patient name (requests spelling of it) and birth date and notes that no match is found in the master patient index. The staff member asks the patient if he has been seen by the practice in the past, and the response is, "No." Additional information, including the patient's address and telephone number, are obtained and still no match is found in the MPI. The staff member then continues adding other registration data to the initial patient information screen(s), including whether the injury was work related; it was, so this is a workers' compensation case. The patient also provides the referral number, the name of the referring physician, and the workers' compensation authorizing information. The computer assigns the patient a health record number, and an initial appointment date is determined. A query to the HIE (health information exchange) in the area yields needed information about the injury and subsequent surgery. Data needed to provide appropriate services is transferred electronically to the practice record.

On the day of the patient's visit, an office staff member collects the referral form and workers' compensation authorization and scans it into the patient record. Those forms contain the information needed to initiate billing. The patient is interviewed in an office in order to gather other patient history and illness information. Because the patient is new to the practice, a Notice of Privacy Practices is shared with the patient, who signs to acknowledge that he has received the document. The receipt is scanned into the EHR. Sharing information with the referring physician and the workers' compensation office does not require patient consent (per HIPAA or other federal and state laws), so authorizations to release information are not necessary. The patient indicates that he has no advance directives, but he is provided a brochure about them for future reference. A notation that no directive exists is made in the EHR by the staff member. Once intake processing is completed, the patient is guided to an examination room where a physical therapy assessment will begin.

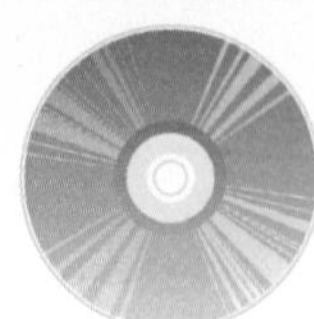

Computer Exploration

Using your e-Medsys® Educational Edition 2.0 access code provided with this text, complete the e-Medsys® Computer Exploration Exercises in Appendix B.

REFERENCES

AAAHC [Accreditation Association for Ambulatory Health Care]. (2011) *Accreditation handbook for ambulatory health care.* Wilmette, IL.

The Joint Commission. (2011). *Standards for ambulatory care.* Oakbrook Terrace, IL.

Petterson, B. J. (2011). Content and structure of the health record. In M. L. Johns (Ed.), *Health information management technology, An applied approach* (3rd ed., pp. 57–130). Chicago: AHIMA.

U.S. Department of Health and Human Services. (2010). *Federal register 42 CFR parts 412, 413, 422 et al. Medicare and Medicaid programs; Electronic health record incentive program. Final rule, 75* (144). Washington, DC: National Archives and Records Administration.

REVIEW QUESTIONS

1. What is the purpose of a master patient/person index?

2. What information might be needed when querying a patient index to determine whether or not a patient has been seen at the practice in the past?

3. List 10 items that can be characterized as demographic information.

4. Which demographic items are used first in patient index searches?

5. What is meant by a "close match" when searching a patient index?

6. Why is it important that different electronic record systems have the same guidelines for identifying patients?

7. What billing-related information is gathered prior to a patient's visit and entered into the practice management component of the EHR system?

8. What types of information must be imbedded in an electronic scheduling system for accurate scheduling to occur?

9. What component of the Notice of Privacy Practices must become part of the EHR? What component of advance directives must become part of the EHR?

____

____

____

10. Accreditation standards of The Joint Commission or of the AAAHC exist for which of the functions discussed in this chapter?

____

____

____

CHAPTER 6 Problem, Medication, and Allergy Lists

CHAPTER OUTLINE

Workflow

Standards: Functional, Content, and Vocabulary

Functional and Content Standards

Vocabulary Standards

KEY TERMS

allergy and adverse reaction list

medication list

problem list

summary lists

OBJECTIVES

Upon completion of the chapter, the learner will be able to:

1. Describe the position of The Joint Commission and that of the Accreditation Association for Ambulatory Health Care (AAAHC) on summary lists in ambulatory patient records.
2. Explain why summary lists are included in the continuity of care record (CCR) and the continuity of care document (CCD) standard.
3. Identify specific capabilities an ONC-ATCB "certified" electronic health record (EHR) must have that support the creation and maintenance of (a) problem lists, (b) medication lists, and (c) allergy and adverse reaction lists.
4. Explain why a reference vocabulary (e.g., SNOMED-CT) is preferred over a classification system (e.g., ICD-9-CM or ICD-10-CM) as the basis for structuring the content of the problem list.
5. Describe an office workflow process that will assure that the summary lists in each patient's EHR are reviewed and updated routinely to maintain their accuracy, completeness, and currency.

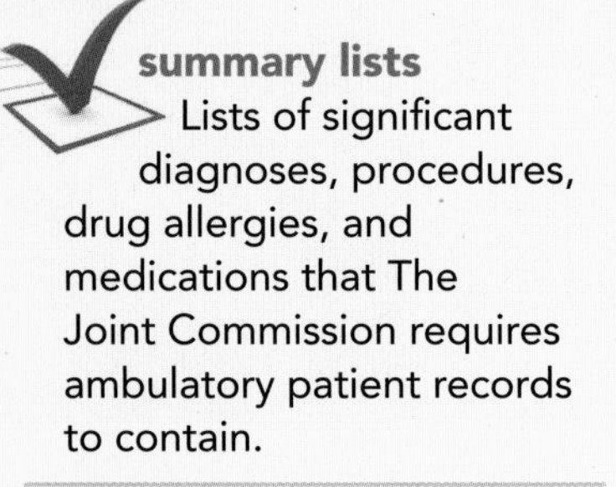

summary lists Lists of significant diagnoses, procedures, drug allergies, and medications that The Joint Commission requires ambulatory patient records to contain.

problem list Summary list of all the major diagnoses that a patient has experienced and been treated for by a health care practice.

allergy and adverse reaction list Summary list of all patient allergies and adverse reactions known to the practice.

medication list Summary list of all the medications a patient has taken or currently is taking.

INTRODUCTION

The Joint Commissions' Ambulatory Care Record of Care, Treatment and Services standard (RC 02.01.07) states that, "the clinical record contains a **summary list** for each patient who receives continuing ambulatory care services" (2011). In addition, the standards in the "Clinical Records and Health Information" section of the AAAHC Accreditation Handbook for Ambulatory Health Care addresses the need for summary lists: "If a patient has had multiple visits/admissions, or the clinical record is complex and lengthy, a summary of past and current diagnoses or problems, including past procedures, is documented in the patient's record to facilitate the continuity of care." (2011.) Summary lists help the health care provider find important clinical information quickly and allow the provider to handle the patient visit more efficiently. In addition, the CCR standard and the CCD standard (see Chapters 4 and 13) both also include the requirement for a **problem list**, **allergy and adverse reaction list**, **medication list**, and immunization list. The data in these lists contributes to the quality and safety of care a patient receives when that patient is transferred from one health care provider to another for continuing care.

For all of these reasons, the ability to create and maintain up-to-date and complete problem, allergy, and medication lists is a standard functional requirement for an ambulatory EHR product. Examples of EHR templates for lists are shown in Figures 6-1, 6-2, and 6-3.

WORKFLOW

Ambulatory EHR products provide the ability to create these important summary lists. At the current time, ambulatory EHR products typically do not generate or revise these lists automatically from data documented in other areas of the record. That is a function associated with the future vision of ambulatory EHRs. For now and the foreseeable future, the actual work processes required

Info | Note

Provider: ADAMS, HOWARD , MD   Department: BARROWS FAMILY HEALTH

Template Type: Established Well   Template: (None)

Folder: Notes

ICD: 784.0 (HEADACHE)
787.01 (NAUSEA WITH VOMITING)

Figure 6-1 Problem list in e-Medsys®.

Allergies: Latex and Dander

Nutritional Assessment

Dietary Intake

EatingHabits/Concerns

Multi-Vitamin/Fluoride Yes ☐ ☐ No Vitamin D Yes ☐ ☐ No WIC Yes ☐ ☐ No Referred ☐

Figure 6-2 Allergy list in e-Medsys®.

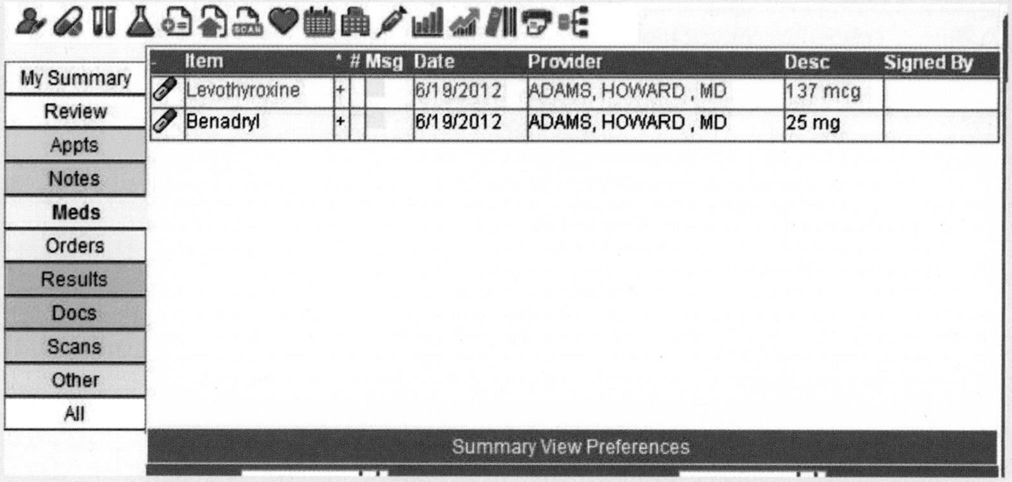

Item	*	# Msg	Date	Provider	Desc	Signed By
Levothyroxine	+		6/19/2012	ADAMS, HOWARD , MD	137 mcg	
Benadryl	+		6/19/2012	ADAMS, HOWARD , MD	25 mg	

My Summary
Review
Appts
Notes
Meds
Orders
Results
Docs
Scans
Other
All

Summary View Preferences

Figure 6-3 Medication list in e-Medsys®.

to create and maintain up-to-date, accurate, and complete summary lists require a continuing effort on the part of health care providers, working collaboratively with their patients, to maintain the currency and accuracy of each summary list.

When a patient arrives for an appointment and is waiting to be seen by a health care provider, the waiting time should be used to give the patient an opportunity to review each of their summary lists for accuracy and completeness. When the patient meets with the health care provider who has the patient's EHR open to these lists, they can discuss any questions the patient may have about content and make changes to the lists. During the examination session and at the conclusion of the office visit, the health care provider may need to make further additions or modifications to the summary lists to reflect the findings and outcome of the visit. When a health care provider interacts with a patient via phone conversation or e-mail communication, any additions or modifications to the summary lists that reflect the findings and outcomes of this "virtual" visit also must be incorporated into the patient's EHR.

Clearly, creating and maintaining accurate, complete, and up-to-date problem lists, medication lists, and allergy lists in each patient's EHR remains the responsibility of the health care provider working collaboratively with the patient. The office workflow processes must be designed to support this effort as an integral activity associated with each patient visit, whether or not that visit is on-site.

STANDARDS: FUNCTIONAL, CONTENT, AND VOCABULARY

The various types of functional, content, and vocabulary standards that are applied to ambulatory EHR systems were introduced in Chapters 3 and 4. Some of these standards speak specifically to the subject of summary lists in the EHR. Of particular importance here are the problem list, the medication list, and the allergy and adverse reaction list.

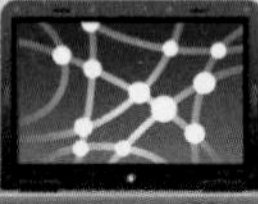

View the functional criteria used by CCHIT to certify ambulatory EHRs at the CCHIT website: http://www.cchit.org/.

Functional and Content Standards

Summary lists are significant components of an EHR because they efficiently convey patient information to health care providers that is needed to make timely and accurate clinical decisions. The CCHIT functional criteria speak to the requirement that the ambulatory EHRs have the ability to provide a problem list, a medication list and an allergy and adverse reaction list.

Examples of the ONC-ATCB certification criteria associated with problem, medication, and allergy/adverse reaction lists in the ambulatory EHR are presented in Table 6-1. Both of these sets of criteria highlight the importance of being able to maintain complete and accurate summary lists in the EHR over time. They do so by specifying that the EHR not only must be capable of capturing problems, medications and allergies, and adverse reactions entered by health care providers but also must be capable of:

- Allowing the removal of these items from a list.
- Allowing the designation of an item as "inactive," "discontinued," or "resolved."
- Entering a specific statement that the patient "has no allergies" or "is on no medication."

Vocabulary Standards

Several standard vocabularies that are being used in EHR systems were introduced in Chapter 3. The clinical concepts entered into an EHR's problem, allergy, and medication lists commonly are entered through the use of standard reference vocabularies such as SNOMED-CT, perhaps in combination with other relevant specialized standard vocabulary systems (e.g., MEDCIN, LOINC, RxNorm, NDC). Both CCHIT and ONC-ATCB criteria specify that the "certified" EHR system must provide the ability to maintain a coded list of problems, medications, and allergies/adverse reactions. When a standard reference vocabulary is used to make entries into these lists, each entry is deposited as coded data (i.e., structured data) into the EHR system's database (data repository). Coded data in the data repository is then readily available to be transmitted electronically to another health care organization when requested, transmitted to the

TABLE 6-1 Example of a Problem List, Medication List, Allergy/Adverse Reaction List Associated ONC_ATCB Certification Criteria for Ambulatory EHRs

§170.302 (c)	Maintain up-to-date problem list. Enable a user to electronically record, modify, and retrieve a patient's problem list for longitudinal care.
§170.302 (d)	Maintain active medication list. Enable a user to electronically record, modify, and retrieve a patient's active medication list as well as medication history for longitudinal care.
§170.302 (e)	Maintain active medication allergy list. Enable a user to electronically record, modify, and retrieve a patient's active medication allergy list as well as medication allergy history for longitudinal care.

Source: National Institute of Standards and Testing (http://healthcare.nist.gov/use_testing/effective_requirements.html)

patient's personal health record, and/or downloaded into a reporting system for quality management.

As mentioned in Chapter 3, ICD-9-CM (and soon ICD-10-CM as of October 1, 2014) and CPT-4 are classification systems that commonly are embedded in the ambulatory EHR and appropriately used to reflect the diagnoses and procedures associated with each patient visit. These classification systems are not, however, the most effective systems to use for creating problem lists. ICD-9-CM and CPT-4 especially are created essentially for administrative purposes and lack the specificity needed by health care providers to communicate clinical concepts clearly. (Note: ICD-10-CM includes a greatly expanded code set in comparison to ICD-9-CM, so it does communicate clinical concepts better than ICD-9-CM). As briefly described in Chapter 3 (see Table 3-2), SNOMED-CT has been mapped to ICD-9-CM and to ICD-10-CM; this makes it possible to translate coded data entered into the EHR problem list with SNOMED-CT terms to ICD-9-CM (or ICD-10-CM) codes when necessary. Examples of vocabulary terms presented within an EHR for use in creating allergy, medication, and problem lists are shown in Figures 6-4, 6-5, and 6-6.

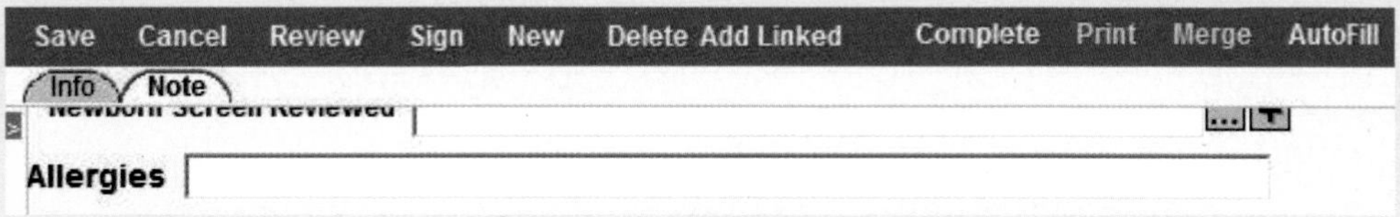

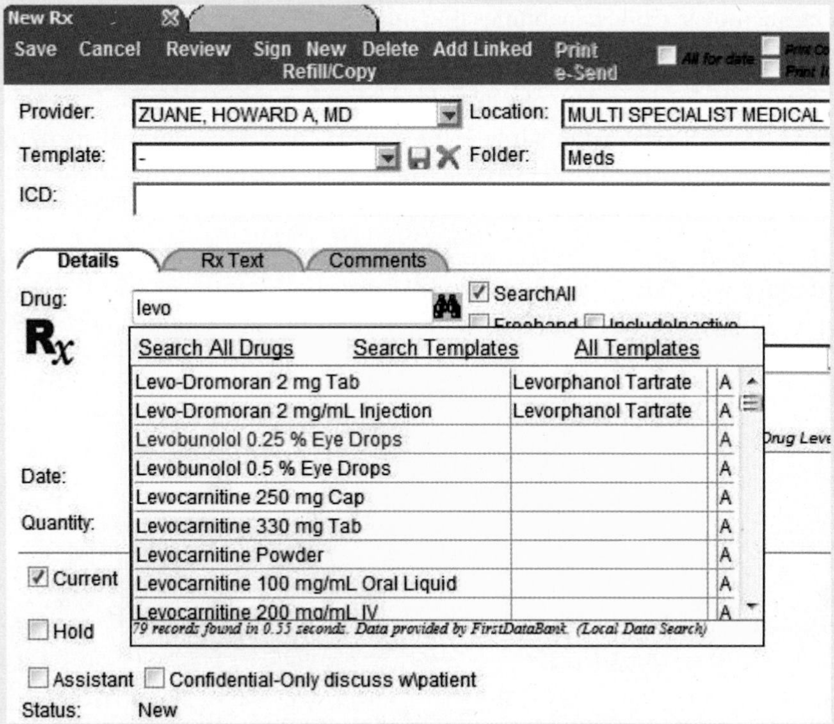

Figure 6-4 Allergy selection list in e-Medsys®.

Figure 6-5 Medication selection list in e-Medsys®.

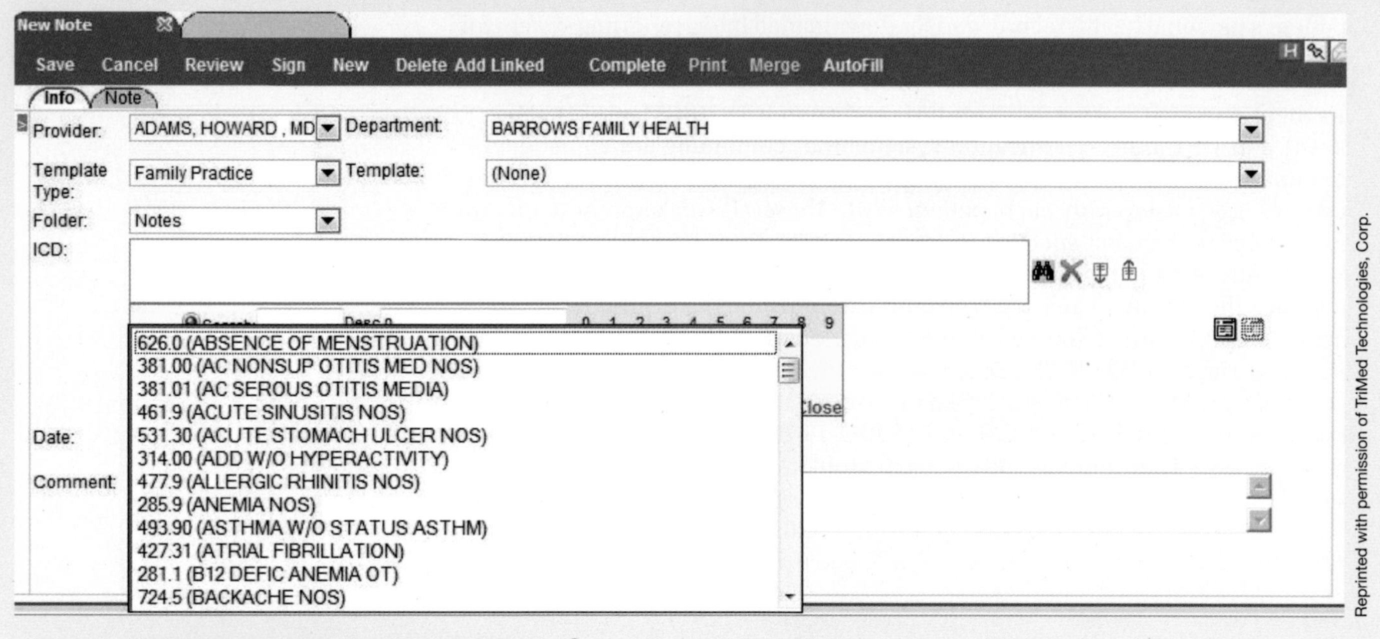

Figure 6-6 Problem selection list in e-Medsys®.

SUMMARY

Just as in paper-based patient record systems, up-to-date, accurate, and complete problem, medication, and allergy/adverse reaction lists are important components of the ambulatory EHR. The CCHIT criteria as well as the ONC-ATCB criteria used to certify ambulatory EHR products include specific capabilities that must be demonstrated through standard test scripts to assure that the "certified" EHRs can support the creation, modification, and removal of items from these summary lists.

Standard reference vocabularies are embedded into EHR systems to support the construction of summary lists that: (a) present clearly understood clinical concepts to health care providers, (b) allow the data in the lists to be stored in coded form in the data repository, and (c) can be electronically transmitted to other health care providers when needed to assure quality and safe continuity of care.

Working collaboratively within an established office workflow process, the patient and the health care provider can ensure that the summary lists within the patient's EHR are reviewed and updated routinely to maintain their accuracy, completeness, and currency.

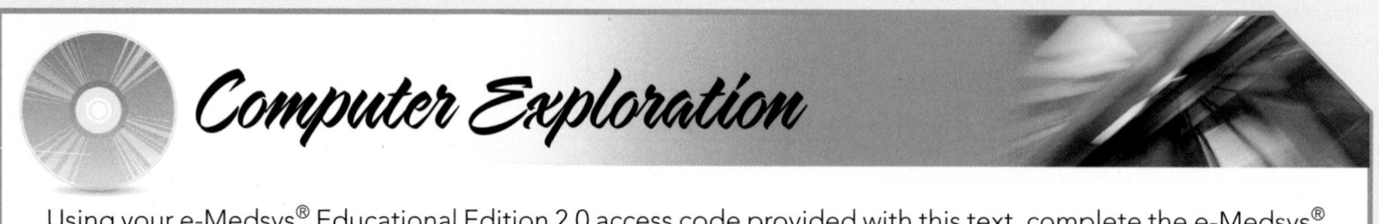

Using your e-Medsys® Educational Edition 2.0 access code provided with this text, complete the e-Medsys® Computer Exploration Exercises in Appendix B.

REFERENCES

AAAHC [Accreditation Association for Ambulatory Health Care, Inc.]. (2011). *Accreditation handbook for ambulatory health care.* Wilmette, IL.

CCHIT Certified 2011 Ambulatory EHR Certification Criteria. Retrieved from http://www.cchit.org.

National Institute of Standards and Technology. (2011). Approved Test Procedures Version 1.1.

The Joint Commission. (2011). *Standards for ambulatory care.* Oakbrook Terrace, IL.

REVIEW QUESTIONS

1. List three types of lists that are described as "summary lists" in The Joint Commission R.C. standards as well as the ONC-ATCB EHR Criteria for Ambulatory EHRs.

____

____

____

2. Explain the reason summary lists are included in the CCR and CCD standards.

____

____

____

3. Which of the following capabilities related to the problem list can be demonstrated by an ONC-ATCB "certified" ambulatory EHR project? (True or False.)

T F Display only the active problems associated with the patient.
T F Maintain the onset date of a problem.
T F Display inactive and/or resolved problems.
T F Record chronicity of a problem.
T F Record user ID and date of all updates to the problem list.

4. Which of the following capabilities related to the medication list can be demonstrated by an ONC-ATCB "certified" ambulatory EHR project? (True or False.)

T F Mark a medication as "erroneous" or "discontinued."
T F Display current medications only.
T F Specify in a discrete field that the patient takes no medications.
T F Enter only coded medications from a standard medication list.
T F Alert the user at the time a new medication is prescribed that drug interaction and allergy checking will not be performed against the uncoded or free-text medication.

5. Which of the following capabilities related to the allergy and adverse reaction list can be demonstrated by an ONC-ATCB "certified" ambulatory EHR project? (True or False.)

T F Capture and store lists of medications and other agents to which the patient has had an allergic or other adverse reaction.
T F Explicitly indicate that a patient has no known drug allergies.
T F Capture non-drug agents to which the patient has had an allergic or other adverse reaction.
T F Remove an item from the allergy and adverse reaction list.
T F Specify the type of allergic or adverse reaction.

6. State the rationale for recommending either SNOMED-CT, ICD-9-CM or ICD-10-CM as the standard terminology to use for recording problems in the EHR.

____

____

____

7. Describe how a patient can be brought into the office workflow process that is established to assure that the summary lists in each patient's EHR are reviewed and updated routinely to maintain their accuracy, completeness, and currency.

____

____

____

CHAPTER 7 Examination/ Assessment Notes, Graphics, and Charts

CHAPTER OUTLINE

Workflow
Standards: Functional and Content
Functional Standards
Content Standards
Documentation
Templates and Free-text Narrative
Graphics and Charts

KEY TERMS

examination protocol
free-text narrative
graphic displays
growth chart
point of care
templates

OBJECTIVES

Upon completion of the chapter, the learner will be able to:

1. Describe the general workflow associated with a health care provider's examination or special assessment activity.
2. Identify common sources for locating examination and assessment content standards applied to ambulatory practice settings.
3. Differentiate structured data from unstructured data by providing examples of each.
4. Explain why using templates to capture documentation in an electronic health record (EHR) generally is preferred over free-text narrative.
5. Describe the purpose and content of the growth chart.
6. Explain why graphing capability is seen as a basic functional criterion for an ambulatory EHR.
7. Explain how the design of the data collection tools used to document examination and assessment findings in an EHR can affect the completeness and timeliness of the data in the patient record.
8. Describe how computer hardware choices and EHR workstation placement can affect the efficiency of the examination or special assessment activity.

INTRODUCTION

As a first step in a clinical interaction with a new or returning patient, each primary health care provider in an ambulatory practice setting engages in an examination or assessment activity. Results of the examination or assessment are the foundation upon which the health care provider makes decisions regarding additional diagnostic tests needed and appropriate treatment options to present to the patient. Well-designed EHRs support the examination or assessment methods of each health care provider and guide the provider in thoroughly documenting an examination or assessment. As a result, well-designed EHR systems introduce efficiencies into the provider's examination or assessment activity and improve the completeness of the provider's documentation of findings.

WORKFLOW

The specific focus of an examination or assessment and the detailed activities involved in the examination will vary significantly based on the health care provider's medical specialty (e.g., obstetrician, orthopedist, cardiologist) or professional discipline (e.g., physical therapy, occupational therapy, speech therapy). However, an overview of the general workflow for an examination or assessment visit to a health care provider is presented in Figure 7-1.

As described in Chapter 5, a patient's visit begins with registration activities, during which personal identification data is collected from the patient (e.g., name, address, birth date) along with a statement regarding the patient's reason for this visit. Then, in most instances, a medical assistant or nurse "rooms" the patient and will ask the patient to explain the reason for the visit (the "chief complaint") and describe any problems or symptoms being experienced. At that time, vital signs (height, weight, blood pressure, temperature, and so forth)

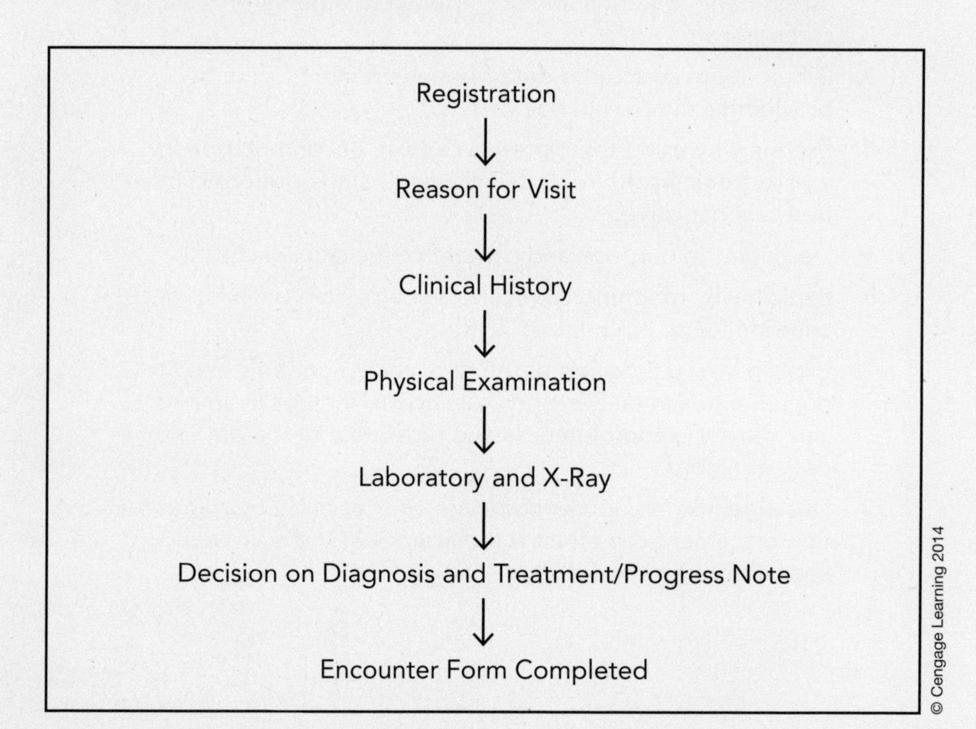

Figure 7-1 General examination or assessment visit workflow.

will be taken as appropriate. All of that data is documented in the EHR so it will be available to the primary health care provider conducting the examination or assessment. The provider will explore further the patient's description of the current problem(s) being experienced (the "reason for visit" or the "chief complaint"). If the patient has been referred by another health care provider for an examination or assessment, the referral letter or the continuity-of-care record also will be available within the EHR for review. The patient's description of the problem, the information in the referral letter, and the data in the continuity-of-care record are significant because they guide the health care provider in selecting a specific focus for the examination or special assessment. As a result, the health care provider will initiate a series of actions designed to gain a better understanding of the potential underlying causes of the patient's problem. This may involve a full or partial review of systems, a full or partial physical examination, and obtaining additional data through various types of diagnostic tests. The data gathered from these activities, along with a review of the patient's problem list, medication list, allergy list, and medical history (diagnoses and procedures), allow the health care provider to establish a diagnosis and to begin treatment planning. In every case, the goal of the examination or special assessment activity is to define the problem and move toward establishing an accurate diagnosis. Then the most effective plan of care can be presented to the patient.

STANDARDS: FUNCTIONAL AND CONTENT

The various types of functional, content, and vocabulary standards that are applied to ambulatory EHR systems were introduced in Chapters 3 and 4. Examination notes, graphics, and various display charts (including flowcharts) are addressed within these standards.

Functional Standards

Well-designed EHR systems function in ways that facilitate the review of existing patient data, the capture of new patient data, and the modification/updating of patient data by authorized health care providers. The Certification Commission for Healthcare Information Technology (CCHIT) functional criteria for ambulatory EHRs address requirements that the EHR must meet to support the health care providers' examination activities.

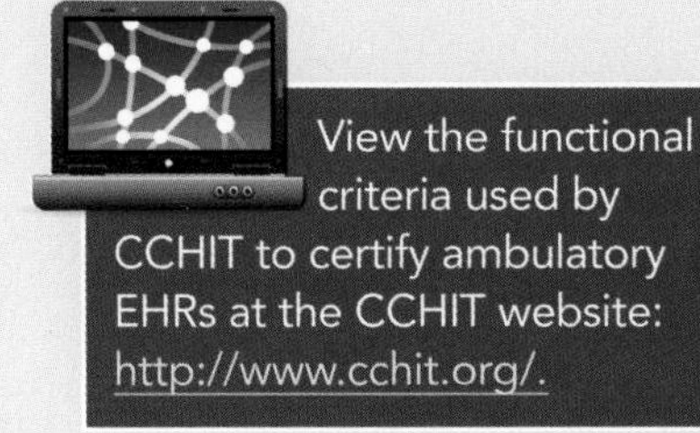
View the functional criteria used by CCHIT to certify ambulatory EHRs at the CCHIT website: http://www.cchit.org/.

Table 7-1 presents a sample of the ONC-ATCB Meaningful Use certification criteria that are focused on supporting the health care provider's examination activities.

Content Standards

As discussed in Chapter 4, there are numerous professional groups, governmental agencies, and accreditation organizations that have established standards regarding the content of health records. The Joint Commission, formerly known as The Joint Commission on Accreditation of Healthcare Organizations (JCAHO), leaves the actual specification of the content required in an assessment to each accredited health care organization, but it does require within its Record Content (RC) Standard RC.02.01.01 that "the clinical record contains any findings of assessments and re-assessments." (2011.) The Accreditation Association for

TABLE 7-1 Examples of Examination Associated ONC-ATCB Certification Criteria for Ambulatory EHRs

§170.302 (f)	Record and chart vital signs (1) Vital signs. Enable a user to electronically record, modify, and retrieve a patient's vital signs including, at a minimum, the height, weight, and blood pressure.
§170.302 (g)	Smoking status. Enable a user to electronically record, modify, and retrieve the smoking status of a patient. Smoking status types must include: current every day smoker; current some day smoker; former smoker; never smoker; smoker, current status unknown; unknown if ever smoked.
§170.302 (h)	Incorporate laboratory test results. (1) Receive results. Electronically receive clinical laboratory test results in a structured format and display such results in human readable format. (2) Display test report information. Electronically display all the information for a test report specified at 42 CFR 493.1291(c)(1) through (7).
§170.302 (j)	Medication Reconciliation. Enable a user to electronically compare two or more medication lists.
§170.304 (a)	Computerized provider order entry. Enable a user to electronically record, store, retrieve, and modify, at a minimum, the following order types: (1) Medications; (2) Laboratory; and (3) Radiology/imaging
§170.304(h)	Clinical summaries. Enable a user to provide clinical summaries to patients for each office visit that include, at a minimum, diagnostic test results, problem list, medication list, and medication allergy list.

Source: National Institute of Standards and Testing (http://healthcare.nist.gov/use_testing/effective_requirements.html).

Ambulatory Health Care (2011) specifies that entries in the patient record made at the time of an examination or assessment include:

- Chief complaint or purpose of visit.
- Clinical findings.
- Discharge diagnosis or impression.

The patient record content requirements specific to examinations or special assessment in the Centers for Medicare & Medicaid Services (CMS) Conditions of Coverage include:

- Identification and social data.
- Pertinent medical history.
- Assessment of health status and health need.
- Physical examination.
- Diagnostic and laboratory test results.
- Physician orders.
- Reports of treatments and medications.

- A brief summary of the episode, disposition, and instructions to the patient.
- Signatures of healthcare professionals involved. (CMS.)

In general, these CMS Condition of Coverage (CoC) health record requirements are quite similar to the basic requirements set forth by other accreditation organizations or licensing bodies. In addition, each type of health care professional engages in examination or special assessment activities using an approach that reflects that profession's unique type of practice and its established methods for evaluating clients. For example, an examination performed by a physician, physician assistant, nurse practitioner, or chiropractor generally is structured first to address the "chief complaint" of the patient and then to follow a standard set of examination steps (**examination protocol**) that specifically eliminate or confirm the potential underlying causes of the "chief complaint." Using the information gained through this process, the health care provider can arrive at a clinical diagnosis and then determine appropriate treatment options accordingly. Other independent health care providers, such as a physical therapist in an independent practice situation, will follow a similar examination or assessment process when a patient presents with a new health complaint.

examination protocol Beginning with the chief complaint, a standard set of examination steps that will specifically eliminate, or specifically confirm, potential underlying causes for the chief complaint.

In spite of some differences among health care providers in the focus and methods of doing examinations or special assessments, there are several similarities. Each type of health care professional begins with reviewing and updating an existing patient history or collecting a new patient history that commonly has medical/surgical, psychosocial, and family components (see Figure 7-2). Each

Info | Note

History

Chronic

Hospitalizations

Surgeries

ER Visits

Current Medications

Family History

Social History

Physical Exam

Wt Ht BMI HC HR RR Temp

Appearance: LMP

	Normal	Abnormal
Head	Normocephalic-no evidence trauma	
Teeth/Gingiva	No obvious caries - no lesions	

Figure 7-2 Patient history in e-Medsys®.

type of health care professional includes a review of patient problems, allergies, and medications, and collects updates on them. Each type also collects current vital signs (blood pressure, temperature, pulse, respiration, etc., (see Figure 7-3) and conducts a general physical examination (see Figure 7-4) of the patient to obtain much of the objective data that contributes to the health care provider's examination or special assessment findings.

Often a health care provider, such as a physical therapist, may receive a client based on a referral for assessment or an order for a specific type of physical therapy treatment program. In that case, the physical therapist will focus on a more in-depth initial evaluation (assessment) of the patient in order to determine muscle strength in each of the extremities, stability and flexibility of all or selected joints, and so forth. The outcome from the assessment is a series of (short-term and long-term) functional goals for the patient. A physical therapy treatment plan based on these short- and long-term goals is developed that reflects specific activities and a timeline for each activity; these allow the patient to achieve progressively the physical capabilities established in the physical therapy goals.

Save Cancel Review Sign New Delete Add Linked Complete Print Merge AutoFill

Info | Pt Info | ROS | Exam | ExamCont

Ht	Wt	BP (sitting/standing)	BP (Supine)	Pulse	RR	Temp
73	210	120/65		67	17	98.6

Figure 7-3 Patient vital signs in e-Medsys®.

Physical Exam

Concern Concern Concern

Wt Lt HC HR RR Temp

Ht Percent. Wt Percent. HC Percent.

Appearance: LMP

	Normal	Abnormal
Head	Normocephalic-no evidence trauma	
Teeth/Gingiva	No obvious caries - no lesions	
Eyes	PERRLA-EOM intact & RR WNL bilat.	
Ears	canals clear-TM's not injected-landmarks WNL	
Nose/Throat	not injected-not congested	
Neck	Supple-no lymphadenopathy	
Lungs	no distress-no rales-no wheeze-clear B.S.	
Heart	regular rhythm-no murmur-S1 &S2 WNL	

Figure 7-4 Patient physical examination in e-Medsys®.

Much the same process as described for the physical therapist would be followed for an occupational therapist's examination of a patient, which generally begins with an already confirmed clinical problem or referral diagnosis and then focuses on more in-depth assessments that specifically address, in this case, the patient's ability to handle activities of daily living: cooking, dressing, bathing, cleaning, driving, shopping, and so on. The outcome of an occupational therapist's initial evaluation (assessment) is also a series of short-term and long-term functional goals for the patient together with an occupational therapy treatment plan.

Figures 7-5A and B are examples from an EHR of the format and content reflecting initial evaluations or assessments from another type of health care provider: physical therapists. When the data collection tools for documenting various types of patient examination or assessment findings are being designed for the

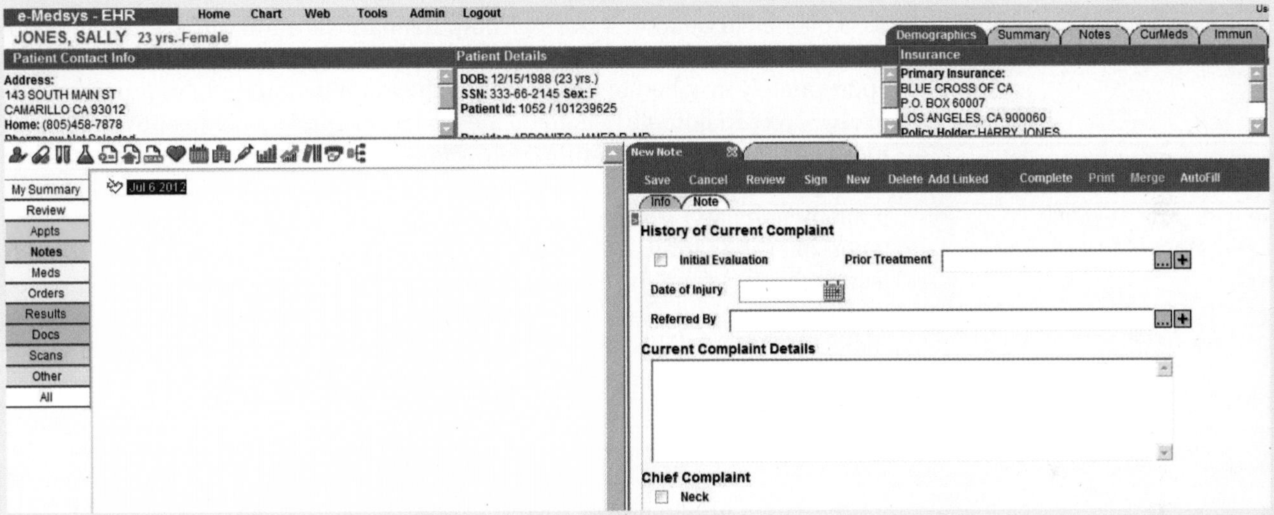

Figure 7-5A Physical therapist initial evaluation in e-Medsys®.

Reprinted with permission of TriMed Technologies, Corp.

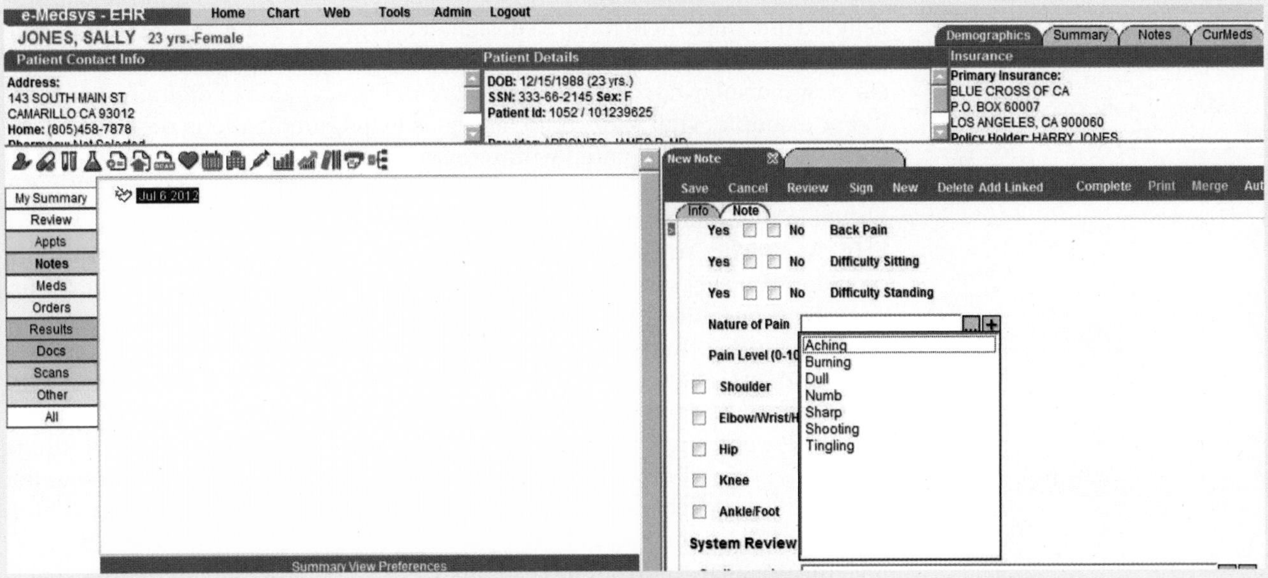

Figure 7-5B Physical therapist initial evaluation with terminology selections in e-Medsys®.

Reprinted with permission of TriMed Technologies, Corp.

practice's EHR, content standards relevant to each type of professional service offered in that specific practice setting should be researched and then incorporated into the documentation tools, as appropriate. Common sources of such data and information content standards are professional associations or specialty societies, accreditation agencies, state licensing agencies, the Center for Medicare/Medicaid Services, and the like.

DOCUMENTATION

Complete, accurate, and timely documentation of the findings from an examination or special assessment is an essential component of a health care practice's legal patient record. A well-designed EHR system will assist the practice's health care providers to meet this expectation.

point of care The time at which treatment is being provided.

As explained in Chapter 3, having computer hardware and workstations that are selected to match the health care provider's documentation needs and that are appropriately installed or positioned in the examination room to promote ease of use plays a major role in helping the health care provider efficiently document in the EHR while also appropriately interacting with or caring for the patient; that is, documenting in the EHR at the **point of care**. Another major factor in implementing an EHR that supports complete, accurate, and timely documentation of examination or assessment findings is well-designed formats for collecting the data from the health care provider. The CCHIT functional criteria for ambulatory EHRs (CCHIT, 2010. Emphasis added) require that the EHR "system shall provide the *ability to enter free-text notes*" and "*provide templates for inputting data in a structured format as part of clinical documentation.*"

Templates and Free-Text Narrative

free-text narrative Unstructured documentation that allows a health care provider to dictate or key text.

It is certainly possible for a health care provider to document the subjective and objective findings from a client examination or special assessment in **free-text narrative** within the EHR. This can be accomplished by directly keying it into a specific area of the EHR designed to receive typed text and scanned documents, or by dictating it and then having the transcribed report electronically fed into the EHR in the area designated to capture such documents. People certainly enjoy reading free-text narrative. Although EHR systems can accept, store, and display narrative text, they are not yet capable of digitally "reading" it. For example, vital signs data, allergies listed, medications described, and laboratory test results stated within the body of a transcribed narrative report cannot be pinpointed as digital or coded electronic data elements and redisplayed in the Vital Signs, Allergy, Medication, or Lab Test display areas of the EHR. As a result, such critical data may not be easily available to a health care provider who accesses the EHR to check on a patient's allergies, medications, vital signs, or lab test results. In addition, data embedded in free-text narrative is not in a form that can be used by the EHR system to trigger important alerts and reminders. (See Chapters 9 and 10 for more information about EHR alerts and reminders.) It is thus not advisable to accommodate large amounts of free-text narrative in an EHR system, because such documentation limits the EHR system's functional ability to display data elements embedded in the narrative to the health care provider when and where it can be most useful. For this reason, when an EHR system is implemented in a provider office setting, the practice group should establish its own policies and guidelines specifying the types of documentation where free-text medical or clinical narrative text is acceptable.

To take full advantage of the capabilities of an EHR system, effective implementations involve the development and use of various types of general examination or special assessment **templates**. These preformatted documentation guides are carefully designed to support each type of examination or special assessment situation that the practice's health care providers commonly perform. Each template contains specific data fields that are required by the health care provider to document a complete set of findings normally associated with a specific examination protocol. Moreover, the data fields are positioned within the template in a sequence that matches the health care provider's preferred examination or special assessment methods. Refer back to Figures 7-4 and 7-5 for examples of examination templates.

templates
Preformatted data collection screens containing specific structured or free-text data fields and designed to support efficient and complete documentation.

Each type of health care provider could have several available templates from which to choose, with each template intentionally designed to support a specific type of examination or special assessment. For example, one template could be a Newborn–Six Week Examination; another template could be an Adult Annual Examination; another could be a High-Risk Obstetric Examination. When the health care provider selects a specific template to use during a patient visit, the provider is presented with a structured set of data fields related to the patient's problem; within each data field, drop-down menus of common findings or free-text options are provided. As the health care provider works through the data fields and makes appropriate selections or free-text entries, the visit (progress) note is simultaneously constructed. Figure 7-6 depicts how a visit (progress) note is developed through the selections made by the health care provider in an examination template.

The subject of structured data elements and unstructured data elements was presented in detail in Chapter 3. When a health care provider documents examination or special assessment findings in templates, the data mostly is entered into structured data fields and also may be entered in some unstructured data fields with a limited character length. As a result, the data entered through structured data fields in templates is capable of triggering alerts and reminders. Also, structured data from the examination or assessment can be deployed electronically for viewing in other areas of the EHR (e.g., in vitals flow sheets, lab result flow sheets, problem lists, allergy lists, medication profiles). Over

Multisysteme

Save Cancel Review Sign New Delete Add Linked Complete Print Merge AutoFill

Info General PFSH/HPI Exam ExamCont Decision

height:	60
weight:	175
BP:(sitting/standing)	120/90
BP:(Supine)	
Pulse:	100
Respiration:	15
Temperature:	99
General appearance	Flush and damp with sweat
CC:	

Figure 7-6 Visit note in e-Medsys®.

time, structured clinical data captured through templates and stored in the EHR database can be accessed for use in the practice's management reporting systems to support its Evaluation and Management (E&M) code assignment, quality management efforts, as well as its long-range business planning activities.

When a practice implements an EHR system, the development of templates is another critically important activity. Templates must be created to support the variety of types of examinations or special assessments commonly performed by each type of health care provider employed in that setting. In order to do this well, template development requires significant input from each type of health care provider. Input is needed to assure that each template is designed to help conduct efficiently and document fully each type of examination or special assessment performed in that practice setting.

graphic displays A format for presenting numerical data that has been entered into structured (coded) data fields, showing trends in clinical data and allowing comparisons over time.

growth chart Graphic display of the height and weight of pediatric patients comparing their data to a developmental standard for the patient's age group.

Graphics and Charts

EHR systems are generally capable of providing **graphic displays** of any piece(s) of numerical data (height, weight, blood pressure, respiratory rates, laboratory test results, etc.) that have been entered into structured data fields within templates. As indicated earlier in this chapter, ambulatory EHRs that are either CCHIT or ONC-ATCB "certified" are systems capable of displaying numerical results in graphic form to assist health care providers observe trends in clinical data and compare results over time.

A **growth chart** is one example of a graphic display of numerical data that is commonly available in ambulatory EHR systems (see Figure 7-7). The growth chart is an important functional component of an EHR used in health care provider settings that serve pediatric patients—for example, family practice and pediatric specialists. The growth chart commonly is available for use with patients between the ages of 2 and 20. It displays height and weight data that has been entered into the EHR through structured data fields within the physical examination template, the vital signs template, or the growth chart itself. It shows the actual height and weight data points of a child as they compare to the expected height and weight data points for a child of the same age. This trended and comparative data allows the health care provider to monitor the child's physical developmental, identify developmental concerns, and initiate early interventions if necessary.

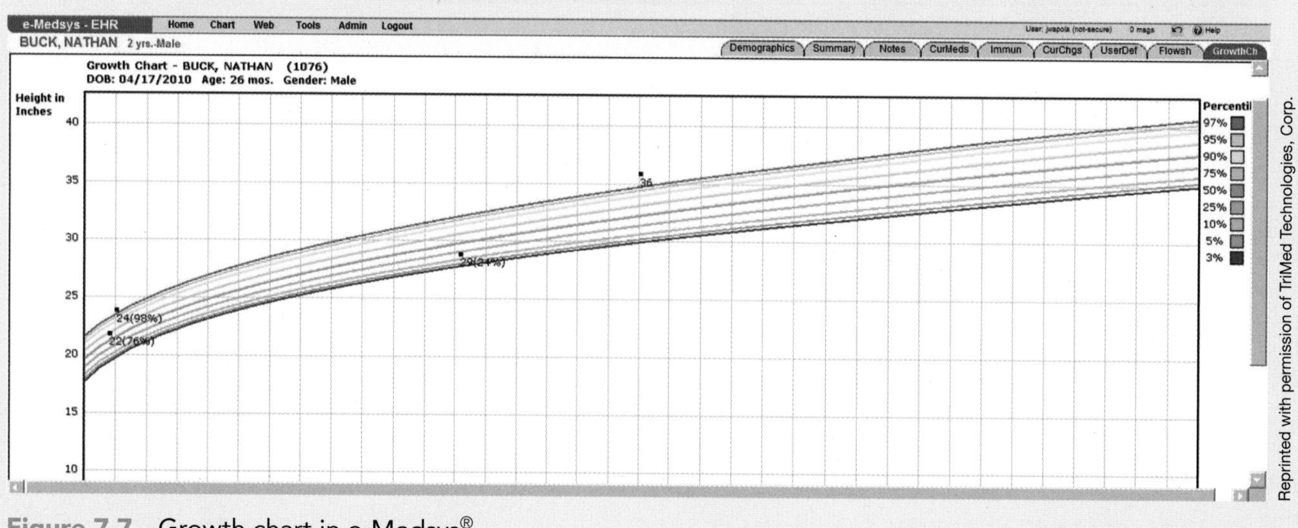

Figure 7-7 Growth chart in e-Medsys®.

SUMMARY

The examinations or special assessments conducted by health care providers in their practice setting establish a foundation from which treatment options and treatment plans are developed for a patient. Well-designed electronic health records systems support the examination or special assessment methods of each type of health care provider. They also guide the provider to complete a thorough examination and to fully document both subjective and objective findings. The large volume of structured data that can be entered into the EHR through well-designed templates makes it possible for the EHR system to generate a variety of patient-specific alerts and reminders and customized reports for both clinicians and administrators to use for quality improvement and business development purposes. There are situations where free-text narrative is an acceptable (and perhaps even a desirable) form of documentation for some examination or special assessment findings; in general, however, the majority of patient examination or assessment findings are best documented in an EHR using templates (incorporating structured data and limited unstructured data). Health care providers who spend much of their time in examination or special assessment activities will find that well-designed documentation templates in the EHR have the capacity to: (a) enhance their productivity, (b) improve the quality of the data collected, which contributes to improved patient-related communication among the health care provider team, and (c) improve the health care provider's ability to monitor and manage the patient's health status carefully over time.

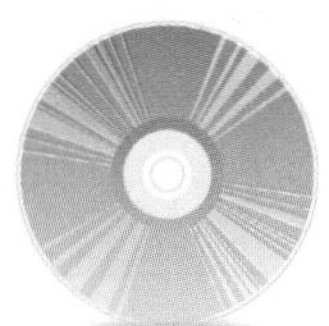

Computer Exploration

Using your e-Medsys® Educational Edition 2.0 access code provided with this text, complete the e-Medsys® Computer Exploration Exercises in Appendix B.

REFERENCES

AAAHC [Accreditation Association for Ambulatory Health Care, Inc.]. (2011). *Accreditation handbook for ambulatory health care*. Wilmette, IL.

CMS [Centers for Medicare & Medicaid Services]. Title 42: Public Health. Part 491—Certification of certain health facilities. CFR491.10: Patient health records.

CCHIT Certified 2011 Ambulatory EHR Certification Criteria. Retrieved from http://www.cchit.org/

National Institute of Standards and Technology. Approved Test Procedures Version 1.1. (2011). Retrieved from http://healthcare.nist.gov/use_testing/effective_requirements.html

The Joint Commission. (2011). *Standards for ambulatory care*. Oakbrook Terrace, IL.

REVIEW QUESTIONS

1. What is the purpose of the examination or special assessment performed by a health care provider when a client presents with a chief complaint or a referral diagnosis?

2. Why is it important for an EHR system to be easy for health care providers to use during an examination?

3. How can computer hardware choices and placement affect the efficiency of the examination or special assessment activity?

4. Why are templates composed largely of structured data fields preferable to free-text narrative for capturing examination documentation in an EHR system?

5. How does the design of the templates used to document examination findings in an EHR affect the completeness and timeliness of the data in the patient record?

6. What type of examination content do the CMS Conditions of Coverage (CoC) require be included in the ambulatory practice's patient record?

7. What is the content and purpose of the growth chart?

8. Why is graphing capability seen as a basic functional criterion for an ambulatory EHR?

CHAPTER 8 Treatment Plan, Orders, and Results

CHAPTER OUTLINE

OBJECTIVES

Upon completion of the chapter, the learner will be able to:

1. Identify common applications associated with an electronic practice-management system (PMS).
2. Explain how an electronic health-record (EHR) system integrated with a practice management system contributes to implementing a treatment plan.
3. List the two basic questions that a treatment plan answers.
4. Describe what a referral letter and the CCR/CCD have in common.
5. Describe how templates contribute to a health care provider's ability to implement a treatment plan efficiently.
6. Describe how the EHR system captures the details of a diagnostic or treatment order.
7. List three common methods used for transmitting a diagnostic or treatment order from one health care practice's EHR system to an external health care provider.
8. Describe how templates contribute to the completeness of treatment or procedure documentation in the EHR.
9. Explain how the practice should handle hard-copy treatment or procedure documentation received from an external health care provider in response to a referral order.

KEY TERMS

daily task list
direct faxing
electronic data interchange (EDI)
order details
order entry templates
procedure notes
procedure notes template
referral letter
results reporting
secure e-mail
treatment notes
treatment plan

treatment plan
A final component of an assessment which specifies any number and variety of actions needed to appropriately address the patient's health care problem(s). In a SOAP note it is the content in the "P" section of the documentation.

INTRODUCTION

At the conclusion of an examination or special assessment, a **treatment plan** is defined for any health problem that has been identified or diagnosed. The plan is included as the final section within the visit note documented in the EHR. The plan can specify any number and variety of actions needed to address the patient's health care problem(s) appropriately. For example, it might include patient education on a health maintenance topic (e.g., dietary instructions), prescribing a medication, ordering monthly laboratory tests to monitor liver function, a referral to another health care provider for a specialized service or procedure, or conducting a nonsurgical or surgical procedure in the health care provider's office setting. To support this process, the EHR system must be capable of: (a) capturing the details of the complete treatment plan, (b) constructing and transmitting orders specified in the treatment plan to the appropriate health care provider so they can be carried out, and (c) capturing the treatment/procedure notes and/or results reported from all other activities that were carried out as specified in the treatment plan.

WORKFLOW

At the conclusion of an examination, the health care provider defines a treatment plan in collaboration with the patient or patient's representative. Based on the plan, the health care provider might immediately conduct some type of treatment session immediately. In addition (or alternatively), the health care provider commonly will write treatment orders and/or new diagnostic orders to request the services of other health care providers to carry out the treatment plan.

When the treatment plan involves the use of a medication, medication orders commonly are created in the form of prescriptions that are delivered electronically through an electronic prescribing ("e-prescribing") module within the EHR system to the pharmacy of the patient's choice. Alternatively, the prescription can, if necessary, be a hard copy printed for the patient to present to their pharmacy or faxed to the pharmacy.

In some cases, the provider may order a medication to be administered to the patient during the office visit. When the medication is administered to the patient it is documented in the medication administration record (MAR) within the EHR. (See Chapter 9 for a full discussion of medication orders and administration in an EHR system.)

daily task list (aka "in basket")
Designation of work that needs to be completed by an employee of a practice.

Non-medication orders for services that will be delivered by another health care provider within the same practice setting are transmitted directly within the EHR system: (a) to the appropriate health care providers' EHR workstations and inserted into their **daily task list** (aka "in basket") if time slots are available on their work schedule, or (b) to the practice's scheduler, who will work with the patient to schedule the service or procedure visit for another date/time. These functions commonly are associated with a practice management system (PMS). The PMS and the EHR system must be implemented in such a way that they share some key data elements. For example, patient demographics, dates of service, diagnoses, and the profiles of health care providers employed by the health care office practice could be gathered in one system and passed along to another system. The PMS and the EHR systems support different functions: the EHR primarily supports clinical activities, and the PMS supports administrative and financial activities. Both are components of a fully functional EHR system in a practice setting.

Common applications within a PMS system include:

- Patient demographics, including their health insurance.
- Appointment scheduling.
- Charge capture and billing.
- Reporting.

When a practice's EHR task distribution ("daily work list" or "in-basket") application and PMS patient-scheduling application are integrated, the workflow becomes more efficient; it electronically links the orders associated with the treatment plan to those health care providers who actually implement the plan by responding to the orders entered into the EHR system. For example, orders for services (lab tests, radiology exams, consultations, etc.) that will need to be delivered by a health care provider outside of the practice setting can be transmitted electronically, along with relevant patient information, through one or a combination of these steps: constructing and electronically delivering a **referral letter**, or the order and a document (e.g., the CCR/CCD), to the other provider through **secure e-mail**; or **direct faxing** from within the EHR; or delivering the documents through some other form of **electronic data interchange (EDI)** set up among health care provider organizations. The continuity of care record (CCR) and the continuity of care document (CCD) contain a standard set of patient data that can be transmitted directly from one health care provider's EHR to another's EHR, in order to facilitate direct communication of important patient information when a patient's care is transferred from one health care provider setting to another. Chapter 13 presents a full discussion of the CCR and the CCD.

If no direct electronic delivery from the EHR to the external provider organization is possible, then a hard copy can be printed from the EHR and delivered by regular fax or mailed to the other provider organization or hand delivered by the patient to the other provider organization.

Figure 8-1 is an example Referral Letter template from an EHR.

referral letter
Request from one health care provider to another to provide specialized services to a patient; includes the transfer of information from one practice to another.

secure e-mail
An e-mail message sent via the Internet that has been encrypted to make it unreadable during transit.

direct faxing
Transfer of health care provider information from one organization to another via facsimile transmission.

electronic data interchange (EDI)
Transfer of health care provider information from one organization to another electronically.

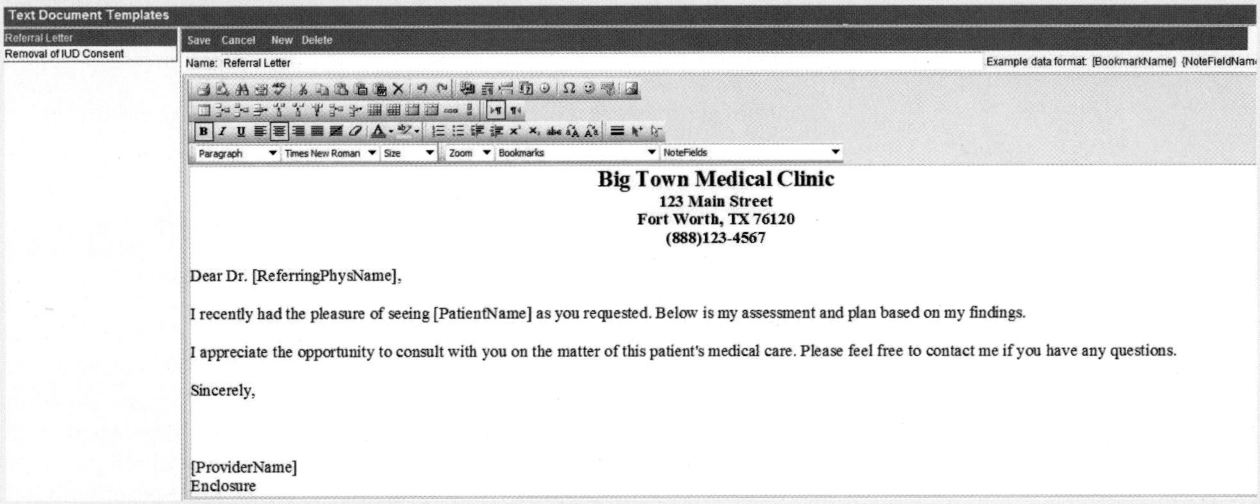

Text Document Templates

Referral Letter
Removal of IUD Consent

Save Cancel New Delete

Name: Referral Letter

Example data format: [BookmarkName] {NoteFieldName

Paragraph | Times New Roman | Size | Zoom | Bookmarks | NoteFields

Big Town Medical Clinic
123 Main Street
Fort Worth, TX 76120
(888)123-4567

Dear Dr. [ReferringPhysName],

I recently had the pleasure of seeing [PatientName] as you requested. Below is my assessment and plan based on my findings.

I appreciate the opportunity to consult with you on the matter of this patient's medical care. Please feel free to contact me if you have any questions.

Sincerely,

[ProviderName]
Enclosure

Figure 8-1 Referral letter template in e-Medsys®.

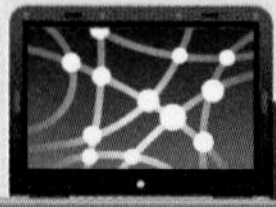

View the functional criteria used by CCHIT to certify ambulatory EHRs at the CCHIT website: http://www.cchit.org/.

STANDARDS: FUNCTIONAL AND CONTENT

Functional and content standards that specifically apply to treatment plans, diagnostic orders, and treatment are discussed in this section.

Functional Standards

EHR systems must capture the details of a patient's treatment plan, efficiently transmit orders and important associated patient data to other health care providers to carry out the treatment plan, and receive reports from all health care providers to document the results of treatment. The functional criteria of the Certification Commission for Healthcare Information Technology (CCHIT) for certification of ambulatory EHRs specifically identify how a certified EHR helps health care providers to manage effectively this entire process of implementing a treatment plan.

Table 8-1 presents a sample of the ONC- ATCB Meaningful Use certification criteria that are focused on supporting the implementation activities associated with the treatment plan.

Content Standards

Chapter 4 included a full discussion of the sources of existing health record data content standards (NCVHS, The Joint Commission, AAAHC, CMS) associated with ambulatory health record systems. In general, every accreditation organization that is focused on ambulatory health care and ambulatory patient records includes treatment plans and therapeutic services provided to the patient as items that must be documented in the patient's record—regardless of whether those record systems are paper based or computer based. The Joint Commission's Record Content (R.C.) Standards for Ambulatory Care specify that the clinical record must contain "plans for care and any revisions to the plan for care" (2011).

The specific content of a treatment plan or specification of what data must be entered into a treatment or procedure note is not clearly defined in any national set of content standards. In combination, the treatment plan and treatment notes, including results reported of all additional tests ordered as part of the plan, must answer these questions:

- What action steps will be taken to address the patient's problem(s)?
- What service(s) were provided and/or what procedure(s) were performed?
- What was the outcome from each service provided and procedure performed?

Each type of health care provider setting determines the data content it wants to include routinely in its treatment plans and notes to fit the particular types of health care treatment plans and services it provides, whether they are rehabilitation therapies, behavioral health therapies, general medical services, or specialty medical/surgical services. As a result, there are ambulatory EHR products that are specialized for particular types of practice settings. Most other ambulatory EHR products are constructed to allow customers to define the specific data content for the practice's treatment plans and treatment/procedure notes.

TABLE 8-1 Examples of Treatment Plan Associated ONC-ATCB Meaningful Use Criteria for Certification of Ambulatory EHRs

§170.302 (h)	*Incorporate laboratory test results.* (1) Receive results. Electronically receive clinical laboratory test results in a structured format and display such results in human readable format. (2) Display test report information.
§170.302 (m)	*Patient-specific education resources.* Enable a user to electronically identify and provide patient-specific education resources according to, at a minimum, the data elements included in the patient's: problem list; medication list; and laboratory test results as well as provide such resources to the patient.
§170.304 (b)	*Electronic prescribing.* Enable a user to electronically generate and transmit prescriptions and prescription-related information.
§170.304 (d)	*Patient Reminders.* Enable a user to electronically generate a patient reminder list for preventive or follow-up care according to patient preferences based on, at a minimum, the data elements included in: Problem list; Medication list; Medication allergy list.
§170.306 (a)	*Computerized provider order entry.* Enable a user to electronically record, store, retrieve, and modify, at a minimum, the following order types: (1) Medications; (2) Laboratory; and (3) Radiology/Imaging.
§170.306 (c)	*Clinical decision support.* (1) Implement rules. Implement automated, electronic clinical decision support rules (in addition to drug-drug and drug-allergy contraindication checking) based on the data elements included in: problem list; medication list; demographics; and laboratory test results.
§170.306 (e)	*Electronic copy of discharge instructions.* Enable a user to create an electronic copy of the discharge instructions for a patient, in human readable format, at the time of discharge on electronic media or through some other electronic means.
§170.306 (f)	*Exchange clinical information and patient summary record.* (1) Electronically receive and display. Electronically receive and display a patient's summary record from other providers and organizations including, at a minimum, diagnostic test results, problem list, medication list, medication allergy list, and procedures. (2) Electronically transmit. Enable a user to electronically transmit a patient's summary record to other providers and organizations including, at a minimum, diagnostic results, problem list, medication list, medication allergy list, and procedures.

Source: National Institute of Standards and Testing (http://healthcare.nist.gov/use_testing/effective_requirements.html)

DOCUMENTATION

All licensed health care providers have a responsibility to document treatment plans, results of diagnostic tests ordered as part of the treatment plan, and treatment/procedure notes when providing services to their patients. The documentation of orders is a fairly structured EHR function. There is little opportunity for clinicians to customize it when the EHR system is implemented. Typically, the only aspects of the EHR ordering function that are customizable are the list of possible orders and the types of data required to complete the order. However, because documentation related to treatment and procedures is highly customizable in most EHR projects, health care providers must give considerable attention to designing this aspect of their EHR system to make sure it meets their practice needs before the system "goes live."

Treatment Plan

The treatment plan generally is documented in the EHR at the end of the clinical note associated with the examination or assessment visit. It may be documented in narrative format within a free-form visit note, documented in narrative within the "P" section of a SOAP-formatted visit note, or constructed from drop-down menu selections presented within one of the practice's many "visit" templates. (See Chapter 4 for a full discussion of SOAP notes and problem-oriented medical records.)

As mentioned previously, another favored method for capturing the treatment plan in an EHR system involves the use of templates to capture more structured visit notes. (See Chapter 7 for a full discussion of templates as a format for documenting examination findings.) When templates are part of a practice's EHR system, the treatment plan is completed as one of the last sections within the template. The treatment plan portion of the template is completed in much the same way as the examination or assessment is documented; that is, the health care provider is presented with a series of possible treatment options associated with the patient's problem. For example, if the patient has hematuria (blood in the urine), the treatment plan section of the template might present the health care provider with options for specifying lab test orders, radiology tests, consultations, prescriptions, in-office medications, patient instructions, and so forth. Then, as the provider selects from the options presented, the treatment plan is documented in the visit note and the provider simultaneously is prompted to place the order or write the prescription within the EHR system. Clearly, the EHRs capability to trigger treatment-related orders at the same time the treatment plan is being constructed by the health care provider makes it possible for the provider to handle this important responsibility for patient care efficiently. The care provider must:

- Decide what to include in the treatment plan.
- Implement the various pieces of the plan through a series of orders placed in the EHR.
- Document the plan along with the treatment actions taken.

Figure 8-2 is an example of a treatment embedded in a visit note template.

order entry templates The format of structured data-entry items required to complete a medical order.

order details Specific items that must be entered by a health care provider to make an order complete.

Diagnostic and Treatment Orders

Orders placed through an EHR system are entered via structured **order entry templates**. The majority of the **order details** (both required and optional) needed to specify the order are completed by the health care provider through selections made from drop-down menus presented within the order template.

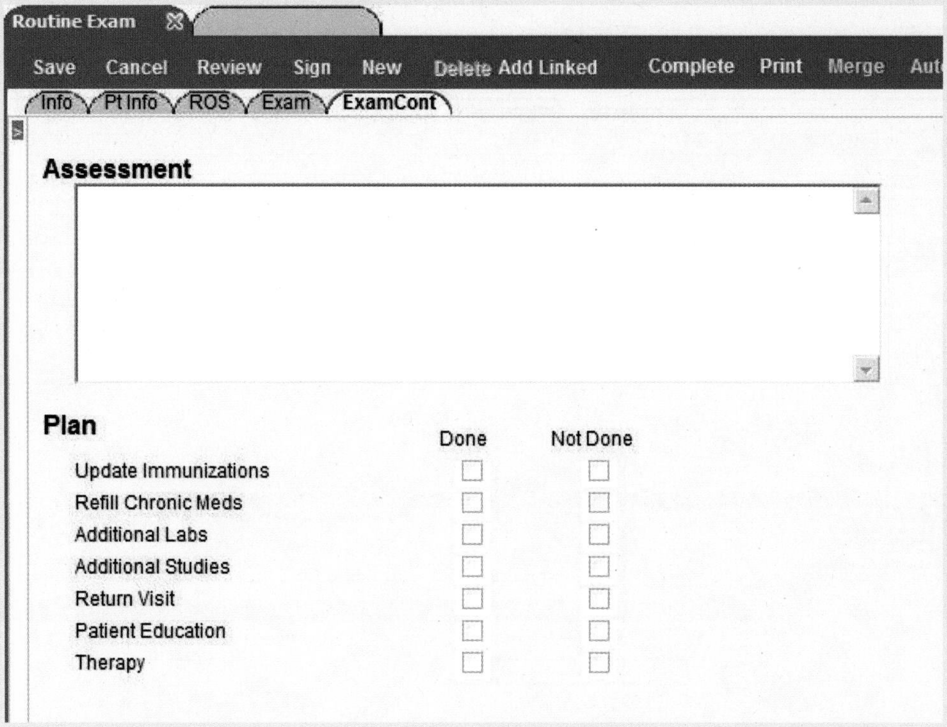

Routine Exam

Save Cancel Review Sign New Delete Add Linked Complete Print Merge Aut

Info Pt Info ROS Exam ExamCont

Assessment

Plan

	Done	Not Done
Update Immunizations	☐	☐
Refill Chronic Meds	☐	☐
Additional Labs	☐	☐
Additional Studies	☐	☐
Return Visit	☐	☐
Patient Education	☐	☐
Therapy	☐	☐

Figure 8-2 Treatment plan as part of a visit note template in e-Medsys®.

Required order details are highlighted within the template to ensure capture of all data needed to describe the specific order being entered into the EHR system accurately and completely. Figures 8-3 and 8-4 are examples of two different types of orders being placed through an EHR system. When the order is signed electronically within the EHR, it is viewable in the appropriate area of the EHR as an open order and remains in that status until a result or report is input or keyed into the EHR in response to the order. At the time the order is signed within the EHR it also is transmitted to the daily task list (the "in basket") of the designated person within the clinic to take action on the order; this designated person is often a nurse, a medical assistant, or a registration/scheduling assistant.

Results Reporting

At the time a treatment service or procedure is performed on a patient in the health care office setting, a description of the service or procedure performed, along with the health care providers assessment of the process and outcomes, must be documented in the EHR. Once again, **treatment notes** (**or procedure notes**) can be done through narrative entries in a free-form report format, or they can be completed through a treatment or **procedure notes template**. Such templates function in much the same way as the visit note templates: the provider selects a treatment or procedure template from those that have been placed in the EHR system. For example, when the skin biopsy template is selected, the health care provider is guided through a series of items to be documented (e.g., procedure performed, specimen removed, specimen disposition, in-office medications given, patient response, prescriptions, patient instructions, follow-up plan). The health care provider also can construct a narrative note within the template or can dictate a procedure note which is transcribed and electronically stored within a designated section of the EHR for transcribed documents. Figure 8-5 shows an example of a procedure note embedded in a template.

treatment notes or procedure notes Unstructured writing by a health care provider describing the patient encounter.

procedure notes template Structured format documentation by a health care provider describing the patient encounter.

Figure 8-3 Order in construction for a diagnostic test in e-Medsys®.

Figure 8-4 Completed order for a consultation in e-Medsys®.

When a diagnostic test order has been carried out and the result is available for review by the patient's primary health care provider, it is entered into the EHR through an electronic feed directly from a test instrument, entered through keyed data entry by an authorized health care provider, or entered through a document-scanning process. There is limited capability for EHR systems to accept data and reports electronically from either medical devices or from the clinical information systems associated with another organization. Considerable national attention now is being given to the interoperability standards that eventually will make direct feed of **results reporting** from medical devices and from the clinical information systems associated with other organizations into the EHR a common system feature. Currently, however, when the results or report come back to the provider from an external health care provider source for incorporation into the practice's EHR, it is quite possible that the report will need to be scanned into the EHR and the associated order within the EHR be updated manually to change its status to complete. The one obvious exception is the electronic communication of laboratory test results from an external organization back to the practice's EHR system. Although universal interoperability does not exist between EHR systems and lab results reporting systems, use of the Logical Observation Identifier Names and Codes (LOINC) terminology standard (see Chapter 3) within both an EHR and a laboratory information system provides a foundation for establishing that type of direct data interchange.

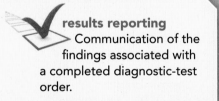

results reporting Communication of the findings associated with a completed diagnostic-test order.

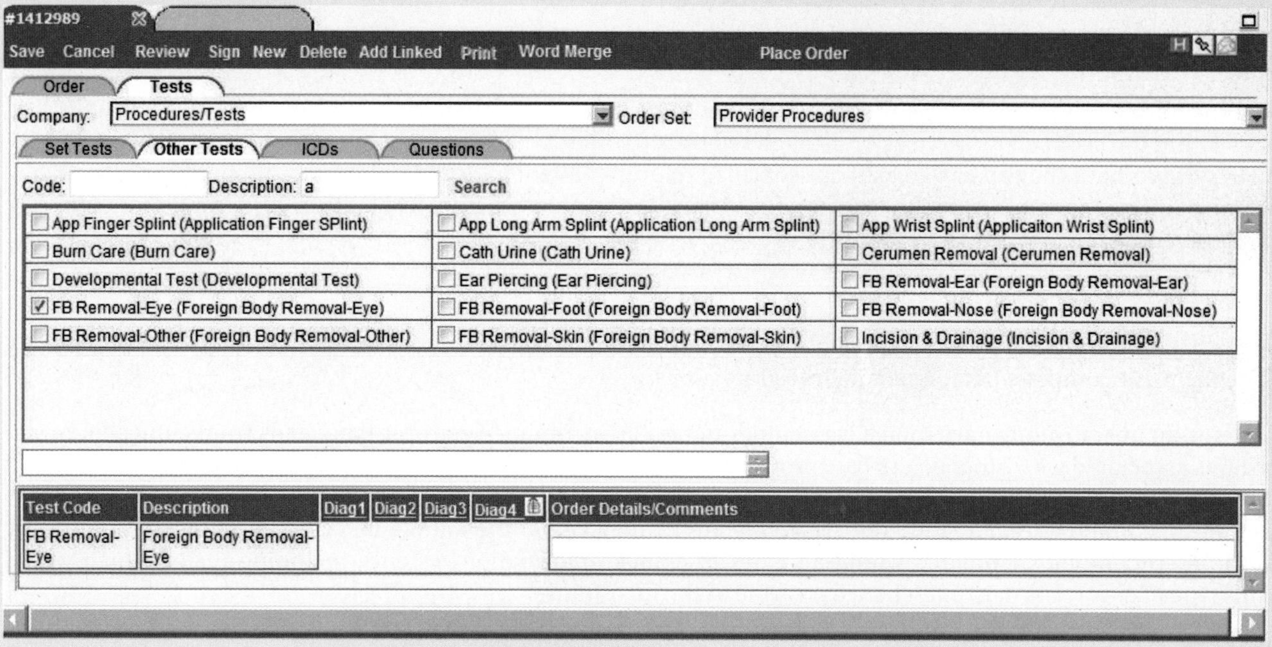

Figure 8-5 Procedure note template in e-Medsys®.

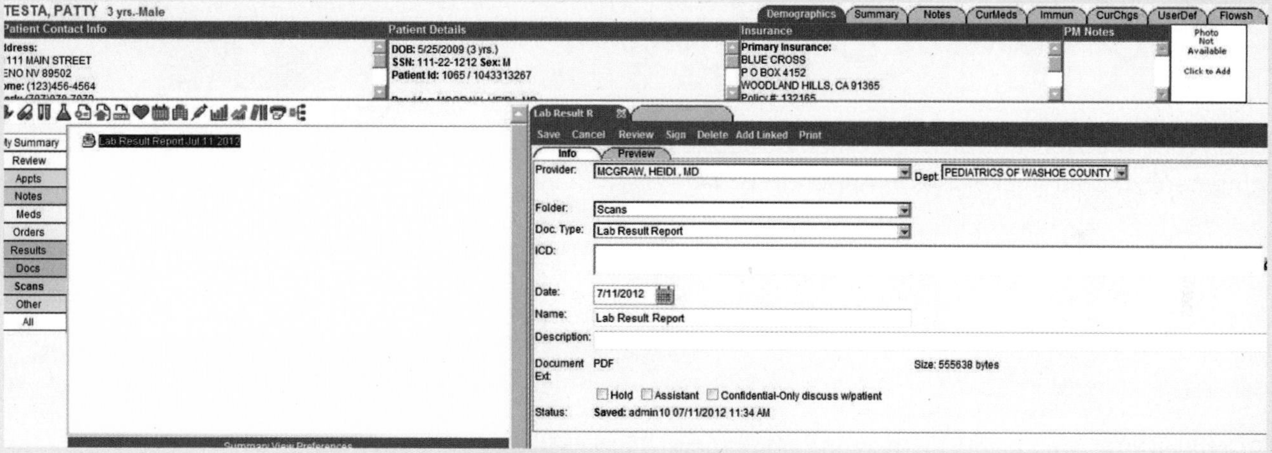

Figure 8-6 Pathology reading results awaiting review in e-Medsys®.

In any case, when a test result is posted into the EHR, the primary health care provider must be notified through an established notification trigger either set up within the EHR itself or one that is initiated by a member of the practice's office staff who monitors incoming results being posted into each patient's EHR. Commonly this is accomplished by an auto-entry of the report, or a manual notification of the report into the provider's daily task list (or "in basket"). Most EHR systems require the primary health care provider who is reviewing the result associated with an order to select a "report reviewed" button within the EHR, which changes the official status of the order and the report from "complete" to "reviewed." This is important for assuring that appropriate follow-up is initiated by the health care provider, including communication of results to the patient, because several days or weeks may have gone by since the original order was placed and the test performed. Figure 8-6 displays a pathology reading result awaiting review by a primary health care provider.

SUMMARY

The health care provider practice has the responsibility to develop a treatment plan for a patient and to implement that plan within the scope of its services or through referrals to other health care providers for continuing care. "Certified" EHR systems have the capacity to extract a subset of relevant patient information to support continuing care when the patient is referred to another health care provider. Using the template feature available in EHR systems, health care providers can efficiently:

- Document complete treatment plans.
- Construct orders and transmit them to others who will be involved with implementing the treatment plan.
- Document complete treatment and procedure notes.

EHR systems do not currently have robust capabilities to handle incoming electronic data feeds from clinical information systems associated with other health care provider organizations, with the notable exception being electronic feeds of test results from laboratory information systems based on the use of the LOINC vocabulary standard for laboratory tests and results. Much attention and effort currently are being given at the national level to adopting and deploying additional interoperability standards within all types of clinical information systems, including EHRs, which would make this type of electronic data interchange possible in the near future.

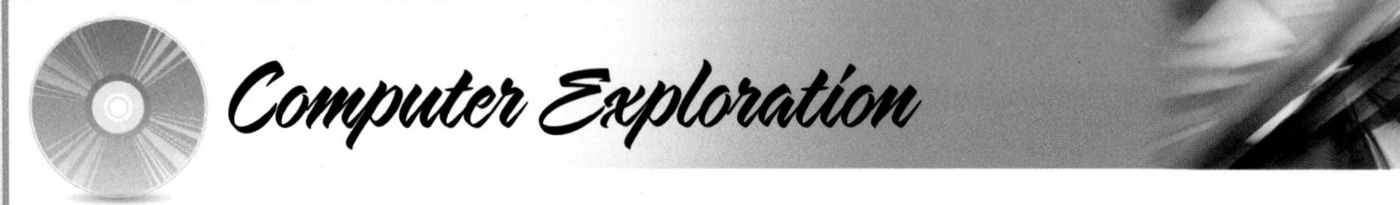

Using your e-Medsys® Educational Edition 2.0 access code provided with this text, complete the e-Medsys® Computer Exploration Exercises in Appendix B.

REFERENCES

CCHIT Certified 2011 Ambulatory EHR Certification Criteria. Retrieved from http://www.cchit.org/

Institute of Standards and Technology. Approved Test Procedures Version 1.1. (2011). Retrieved from http://healthcare.nist.gov/use_testing/effective_requirements.html

The Joint Commission. (2011). *Standards for ambulatory care*. Oakbrook Terrace, IL.

REVIEW QUESTIONS

1. What types of software applications are common components of an electronic practice-management system (PMS)?

2. How does an EHR system integrated with a practice management system contribute to implementing a treatment plan?

3. What two questions does a treatment plan answer?

4. What do a referral letter and the CCR/CCD have in common?

5. Where is the treatment plan documented in an EHR that uses templates for documenting visit information?

6. How are the details of a diagnostic or treatment order captured within an EHR?

7. How does a standard terminology such as LOINC support the EHR's ability to exchange orders and results with an external health care provider?

8. In what way does a template improve the completeness of a treatment or procedure note in the EHR?

9. In what way does a template contribute to a health care provider's ability to implement a treatment plan efficiently?

____

____

____

10. What process should a practice implement to incorporate properly the treatment or procedure documentation received from an external health care provider in response to a referral order?

____

____

____

CHAPTER 9 Medication Orders and Administration

CHAPTER OUTLINE

KEY TERMS

computerized provider order entry (CPOE)
drug vocabularies
medication (drug) alerts and reminders
medication (drug) reference information
order format and details (order sentence)

OBJECTIVES

Upon completion of the chapter, the learner will be able to:

1. Identify common root causes of medication errors.
2. Explain how an electronic health record (EHR) can address some of the root causes of medical errors.
3. Identify specific capabilities that a "certified" EHR must have in order to create prescriptions that support correct medication administration.
4. List the minimum patient-specific data required to support safe medication ordering and administration as defined by The Joint Commission.
5. Describe at least three sources for standard drug terminologies used in EHRs.
6. List the elements included in a standard medication order format.
7. Distinguish a drug-terminology from a drug-reference information system.
8. Explain what causes medication alerts to be triggered within an EHR or **computerized provider order-entry (CPOE)** system.
9. Explain how reminders generated from an EHR system can positively affect medication management.
10. Describe the preferred and common alternate methods for electronically submitting a prescription from the EHR to the pharmacy.

computerized provider order entry (CPOE) A software application that allows health care providers to enter orders electronically to carry out a patient's treatment plan and electronically communicates the orders over a computer network to other individual(s) responsible for carrying out the order(s).

INTRODUCTION

The Institute of Medicine (IOM) report entitled *To Err Is Human: Building a Safer Health System* (Kohn, Corrigan, & Donaldson, 2000) sounded an alarm regarding patient safety issues in the nation's health care system. The IOM estimated that 44,000 to 98,000 Americans die each year from preventable medical errors, making medical error the eighth-leading cause of death among Americans. Although there are numerous types of errors that occur in all types of health care organizations, the one type that is most likely to occur in a health care provider setting is a medication error. The IOM estimates that preventable medication errors result in tens of thousands of deaths associated with care in outpatient facilities, including the clinic setting. Table 9-1 lists some common causes of medication errors that have been identified by the American Hospital Association. EHR systems have the capacity to support good medication ordering (prescribing) and administration practices, which can contribute to significant reductions in medication errors.

WORKFLOW

Medication ordering—the health care provider's treatment order for a medication—in a health care provider office that uses EHRs involves the creation of prescriptions through the EHR system and electronic submission of the prescription to a pharmacy for dispensing to the patient. The prescription may be created as the result of a patient visit to the office or it may be created as the result of a telephone, e-mail, or patient portal interaction with a continuing patient. In all cases, the health care provider involved with preparing the prescription will access the patient's EHR to review the problem together with allergy and medication lists and any other relevant data (e.g., age, gender, height/weight, pregnancy status) before initiating the process of preparing the prescription itself. In addition, the health care provider might click into the drug reference information that is accessed through the EHR system. Drug reference information embedded in the EHR system will assist the health care

TABLE 9-1 Some Common Causes of Medication Errors
Incomplete patient information (e.g., not knowing about patients' allergies, other medicines they are taking, previous diagnoses, or lab results)
Unavailable drug information (e.g., lack of up-to-date warnings)
Miscommunication of drug orders, which can involve poor handwriting, confusion between drugs with similar names, misuse of zeroes and decimal points, confusion of metric and other dosing units, and inappropriate abbreviations
Lack of appropriate labelling as a drug is prepared and repackaged into smaller units
Environmental factors (e.g., lighting, heat, noise, and interruptions) that can distract health professionals from their medical tasks

Source: Nordenberg (2002).

TABLE 9-2 Examples of Potential for Name Confusion in Drugs

DRUG	DRUG	RESULTS FROM CONFUSION
Lamictal, an epileptic drug	Lamisil, an antifungal drug	Epileptic patients receiving the antifungal drug Lamisil by mistake could experience continuous seizures. Patients erroneously receiving the antiepileptic drug Lamictal might experience a serious rash, blood pressure changes, or other side effects.
Celebrex, prescribed for arthritis	Cerlexa, an antidepressant	No serious clinical harm, but increased cost and reduced quality of patient care.

Source: Nordenberg (2002).

provider to distinguish medications with similar names. Table 9-2 provides two examples of drug names that easily can be confused, along with an explanation of the type of patient response that could result from such confusion.

In addition, drug reference information embedded in the EHR provides the health care provider with the most up-to-date information about when the medication is contraindicated, dose and form options, and normal dose ranges.

When the health care provider is ready to create the prescription, the EHR provides a template that structures the prescription in a standard format and provides appropriate drop-down menus that guide the selection of the specific medication (by either generic or brand name), the dose strength and dose units, the form, the route of administration, and the frequency with which it must be taken. A completed prescription is shown in Figure 9-1.

When all of the required medication order details have been entered into the prescription templates, the order is submitted to be checked by the EHR system's drug interaction rules engine. If no alerts are produced, then the prescription is submitted to a specified pharmacy, and the patient's medication list (medication profile) in the EHR is updated to reflect the relevant prescription details.

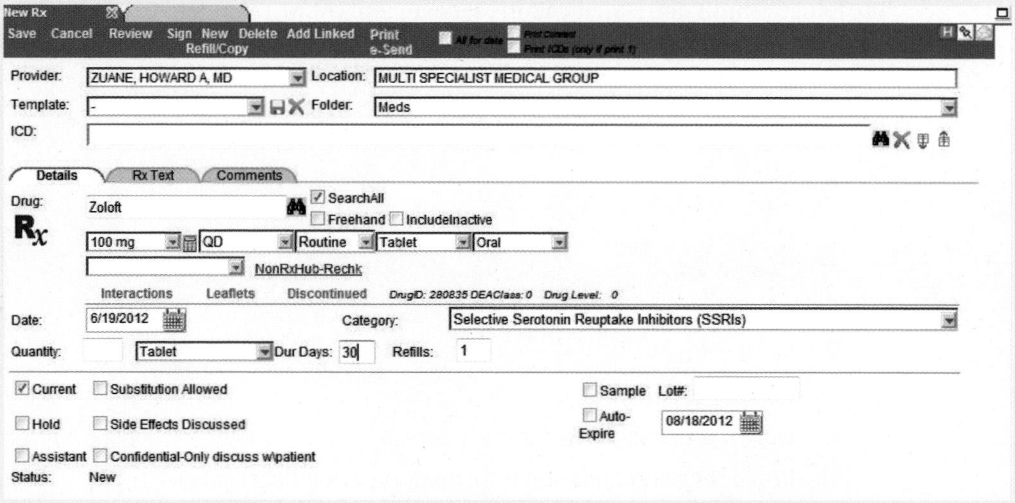

New Rx
Save Cancel Review Sign New Refill/Copy Delete Add Linked Print e-Send
Provider: ZUANE, HOWARD A, MD Location: MULTI SPECIALIST MEDICAL GROUP
Template: - Folder: Meds
ICD:
Details Rx Text Comments
Drug: Zoloft SearchAll Freehand IncludeInactive
100 mg QD Routine Tablet Oral
NonRxHub-Rechk
Interactions Leaflets Discontinued DrugID: 280835 DEAClass: 0 Drug Level: 0
Date: 6/19/2012 Category: Selective Serotonin Reuptake Inhibitors (SSRIs)
Quantity: Tablet Dur Days: 30 Refills: 1
Current Substitution Allowed Sample Lot#:
Hold Side Effects Discussed Auto-Expire 08/18/2012
Assistant Confidential-Only discuss w\patient
Status: New

Reprinted with permission of TriMed Technologies, Corp.

Figure 9-1 Completed medication (prescription) order in e-Medsys®.

As described in Chapter 8 in relation to some diagnostic orders, electronic submission of the prescription may involve a literal transmission of electronic data from the provider office's EHR system to the pharmacy's electronic information system. This type of electronic data interchange (EDI) is the most efficient and desirable approach for communicating a prescription from the health care provider office to the pharmacy, because it minimizes the potential for any miscommunication about prescription details. EDI requires transmission of electronic data directly from one computer system into another computer system. In situations where direct electronic data interchange capability is not established between the provider's office EHR system and a pharmacy's electronic information system, the electronic prescription may be faxed to the pharmacy directly from the EHR.

STANDARDS: FUNCTIONAL, CONTENT, AND VOCABULARY

The subject of medication ordering and medication administration is a hot topic within the various groups that are involved with establishing standards for EHR systems. The existing functional, content, and vocabulary standards associated with this topic are discussed here.

Functional Standards

View the functional criteria used by CCHIT to certify ambulatory EHRs at the CCHIT website: http://www.cchit.org/.

The large volume of Certification Commission for Healthcare Information Technology (CCHIT) functional criteria that is focused on the EHR's ability to support medication ordering is a strong indication of its potential for significantly contributing to a reduction in the number of errors in medication ordering and administration. CCHIT functional criteria for certification of ambulatory EHRs specifically require that a certified EHR supports medication ordering.

Table 9-3 presents a selection of ONC-ATCB Meaningful Use criteria that relate to medication ordering.

Content and Vocabulary Standards

The Joint Commission's Medication Management (M.M.) standard 01.01.01 identifies a set of patient-specific data required to "safely order, prepare, dispense, administer and monitor medications." (2011, p. MM-4.)

This patient-specific data set includes, at minimum:

- Age.
- Sex.
- Diagnoses.
- Allergies.
- Sensitivities.
- Current medications.
- Height and weight (when necessary).
- Pregnancy and lactation information (when necessary).
- Laboratory results (when necessary).

TABLE 9-3 Examples of Medication Order Associated ONC-ATCB Meaningful Use Criteria for Certification of Ambulatory EHRs

§170.302 (a)	Drug-drug, drug-allergy interaction checks (1) Notifications. Automatically and electronically generate and indicate in real-time, notifications at the point of care for drug-drug and drug-allergy contraindications based on medication list, medication allergy list, and computerized provider order entry (CPOE).
§170.302 (b)	Drug-formulary checks. Enable a user to electronically check if drugs are in a formulary or preferred drug list.
§170.302 (d)	Maintain active medication list. Enable a user to electronically record, modify, and retrieve a patient's active medication list as well as medication history for longitudinal care.
§170.302 (e)	Maintain active medication allergy list. Enable a user to electronically record, modify, and retrieve a patient's active medication allergy list as well as medication allergy history for longitudinal care.
§170.302 (j)	Medication Reconciliation. Enable a user to electronically compare two or more medication lists.
§170.304 (a)	Computerized provider order entry. Enable a user to electronically record, store, retrieve, and modify, at a minimum, the following order types: (1) Medications; (2) Laboratory; and (3) Radiology/imaging
§170.304 (b)	Electronic prescribing. Enable a user to electronically generate and transmit prescriptions and prescription-related information.

Source: National Institute of Standards and Testing (http://healthcare.nist.gov/use_testing/effective_requirements.html)

This specified data content resides in the patient EHR and must be easily accessible to the health care provider when medication orders (prescriptions) are being placed into the EHR. For this reason, the design of the EHR should bring forward the summary lists (including problems/diagnoses, allergies, and medications), the patient age, gender, and height/weight, and laboratory test results for review at the time a prescription is being created.

Another key aspect of safe medication ordering and administration is related to the use of a standard vocabulary when specifying the medication being ordered. Standard terms assure accurate and complete communication of the details of the medication order or prescription to the pharmacy as well as to the individual who actually will be administering or taking the medication. At times the medication will be administered by a health care provider, but most commonly medications ordered for a patient during an office visit will be administered by the patient or a member of the patient's family, both outside the health care provider's control.

drug vocabularies National terminologies associated with pharmacy information systems to support accurate communication of prescriptions and assure correct drug labeling.

The National Drug Codes (NDCs) and RxNorm were introduced briefly in Chapter 3 as two of the national **drug vocabularies** associated with pharmacy information systems to support accurate communication of prescriptions and assuring correct drug labeling.

RxNorm provides standard names for both branded and generic medications. These medication names include the active ingredients in the medication, the dose strength, the dose form, and the related brand name(s); for example:

- Acetominophen 500 mg. Oral tablet—generic name
- Acetominophen 500 mg. Oral tablet (Tylenol)—brand name (U.S. National Library of Medicine)

NDCs serve as universal product identifiers for prescription drugs and for a limited number of over-the-counter drugs. The NDC associated with a specific drug product is a unique number that identifies the company producing the drug, the drug product, and the package size. The NDC will be a 10-digit number separated into three sections configured as follows: either 4-4-2, 5-3-2, or 5-4-1.

RxNorm drug names are linked to NDCs and also to several other drug vocabularies commonly used in pharmacies and in drug interaction software. As a result, RxNorm can be used to translate drug names that must be passed between computer systems that are not using the same software or the same drug vocabulary.

Multum is an example of a drug vocabulary being used in the health information technology marketplace. It can be embedded in an EHR product to provide a vocabulary and formats for medication orders. Multum also includes up-to-date drug product information that is accessible by the health care provider (and printable in the form of an educational leaflet for the patient) at the point of care. This drug product information in electronic form also provides the knowledge base underlying the EHR system's drug interaction alerts and reminders function. Medication (drug) alerts and reminders will be discussed later in this chapter.

order format and details (order sentence)
General sequence for the detailed information passed from the prescribing provider to the pharmacy.

Using the specific drug vocabulary embedded in the practice's EHR system, the system will present a standard order format and an established medication selection list to the health care provider at the time a medication order or a prescription is being entered into the EHR. The standard **order format and details** (also known as the **order sentence**) for a medication (drug) is generally: drug name (generic and/or brand), dose, units, route of administration, form, frequency—including PRN (pro rata, or "as needed") and PRN reason—and start date. When the drug order is in prescription form, the number of refills allowed is included in the order as well. For a health care provider ordering acetaminophen for the patient, Table 9-4 shows an example of the order detail that

TABLE 9-4 Medication Order Detail

INGREDIENT	STRENGTH	UNIT	ROUTE	DOSE FORM	FREQUENCY	PRN REASON	DATE
Acetaminophen	325	Mg	Oral	Tablets	PRN	Pain	09/11/2006
Acetaminophen	325	Mg	Rectal	Suppository	Twice daily		09/11/2006
Acetaminophen	650	Mg	Oral	Capsule	Once daily		09/11/2006
Acetaminophen	120	Mg/5ml	Oral	Elixir	Three daily		09/11/2006

would be necessary for the EHR system to accept it as complete. If the order were a prescription, then the number of refills allowed also would be required for EHR acceptance as complete.

MEDICATION REFERENCE INFORMATION

One of the CCHIT ambulatory EHR functionality criteria (FN 07.05) states that the system shall "provide the ability to access reference information for prescribing/ordering." (2010.) Currently **medication (drug) reference information** is readily available in published hard-copy reference texts such as the Physician Desk Reference (PDR) and is also available in the form of software that can be loaded on desktop computers, laptop computers, or even handheld (PDA) devices that health care providers can carry with them. EHR product vendors who include up-to-date drug reference information software (such as Multum, discussed earlier) into the EHR itself are taking a major step to make sure that health care providers have easy access to this important reference content, as well as relevant patient-specific data (age, gender, weight, allergies, current medications, laboratory test results, etc.) at the time it is needed—that is, at the point of care.

medication (drug) reference information
Published texts that provide details on drugs approved for use in the United States; often available in hard copy or via software.

Medication (drug) reference information software typically provides the health care provider with a description of the drug, including its effects, the status of its approval, and approved uses. The medication (drug) reference information also includes details about specific warnings associated with use of a medication, side effects associated with its use, and dosage recommendations for various age groups (pediatric, adult, geriatric). In addition, medication (drug) reference information software may provide drug education leaflets that present important information about the drug in a way that it is useful to the patient or the patient's family.

MEDICATION ALERTS AND REMINDERS

The case situation presented at the start of this chapter highlighted ways that an EHR system can help prevent medication errors. The EHR does so by comparing the standardized drug order details entered into the system by the health care provider against the appropriate rules and guidelines embedded in the EHR system. Most important, the EHR compares the drug order details with the system's rules *before* it allows the health care provider to sign the order for processing. As a result, the EHR can generate **medication (drug) alerts and reminders** to the health care provider which will call attention to any potential adverse effects that could result if the intended medication order is carried out.

medication (drug) alerts and reminders
Messages sent to a health care provider that call attention to any potential adverse effects that could result if the intended medication order is carried out.

For example, a health care provider inadvertently may order a dose of a medication for a 10-year-old boy that is inadvisable for a person in that age group, or may order a drug that is known to create an undesirable clinical state (e.g., irregular heart rhythm) when used in combination with a current, previously prescribed medication. The particular medication (drug) reference information database that is embedded in the practice's EHR system, coupled with the patient specific information in the EHR (e.g., age, allergies, current medications, lab test results), is the source that trigger this type of alert function. To activate the alert, these two sources of information (the drug reference information database and the patient-specific information) work in conjunction with a set of decision rules that have been built into the EHR system. Generally, the health care provider is allowed to act on the alert in any way the provider deems appropriate: accept the advice offered through the alert and change the order, or consider the advice but decide to continue with the order. In the latter case, the EHR system generally will require the provider to enter the reason for deciding to proceed with the order in spite of the alert, so that the decision's rationale becomes a part of the legal patient record.

It is important to know that this type of medication alert can be triggered only when the drug being ordered has been selected from the standardized medication (drug) terminology built into the EHR system. If the health care provider enters the order in free text, which often is allowed in an EHR system to accommodate special use cases, then the drug-interaction-alerts function cannot be triggered. In such cases, the EHR should have the capacity to send a warning message to the health care provider that clearly states that normal drug-interaction checking will not be performed against this free-text (uncoded) medication order.

One of the CCHIT's functional criteria (AM 11.20) states that "the system shall provide the ability to add reminders for necessary follow-up tests based on medication prescribed." (2010.) This type of reminder helps the health care provider determine the effectiveness of a patient's medications. For example, a routine follow-up testing reminder would allow the health care provider to identify an undesirable decrease in the patient's potassium level or identify a desirable decrease in the patient's cholesterol level. Then the health care provider can make a timely decision concerning whether or not to continue that particular medication treatment.

Clearly the alerts and reminder capabilities of ambulatory EHR systems have great potential for reducing the number of medication errors that occur in health care provider practices, improving the quality of patient care outcomes through effective medication management and reducing the costs associated with ineffective medication management.

SUMMARY

The nation is focused on improving the cost, quality, and safety of health care. The Institute of Medicine has identified the frequency of medication errors as a major factor that must be addressed in that effort. Several of the root causes associated with common and preventable medication errors in health care provider office practices can be addressed effectively through EHR systems that support good medication-ordering (prescribing) and administration practices. The CCHIT's functional criteria for ambulatory EHRs and the criteria for an ONC-ATCB "certified" EHR both place significant emphasis on specific medication- (prescription-) ordering capabilities. An EHR system into which a standard drug vocabulary, medication (drug) reference, and drug interaction rules have been embedded can reduce common medication errors significantly. Reminders triggered through the EHR system and delivered to health care providers (or directly to patients) also have the potential to reduce the cost and improve the quality of patient care by increasing the health care provider's ability to manage patients' medications effectively and increase patient compliance.

Computer Exploration

Using your e-Medsys® Educational Edition 2.0 access code provided with this text, complete the e-Medsys® Computer Exploration Exercises in Appendix B.

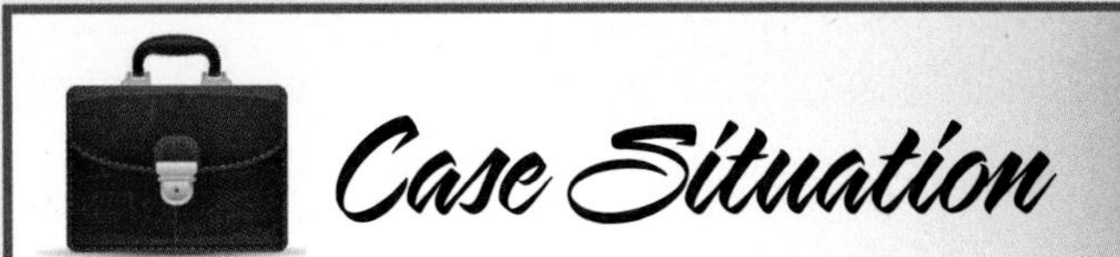

Case Situation

Two women received poisonous doses of chemotherapy while being treated for recurrent breast cancer at a prestigious cancer clinic in the United States. One of the women, age 39 at the time, died as a result of the error, and the second patient suffered permanent heart damage and died from cancer several months after the mistake. The reason for the error: instead of prescribing the daily dose of the powerful anticancer drug cyclophosphamide to be given on each of four days, as planned, the doctor ordered the drug's combined four-day dose so that the total was given to the patients each day.

Since the fatal miscommunication, the cancer clinic has updated its systems to avoid errors. The clinic has installed a computer system to support many clinical tasks, including medication ordering and administration. Physicians no longer hand-write prescriptions but instead fill out an electronic form with the patient's personal information as well as the name of the drug, the dose, and the number of days for which the medicine is to be given. The information goes into the institute's computer system, which compares the information with upper dose limits for the drug and other preprogrammed guidelines. If the doctor seems to have made a mistake, the computer signals the error.

Additionally, upon receiving the order from the patient or the patient's representative, the pharmacist conducts yet another computerized review for potential drug interactions with other drugs, foods, or patient allergies in the pharmacy database. After being prepared at the pharmacy, a pharmacy technician verifies the name and address of the patient to make sure the right person gets the drug. Additionally, the cancer center began a system of nonpunitive error reporting to encourage open discussion of medical mistakes. The change effectively brought about what the clinic has described as a "dramatic increase" in error reporting. (Case adapted from Nordenberg, 2002.)

REFERENCES

Kohn, L. T., Corrigan, J. M., & Donaldson, M. S. (2000). *To err is human: Building a safer health system* (Institute of Medicine Committee on Quality of Health Care in America). Washington, DC: National Academy Press.

Cerner Corporation. Multum. http://www.multum.com/

CCHIT Certified 2011 Ambulatory EHR Certification Criteria. Retrieved from http://www.cchit.org/

Federal Drug Agency. *National drug code (NDC) directory*. Washington, DC: Author.

National Institute of Standards and Technology. Approved Test Procedures Version 1.1. (2011). Retrieved from http://healthcare.nist.gov/use_testing/effective_requirements.html

The Joint Commission. (2011). *Standards for ambulatory care*. Oakbrook Terrace, IL.

Nordenberg, T. (2002). Make no mistake: Medical errors can be deadly serious.

U.S. National Library of Medicine. An Overview to RxNorm. Retrieved from http://www.nlm.nih.gov/research/umls/rxnorm/overview.html

REVIEW QUESTIONS

1. What are the common root causes of medication errors?

2. How can an EHR system eliminate some of the root causes of medical errors?

3. Are the following medication-ordering capabilities required of "certified" ambulatory EHR products? (True or False)

   T F The system shall create prescription or other medication orders with sufficient information for correct filling and administration by a pharmacy.
   T F The system shall use Multum to provide the knowledge source for its drug-interaction databases.
   T F The system shall capture common content for prescription details as specified by the federal government.
   T F The system shall update the medication history with the newly prescribed medications.
   T F The system shall maintain a coded list of medications.

4. What patient-specific data should be readily accessible to a health care provider for assuring correct medication decisions for a patient?

5. What role(s) can Multum play in EHR systems?

6. Provide an example of a medication order that includes all of the elements in the standard medication order format.

7. Provide two examples of significantly different situations that would cause a medication alert to be triggered within an EHR or CPOE system.

8. What alternative actions can a health care provider take when a medication alert is triggered within an EHR?

9. What specific type of EHR system capability can assist the physician in managing a patient's medications more effectively?

____

____

____

10. How are prescriptions that are generated from an EHR system communicated to the pharmacy to be filled?

____

____

____

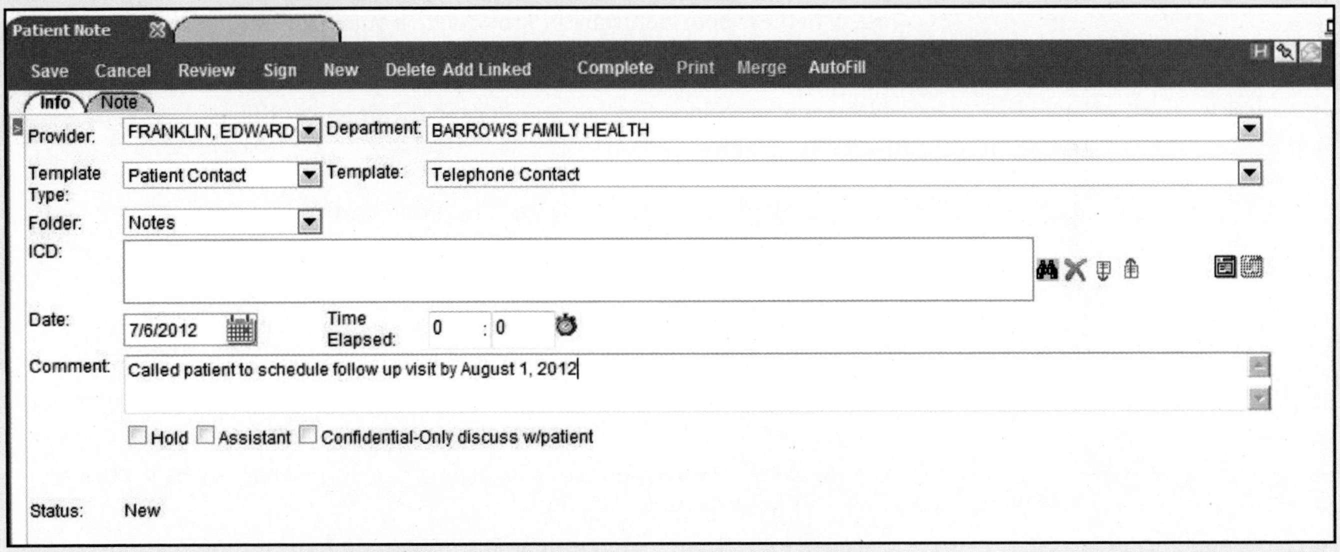

Patient Note

Save Cancel Review Sign New Delete Add Linked Complete Print Merge AutoFill

Info Note

Provider: FRANKLIN, EDWARD Department: BARROWS FAMILY HEALTH

Template Type: Patient Contact Template: Telephone Contact

Folder: Notes

ICD:

Date: 7/6/2012 Time Elapsed: 0 : 0

Comment: Called patient to schedule follow up visit by August 1, 2012

Hold Assistant Confidential-Only discuss w/patient

Status: New

Figure 10-2 EHR message template in e-Medsys.

the document received as a "communication." A patient identifier is entered into the scanner to indicate the correct patient along with a code so it is inserted in the communication section of the record. Once processed, the message will be digitally identified with the patient and that part of the EHR. In this instance, a message alert can be initiated by the office staff for the receiver's attention. Although interpretation errors would not occur, staff time for accessing the patient index and scanning are required. Until a direct interface exists for incoming messages between a fax machine and the EHR, incoming fax messages will be processed in the same manner as paper documents. When a fax does have a direct incoming interface, some sort of patient identification will be required so that the information is transferred to the correct patient record. This ID number could be assigned by the office or agreed upon by the patient and provider. Then the message alert follows in a manner similar to that described for telephone messages.

Another alternative is to communicate to and from the practice via e-mail or text messaging. An e-mail system could have a direct interface with the EHR using patient identifiers, but text messaging requires downloading to the EHR. Once the correct patient is identified, electronic entry of the message in the EHR and workflow queue of the correct recipient occurs. This type of electronic exchange of information has advantages as well as limitations. Health care providers note that:

- Messaging is often not reimbursable.
- Messaging can be time consuming.
- E-mails can be intercepted, compromising confidentiality.
- Errors in addresses can compromise confidentiality.
- There is no assurance that the sender is actually the patient.
- Viruses might be introduced if e-mail attachments are opened.
- Misfiles or lost messages can occur.
- Messages can be misinterpreted.
- Time could be wasted if messages are returned or are used in emergencies.
- Some states may not allow this type of communication in patient-care situations. (AHIMA eHIM Work Group, 2003.)

Many of these comments are not unique to e-mail communications, but special care must be taken because of the increased risk of misdirected messages.

Electronic messages also offer benefits to the practice. They:

- Reduce time spent on telephone calls.
- Allow individuals to respond to messages at scheduled, convenient times.
- Provide another communication alternative to improve health care.
- Expand the amount of information that can be provided through attachments or web links included in the message.
- Provide written evidence of communication for use in treatment or, if needed, for legal purposes.
- May save a patient the cost of an office visit. (AHIMA eHIM Work Group, 2003.)

e-mail and electronic text messages Scripted messages entered on one computer, cell phone, or PDA and then sent to another computer or receiving device.

Because **e-mail and electronic text messages** are becoming such a common mode of communication, their use in health care now or in the future is certain. However, they involve some unique challenges, requiring that practices develop some additional policies and procedures for their use. It may be desirable, for example, to have a special patient authorization form permitting e-mail communications; in addition to authorizing e-mails, it might list risks of electronic communication so that patients can make informed decisions. The authorization form also might indicate the patient's responsibility to update the address, should it change. Guidelines could be provided to the patient on the appropriate use of e-mails. The patient's e-mail address should become part of the patient identifying information in the master patient index of the EHR. Regular verification of the e-mail address is also important. As is true with other types of patient communications, electronic communications themselves must become part of the EHR. Because they are received electronically, however, the step of transcription or scanning is not needed. Workflow queues are updated electronically.

Responding to Patients

Information provided to patients and the results of message interactions must be recorded in the EHR. Health care providers may enter response information into the EHR for follow-up by other office personnel or may contact the patient themselves. In fact, the Accreditation Association for Ambulatory Health Care (AAAHC) supports documentation of specific types of communication in its Clinical Record and Health Information standard:

> M. Significant medical advice given to a patient by telephone or online is entered in the patient's clinical record and appropriately signed or initialed, including medical advice provided after-hours. (AAAHC, 2011, p. 42.)

Usually the EHR message template (see Figure 10-2) provides a means of documenting the information shared in free-text form. The actual response to the patient can be in whatever communication mode the patient prefers (e.g., phone, letter, e-mail). In order to preserve confidentiality, practice personnel must be careful to identify the receiving party as the patient or as someone authorized by the patient to receive restricted information.

Return written (paper) communications from the provider to the patient can originate in the record system via letter templates housed there or can be scanned into the record to become a permanent part of it if initiated outside

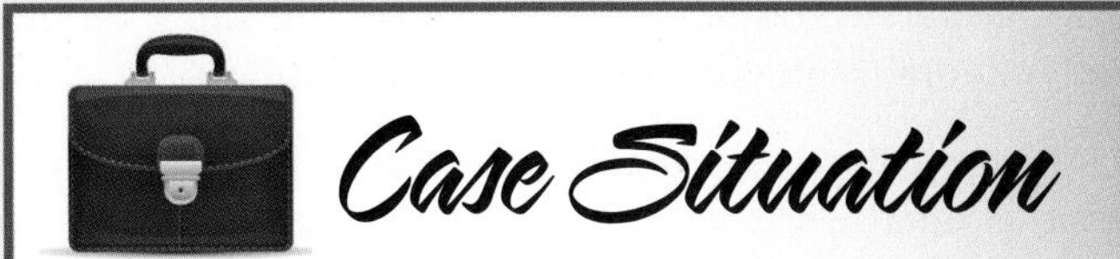

When the gynecology group practice adopted an EHR, the office manager put the following steps in place for patient communications:

In Person/Telephone:

1. Identify the correct patient in the MPI.
2. Access the correct patient's EHR.
3. Add a note to the "Communication" section of the patient's record with information about the request.
4. Send an alert to the provider/staff member involved.

Paper/Facsimile:

1. Identify the correct patient in the MPI.
2. Add both document and patient identification codes to the document(s).
3. Scan and verify the clarity of the documents.
4. Send the documents to the "Communication" section of the patient's record.
5. Send an alert to the provider/staff member involved.

E-mail/Text Messages:

1. Identify the correct patient in the MPI.
2. Download/send the message directly to the "Communication" section of the patient's record.
3. Send an alert to the provider/staff member involved.

the system. Fax machines commonly have a direct interface with the EHR for sending information. The EHR components to be sent are identified to the computer system and the correct fax number entered with a command to "send." It is best if this release of information function is performed only by those specifically authorized within the practice. Transposition of numbers in a fax address is not uncommon, so care must be taken. E-mail responses can be done in free text using the "Reply" function or via templates created by the practice for this purpose. Templates used in replying to e-mails need to include a confidentiality notice and consistent signature formats. Practice policies should include guidelines about what can and cannot be shared via e-mail. As with all electronic systems, computer system security must be addressed.

To ensure the confidentiality of protected information, messages that include medical information—especially sensitive information such as data relating to sexually transmitted diseases or psychiatric conditions—may be processed differently. Unless a patient has given consent to receive confidential medical information via e-mail, an alert is generated in the patient's e-mail system that important information is available from the practice office. In that e-mail message, the patient is instructed to contact the office for specific information. A telephone call to the practitioner's office most likely would result.

E-mails and text messages are a step into the world of electronic communications. Another option for a practice's electronic communications adds more capabilities: a patient portal.

PATIENT PORTALS

patient portal Secure Internet connection to a practice for communication and access to practice databases by patients.

A **patient portal** is a secure Internet-based interactive web site for patient-provider communication and access to practice databases. Portals link a number of systems to receive and present information. To access the practice portal, the patient must have the correct web address (URL), a password, and a distinctive patient number or other identifier as in Figure 10-4. These pieces of information are entered by the patient to begin a portal session.

Once allowed access to the secure portal, the patient may be able to do some or all of the following by choosing the appropriate item from a practice portal menu:

- E-mail office personnel directly with questions (correct individual indicated by selecting from a drop-down menu of personnel names).
- Complete required paperwork.
- Request prescription refills/renewals.
- Obtain test results.
- Access a treatment record or portions of a treatment record, including images as permitted by practice policy.
- Dispute information found in a record.
- Provide or transfer medical information from a personal health record or one from another provider outside the practice.
- Request sharing of information with other practitioners or individuals outside the practice.
- Update demographic, financial, or other information.
- Report medical home test results or results of medical monitors to the provider.
- Schedule or change appointments by linking to the practice management component.
- Check billing statements by linking to the practice management component.
- Complete patient surveys and questionnaires.
- Access patient education material that is supplied by the practice, from specialists associated with the practice, or via links to web sites from the practice.
- Compare health status to national norms. (Koprowski, 2006; Burrington-Brown, 2005; Friedman, 2005; AHIMA eHIM Task Force, 2004.)

An example of a practice portal menu is shown in Figure 10-4.

Menu options need not be introduced all at once; they can be added over time as the practice desires. Depending on the menu choice, the practice electronic

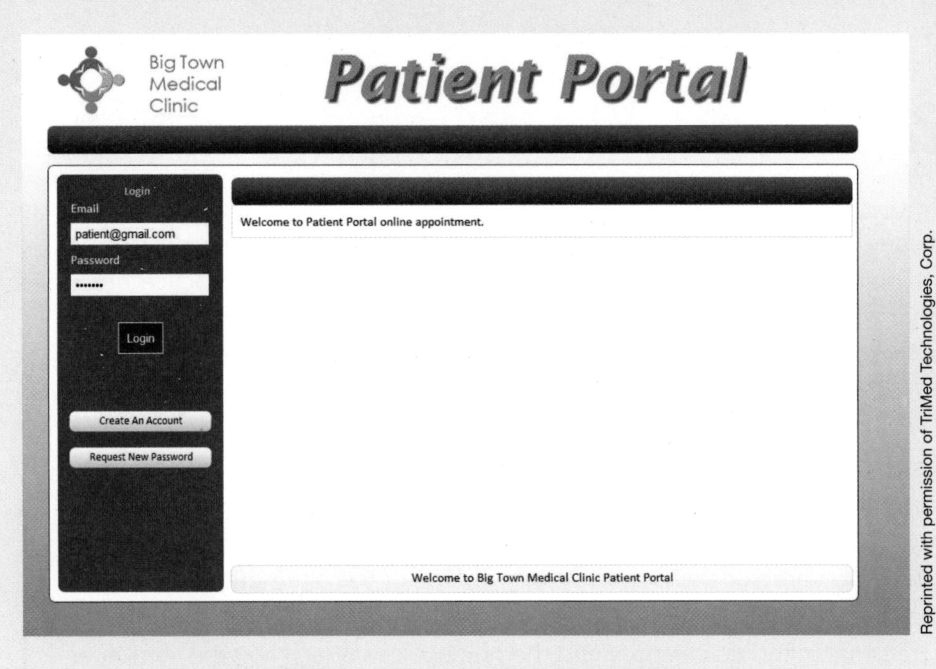

Figure 10-3 Home page for a patient portal in e-Medsys.

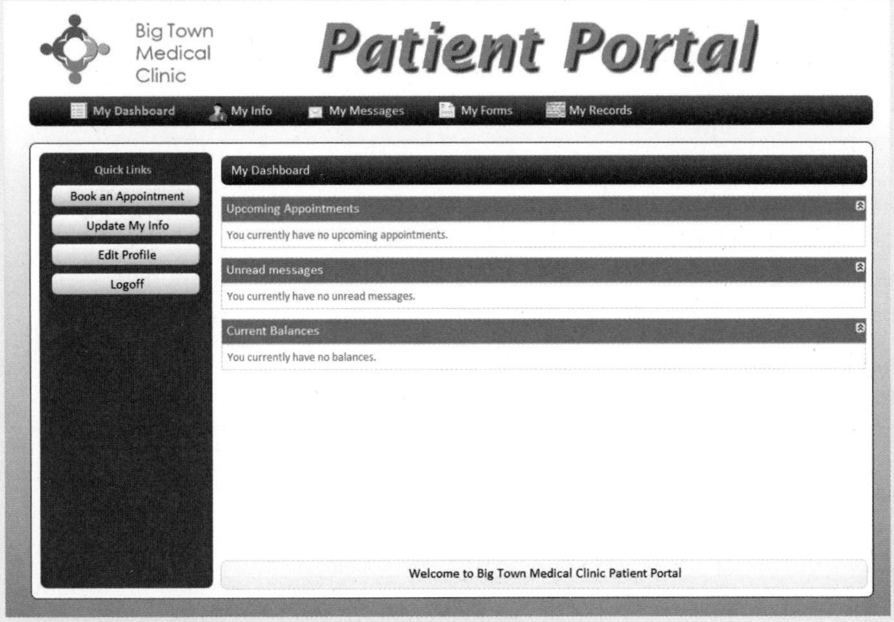

Figure 10-4 Patient portal menu in e-Medsys.

system accesses the correct patient information from its health records, practice management database, or individual providers in the practice. All information added to a record is identified automatically by date, time, and author name, the latter through linkage to the patient identifier used when entering the system.

Practice portals also permit communication from a provider or staff member to the patient. Reminders can be sent directly to a patient's e-mail address if an appointment, a screening, or other service is needed. This function is part of the CCHIT criteria for EHR product certification. If further confidentiality is

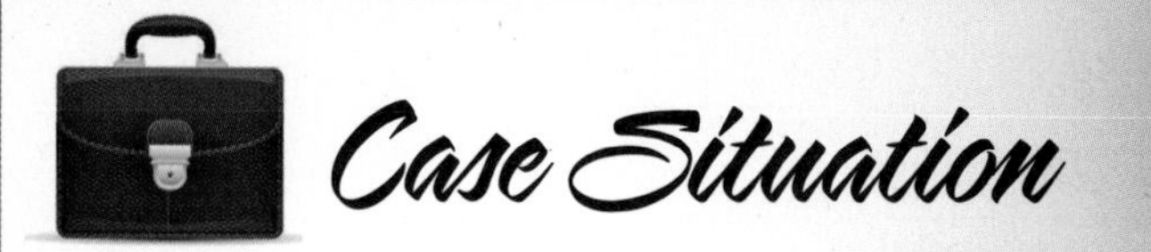

When reviewing e-mails after dinner one evening, a patient discovered a message from her physician's office that she was due for her annual Pap test and physical examination. Her physician's practice has a patient portal, and she received her access code for the portal at her last visit. She entered the URL for the portal and, upon reaching the entry screen, entered her name and code in the locations noted. Once the computer system had verified the information she had entered, she arrived at the menu screen for the portal. She chose "Make an Appointment" and her physician's name from a drop-down menu listing practice care providers. Because there is a link built into the EHR between messages sent regarding appointments and the appointment screen, the patient immediately was presented with the next three available open appointment times for a female physical examination. None of the three fit her work schedule, so she requested "More Options" by clicking on a box next to the statement. One of the alternatives presented this time was fine, so she checked the box in front of that date and time; the appointment was automatically logged into the physician's personal schedule calendar and the practice calendar. Next the computer screen showed her address, telephone numbers, and payment information, as well as a prompt asking if there were any changes. Her contact information was correct, but she had chosen a new payer during her employer's last open enrollment period. She checked "Change" next to the payment information indicating that a change was needed. A screen then was presented asking for the new information. She pulled out her insurance card and provided what was needed. The EHR then transferred the new payment information to the practice management payment database. Office staff would validate all the information provided at the time of the patient's appointment.

While she was in the portal, she decided to check to see if all charges from a visit a month ago had been paid by her prior insurer. She returned to the portal menu screen and selected "Billing and Accounts." There she found the drop-down menu where payments were recorded and noted that a payment had been made, leaving a zero balance. All payments had been received. With that information, she exited or logged out of the portal.

desired, the e-mail message can instruct the patient to access the patient portal in order to retrieve information. Usually the portal menu item requiring patient attention will be highlighted in some manner to ensure that it is noticed. Such information can include test results, medication renewal information, and instructions for tests or other services. Once accessed and read by the patient, the EHR has the capacity to document access by the patient. The date and time of system access and the identity of the patient are recorded automatically.

PERSONAL HEALTH RECORDS

As patients become more focused health care consumers, they may decide to maintain health records of their own. In addition, a number of national groups are encouraging individuals to become more active participants in their health care by documenting medical information. These records generally are referred to as personal health records (PHRs). This record may be maintained in a variety of formats (see Chapter 13), but electronic versions are receiving the most attention. Because they are maintained by the patient, control of and access to the PHR is determined by the patient. Thus it is not part of the practice's EHR. At times patients may want to share information from their PHR with care providers or may want to add information from the provider's record to their PHR. When PHR information is shared, it needs to be documented in the appropriate area of the practice EHR with an indication that the information was provided by (or given to) the patient. Information can be received or shared by the practice electronically or via any of the other communication modes discussed in this chapter. Steps in the record-documentation process will be determined by the format of the personal health record. For example, information maintained by a patient on paper files could be indexed and scanned into the practice's EHR. Files maintained on computers permit electronic transfer of information. The electronic system does the work of appropriately routing the information to and from the patient, thus saving practice personnel time and effort. Patient satisfaction is improved by providing information when and where the patient desires, the patient becomes a partner in health care, and a preventive care focus is encouraged. PHRs will be discussed in more detail in Chapter 13.

SUMMARY

Patient communications are an important part of a practice and must be documented for continuing care and legal purposes. In support of this activity, a number of standards including those of the CCHIT, The Joint Commission, the AAAHC, and "meaningful use" criteria include references to patient/provider communications. Patients may communicate with health care practices by telephone, mail, fax, and e-mail or other electronic devices. These communications require documentation in the EHR as legal evidence of the interaction. Each communication mode has advantages and disadvantages. Whether the information is received directly into the EHR, or must be scanned into it, or transcribed by personnel to become part of it, the EHR has the capacity to track messages until responses have been made. Once entered into the EHR, the messages received and responses by office personnel usually can be accessed via a "Communication" or "Patient Communication" section of the EHR.

Alerts and reminders ensure that appropriate medical care decisions, the responses to care, and appointments to support that care are brought to the attention of the correct individuals in a timely way. A practice's own web-based patient portal can provide another secure means for patient communication. Portals are used for receiving and sending messages as well as for providing information to patients and allowing them to access their medical and financial records. Although not a part of the practice record, a patient's personal health record may be used to contribute information to the practice health care database or receive information from it.

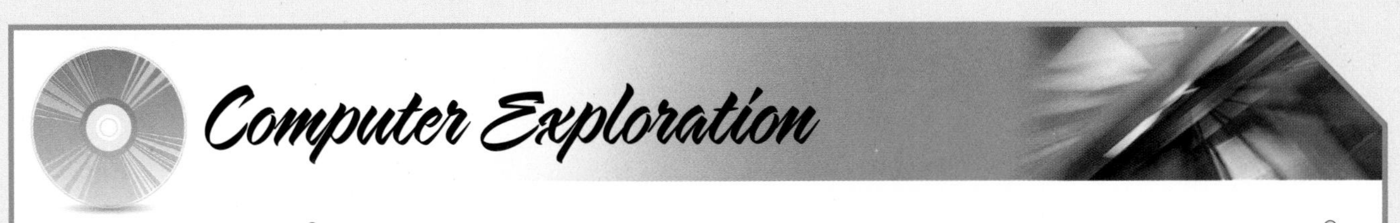

Using your e-Medsys® Educational Edition 2.0 access code provided with this text, complete the e-Medsys® Computer Exploration Exercises in Appendix B.

REFERENCES

AAAHC [Accreditation Association for Ambulatory Health Care, Inc.] (2011). *Accreditation handbook for ambulatory health care.* Wilmette, IL.

AHIMA e-HIM Task Force. (2004). The strategic importance of electronic health records management. *Journal of AHIMA, 75(9)*, 80A–B.

AHIMA e-HIM Work Group. (2003). E-mail as a provider-patient electronic communication medium and its impact on the electronic health record. (AHIMA Practice Brief.) Retrieved March 3, 2005, from http://library.ahima.org

Burrington-Brown, J. (2005). The power of patient access. *Journal of AHIMA, 76(5)*, 58–59.

Friedman, B. (2005). Health records get personal: A technology outlook for consumer access to personal health information. *Journal of AHIMA, 76(1)*, 42–45.

The Joint Commission. (2011). *Standards for ambulatory care.* Oakbrook Terrace, IL.

Koprowski, G. (2006). Networking: Portals for medical care. *Hi-Tech.* Retrieved from http://www.upi.com/Hi-Tech/view.php?StoryIC=20060626-092227-4555r

REVIEW QUESTIONS

1. What are ten reasons that patients or health care providers may need to communicate with one another?

2. In which areas have "meaningful use" criteria been written?

3. What methods/formats are used by patients to send messages to a practice?

4. How are each of those types of communication processed for entry into an EHR once they arrive at the practice?

5. What are the advantages and disadvantages of processing each communication type?

6. How does a scanner identify the correct patient and location for data it processes?

7. What methods/formats are used by providers to communicate with patients?

8. What special precautions must be taken when contacting patients by e-mail? Why must they be taken?

9. What special precautions must be taken when communicating sensitive or restricted patient information?

____

____

____

10. Give examples of several treatment events that would trigger a provider-message alert or a patient reminder in an electronic record system.

____

____

____

11. For what applications can a patient portal be used?

____

____

____

12. How might a patient's PHR be used in practice communications?

____

____

____

CHAPTER 11 Coding, Billing, and Practice Reports

CHAPTER OUTLINE

OBJECTIVES

Upon completion of the chapter, the learner will be able to:

1. Describe the basic workflow of the coding and billing functions in a practice electronic health record (EHR) environment.
2. Identify the code sets mandated by the Health Insurance Portability and Accountability Act (HIPAA) for use in electronic bill submission.
3. Differentiate between a classification system and a nomenclature.
4. Identify the groups responsible for updates to ICD, CPT, and HCPCS Level II.
5. Describe appropriate uses of ICD, CPT, HCPCS Level II, and the Diagnostic and Statistical Manual of Mental Disorders (DSM) in the office practice.
6. Describe the role of Systematized Nomenclature of Medicine—Clinical Terminology (SNOMED-CT) in the EHR and the importance of mapping it with code sets.
7. Differentiate between encoders and computer-assisted coding and describe how each is used with the EHR.
8. Describe the bill-submission sequence, including the role of scrubbers and the interface with EHRs.
9. Provide examples of the report-generation functions of a comprehensive EHR system.

KEY TERMS

American Hospital Association (AHA)

American Medical Association (AMA)

classification system

code sets

computer-assisted coding (CAC)

Cooperating Parties

Current Dental Terminology (CDT)

encoder

encounter form

evaluation and management codes (E/M codes)

Explanation of Benefits (EOB)

Healthcare Common Procedure Coding Systems (HCPCS)

International Classification of Diseases—10th Revision, Clinical Modification (ICD-10 CM)

mapping

National Center for Health Statistics (NCHS)

natural-language processing

nomenclatures

remittance advice (RA)

scrubber

INTRODUCTION

Diagnostic and procedural codes, via numbers or letters, represent the reason for a patient's visit and the major treatment required to respond to it. Codes are required for reimbursement for the care provided, and payment based upon them may determine the financial success of the practice. In addition, codes can be used for clinical decision support, research, disease-incidence monitoring by public health agencies, planning by the practice, evaluating reimbursement trends, identifying practice patterns, or other purposes (AHIMA, 2004b). Quality-of-care monitoring often is tied to diagnostic or procedural codes. Comparisons cannot be made between practices or care providers if coding is inconsistent or inaccurate. For all these reasons, quality coding is important to a practice. Code assignment must follow established rules and guidelines. Evidence must be found in the patient's record to support the codes assigned.

The electronic health record (EHR) makes the coding and billing processes more efficient by tying documentation completed during the patient visit directly to coding and billing. Reentry of data is eliminated, speeding the timeline from service to submission of the bill and, it is hoped, resulting in more timely payment as well as fewer errors. Efficiency in reporting service or financial data for other purposes also is enhanced. The ability to blend information from the medical record component of the EHR system and the practice management component enables production of almost unlimited types of reports. Practice decisions can be supported with sound, current data.

CODING AND BILLING WORKFLOW

The coding and billing workflow usually begins prior to the patient visit, when basic patient payment information is collected and eligibility for health care services is determined by accessing payer information about patient benefits. During the registration process, practice office personnel record or verify patient demographic data and service-payment information on pertinent EHR screens (see Chapter 5). As the patient visit progresses, the health care provider documents objective and subjective findings, interprets those findings, establishes a plan of care, and provides directions for further care via diagnostic and treatment orders. All the information gathered is evaluated to determine a patient diagnosis. The diagnosis is recorded on the patient's problem list (see Chapter 6). Procedures performed and supplies provided also are recorded via documentation elsewhere in the care record. Once the provider's recording is in place, codes can be assigned. Encoder software can assist personnel in code selection or, if computer-assisted coding software is used, the software can search for and access diagnostic and procedure data fields in the EHR and apply codes without assistance. Designated office staff then can review the codes that have been assigned, clarify codes when needed, and perform coding quality reviews. Once codes are assigned, they can be applied to the patient's bill for services via transfer of the coded data from one location to another in the EHR and its practice management partner. If the codes are entered in designated data fields and the software meets established guidelines for interoperability, codes can be transferred even when the electronic medical record and the practice management EHR software are separate systems from different vendors.

The remainder of the information required for the bill, including patient and provider information, most likely has been generated already via data transfer from the EHR or preset categories in the billing component of practice management software. In fact, proposed federal government changes in its uniform billing form have been designed with data transfers in mind. Then the bill's content is evaluated for inconsistencies or inappropriate information. If all data meets established criteria, the bill is submitted electronically either directly to the third-party payer or to a claims clearinghouse that performs additional edits before submission to the payer. Defined supporting information also may be sent to the payer electronically. In turn, electronic communication such as an **Explanation of Benefits (EOB) or remittance advice (RA)** from the payer can indicate payment and transfer of funds, provide information about claim problems for follow-up action, or indicate noncoverage of services. An example of this type of notice is shown in Figure 11-1A and Figure 11-1B.

Explanation of Benefits (EOB) or remittance advice (RA)
Communication from a third-party payer to a practice indicating payment for services, claim problems for follow-up action, or noncoverage of services.

Questions that arise from the EOB or RA and follow-up actions also can be communicated and transmitted electronically. Of course, payment for services also can include billing additional third-party payers or the patient for legitimate costs not covered by other payment sources. Once information from the primary payment source is received, contacting other payers also can occur electronically via online submission or template letters generated by the practice management component of the system to the patient. Diagnostic and treatment information—including codes required for reporting for other purposes, such as quality of care monitoring and to meet public health requirements—can be

EXPLANATION OF BENEFITS - THIS IS NOT A BILL

Date:

MEMBER #:
CLAIM NO:
PATIENT NAME:
POLICY HOLDER NAME:

GROUP ID	CHECK NUMBER	DATE	ANY QUESTIONS - PLEASE CONTACT
			Payer name and address
GROUP NAME			
SERVICING PROVIDER			
ISSUED TO			

CLAIM SUMMARY INFORMATION

Charge	Not Covered Amount	Exceed Benefit	Allowed Amount	Deductible	Co-pay	Co-insurance	Benefit Amount
OTHER INSURANCE CARRIER PAID =		AMOUNT PAID BY GHC =			MEMBER RESPONSIBILITY =		

Benefit Information	Annual		Used		Remaining	
	Patient	Family	Patient	Family	Patient	Family

CLAIM DETAIL INFORMATION

DATE OF SERVICE		SERVICE	CHARGE AMOUNT	NOT COVERED	EXCEED BENEFIT AMOUNT	ALLOWED AMOUNT	DEDUCTIBLE	CO-PAY	CO-INSURANCE	BENEFIT AMOUNT	REASON CODE
From	To										

Reason Code Summary

Code	Reason
41	HEALTHEOS OR MULTIPLAN ADJUST

Please keep a copy of the Explanation of Benefits for your records

Figure 11-1A Example of an explanation of benefits (EOB). *(Continues)*

(Continued)

Your ERISA Rights

The following applies to plan participants subject to the Employment Retiree Income Security Act of 1974.

If ABC up holds a denial following completion of ABC's appeals process, you may be entitled to certain rights and protection under section 502 (a) of the Employee Retirement Income Security Act of 1974 (ERISA), including rights to file suit in a state or federal court. If you have any questions about his statement or about your rights under ERISA, or if you need assistance in obtaining documents form the plan administrator, you should contact the nearest office of the Pension and Welfare Benefits Administration, U.S. Department of Labor, listed in your telephone directory or the Division of Technical Assistance and Inquires, Pension and Welfare Benefits Administration, U.S. Department of Labor, 200 Constitution Avenue N.W., Washington, D.C. 20210. You may also obtain certain publications about your rights and responsibilities under ERISA by calling the publications hotline of the Pension and Welfare Benefits Administration.

Copies of any internal rules, guidelines or protocols relied upon in making this determination are available to you, free of charge, upon written request. An explanation of any scientific or clinical judgment relied upon for denials based on medical necessity or experimental treatment is also available to you, free of charge upon written request.

Review and Appeal Process

If you have questions or disagree with the payment issued on this claim, please call our Member Services Department at the phone number listed on the front of this explanation of benefit.

You may appeal this claim by sending a written request to the ABC's Member Services Department as PO Box 55555, Eagle River, WI 55555. Include the reasons for your appealing decision and all pertinent information and documentation related to your appeal.Please refer to your Certificate or other documentation for specific information on your appeal rights.

ABC will acknowledge receipt of your appeal within five (5) business days of receipt. You will be notified, in writing, of the plan's decision within 30 calendar days. In certain cases, ABC may extend this period one time by up to 30 calendar days. If an extension is necessary, you will be notified prior to the expiration of the initial 30-day period.

HELP STOP INSURANCE FRAUD! If you know or suspect any illegal activity concerning insurance claims, contact our Member Services Department at (555) 555-5555. ***You do not need to identify yourself.***

Figure 11-1A

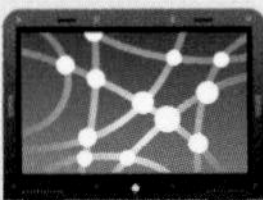

View the functional criteria used by CCHIT to certify ambulatory EHRs at the CCHIT website: http://www.cchit.org/.

abstracted from the EHR in a similar manner and submitted via confidential electronic networks. This workflow is supported by functional standards for ambulatory care EHRs developed by the CCHIT.

CODE SETS AND CLINICAL VOCABULARIES

code sets—coding systems a term particularly used for those codes approved by HIPAA regulations for use in electronic transactions.

Performing the coding and billing function accurately requires that the care provider, payer, and other entities who may be contracted to assist with the process all use the same clinical terminology and **code sets** or coding systems. Defined clinical terminology and coding systems permit linkage of patient data to medical research, to decision-support systems, and to quality-of-care standards. They also enable the exchange of information between providers, alerts and reminders that reduce treatment errors, and uniform reporting for research, public health, quality reviews, and reimbursement for services provided. When defined terminologies and code sets are adopted, data can be entered once but used for multiple purposes, saving time and increasing efficiency.

Regulations resulting from the federal government's Health Insurance Portability and Accountability Act (HIPAA) initiated standards in this area by

Key to ABC's Explanation of Benefits.

EXPLANATION OF BENEFITS – THIS IS NOT A BILL

John Q Customer
123 Made Up Lane (1)
Anywhere, USA 55555
Xxxxxxxx
xxxxx

(4) **Date: 10/17/06**
(5) **MEMBER #: 0000000**
CLAIM NO:
0000000
(1) **PATIENT NAME:**
CUSTOMER II, JOHN Q
(6) **POLICY HOLDER NAME:**
CUSTOMER II, JOHN Q

GROUP ID (7)	CHECK NUMBER (2)	DATE (3)	ANY QUESTIONS – PLEASE CONTACT
0000000	Xxxxxxx	xx/xx/xxxx	Payer name and address
GROUP NAME Payer name (8) XXXXXXXX(50)XXXXXX			
SERVICING PROVIDER HCO name (9) XXXXXXXXXX(50)XXXXXXXX			
ISSUED TO HCO name (10) XXXXXXXXX(50)XXXXXXXX			

CLAIM SUMMARY INFORMATION

Charge (11)	Not Covered Amount (12)	Exceed Benefit (13)	Allowed Amount (14)	Deductible (15)	Co-pay (16)	Co-insurance (17)	Benefit Amount (18)
$0,000.00	$0,000.00	$0.00	$000.00	$0.00	$000.00	$0.00	$000.00
OTHER INSURANCE CARRIER PAID =		(19) $0.00	AMOUNT PAID BY GHC =	$000.00 (20)		MEMBER RESPONSIBILITY =	$00.00 (21)

Benefit Information (if applicable to your plan)	Annual Patient Family	Used Patient Family	Remaining Patient Family
In Network – Individual Year to Date Deductible In Network – Individual Year to Date Maximum Out of Pocket In Network – Family Year to Date Deductible In Network – Family Year to Date Maximum Out of Pocket Out of Network – Individual Year to Date Deductible Out of Network – Individual Year to Date Maximum Out of Pocket Out of Network – Individual Year to Date Deductible Out of Network – Individual Year to Date Maximum Out of Pocket	(22) (28)	(22A)	(22B)

CLAIM DETAIL INFORMATION

DATE OF SERVICE From	DATE OF SERVICE To	SERVICE	CHARGE AMOUNT	NOT COVERED	EXCEED BENEFIT AMOUNT	ALLOWED AMOUNT	DEDUCTIBLE	CO-PAY	CO-INSURANCE	BENEFIT AMOUNT	REASON CODE
(23)	(24)	(25)	(11)	(12)	(13)	(14)	(15)	(16)	(17)	(18)	(26)

Reason Code Summary (27)

Please keep a copy of the Explanation of Benefits for your records.

Figure 11-1B Example of an explanation of benefits (EOB) with data. (*Continues*)

requiring specific code sets for use in electronic transactions, including submission of electronic bills. The International Classification of Diseases—9th Revision—Clinical Modification (ICD-9-CM) is the designated coding system for reporting diagnoses until October 2014 when the **International Classification of Diseases, 10th Revision, Clinical Modification (ICD-10 CM)** will take its place. The **Healthcare Common Procedure Coding Systems (HCPCS)**, including Current Procedural Terminology (CPT), is required for procedures in the medical office environment. The designated coding standard for dental services is **Current Dental Terminology (CDT)**. A data set for drug reporting also was identified but has since been repealed. Updates to these systems (for example, ICD-10 CM replacing ICD-9-CM) require legislative approval by the federal government to become acceptable replacements. These defined code sets were mandated for electronic submission of bills for federally funded programs and have been adopted across the United States by other third-party payers as well.

International Classification of Diseases—10th Revision, Clinical Modification (ICD-10 CM)
An international update to the ICD-9 disease classification coordinated by the World Health Organization; to be initiated in the US in 2014.

Healthcare Common Procedure Coding Systems (HCPCS)
Coding system designated by HIPAA for electronic transactions relating to procedures performed in the ambulatory setting.

Current Dental Terminology (CDT)
Coding standard for dental services and the HIPAA-designated coding system for electronic transactions.

(Continued)

1) **Patient Name**

2) **Check Number** – if a check is issued, this is the ABC check number.

3) **Date of Check** – issued by ABC

4) **Member Number** – unique number issued by ABC to each patient.

5) **Claim Number** – ABC's unique claim number for this charge.

6) **Policy Holder Name** – Name of the person whom has the insurance. Also known as the subscriber.

7) **Group ID** – this is the number of the Employer or individual's plan number.

8) **Group Name** – this is the name of the Employer or individual plan.

9) **Servicing Provider** – This is the provider whom is billing the charge.

10) **Issued To:** - This is the provider or individual to whom payment is being made.

11) **Charge Amount** – This is the amount of the charge for the service(s)

12) **Not Covered Amount** – This is the amount of the service that is not covered by your plan.

13) **Exceed Benefit** – This is the amount which is over your benefit maximum limit and therefore is not covered.

14) **Allowed Amount** – This is the amount allowed for your services, after any discounts have been deducted by your plan. It may also the maximum allowed for Reasonable and Customary charge.

15) **Deductible** – If your plan has a deductible, this is the amount applied to your service(s)

16) **Co-Pay** - If your plan has a co-payment, this is the amount applied to your service(s)

17) **Co-insurance** - If your plan has co-insurance, this is the amount applied to your service(s)

18) **Benefit Amount** – This is the amount of benefits paid by your plan.

19) **Other Insurance Paid** – If you have another insurance plan, this is the amount they have paid for this service(s).

20) **Amount Paid by GHC** – This is the amount paid by your ABC plan.

21) **Member Responsibility** – This is the amount owed by you to the provider. This includes any not covered amounts, exceed benefits amounts, deductibles, co-payments and co-insurances.

22) **Benefit Information Annual** – If you have ABC's Preferred Provider Organization (PPO) plan, this indicates your annual In-network and Out-network maximums. (Note: This does not apply to an HMO plan)

22A) **Benefit Information Used** – If you have ABC's Preferred Provider Organization (PPO) plan, this indicates your annual In-network and Out-network amounts used. (Note: This does not apply to an HMO plan)

22B) **Benefit Information Remaining** – If you have ABC's Preferred Provider Organization (PPO) plan, this indicates your annual In-network and Out-network amounts left for the calendar year. (Note: This does not apply to an HMO plan)

23) **Date of Service From** – This the beginning date of service

24) **Date of Service To** – This the ending date of service

25) **Service** – This is a brief description of the service(s)

26) **Reason Code** – this is an indicator or key to a more detailed explanation for this line of service and it is listed after the claim detail information.

27) **Reason Summary Code** – this is a description of the indicator listed in #26

28) **MOOP** – this is Maximum Out of Pocket

Figure 11-1B

CODING, BILLING, AND THE EHR

encounter form Preprinted paper template designed to record the diagnoses and procedures completed during an office visit along with their ICD or CPT codes.

In the past, the **encounter form** has been the link between diagnostic and procedural information associated with an office visit and the service payment (billing) function associated with that same visit. Often a practice preprinted encounter forms that contained the most common diagnoses and procedures of the practice along with their respective codes from the ICD or the CPT systems. Sections for open text on the form allowed the provider to add diagnoses or procedures that were not preprinted. During the office visit, health care providers checked off the appropriate items on the encounter form that described a particular patient's condition and treatment. The coded data from the encounter form then was entered into the billing software program. Open-text additions to the form require manual coding or the use of a specialized computer program to assist in assigning codes. Then the coded data was entered into the billing software program. Medical billing software is typically a part of a practice management system.

In the EHR/practice management interoperative system, medical billing systems and coding systems both can interface with the EHR system so that data can be shared by the systems electronically. As discussed earlier in this chapter, this type of interoperability among computer systems to achieve data sharing is a goal for health care provider practices to strive for as they implement their health information technology plan. It saves manual system steps that are time consuming and that create the possibility of errors when data is transferred from one to another.

Diagnostic Coding

The ICD is an international **classification system** coordinated by the World Health Organization. Classification systems group similar diagnoses or procedures together for reporting purposes—they classify them. Classification systems are effective for payment and most other uses of coded information, but, because of the grouped data, they are not explicit enough to be applied as a clinical terminology or vocabulary for other purposes. The Clinical Modification of ICD (ICD-9-CM and ICD-10) used in the United States adds codes for more accurate monitoring of diseases and for the "cause of death" data not supported by the international ICD version. Only Volumes 1 and 2, the listing of diagnostic codes and its related alphabetic index, are used by practice providers.

At the current time in the United States, code modifications and additions are recommended by a group called the **Cooperating Parties**. Members of the Cooperating Parties are representatives of four national stakeholder groups: The **National Center for Health Statistics (NCHS)**, the **American Hospital Association (AHA)**, the American Health Information Management Association (AHIMA), and the Centers for Medicare and Medicaid Services (CMS). After discussion, the co-chairs of the group make the final decision on all revisions. ICD codes can be updated twice a year, in April and October. All coding software must have the capability of incorporating these regular updates.

Other nationally recognized coding systems may be used by certain health care specialists but are not mandated by HIPAA. For example, the codes from the current edition of the Diagnostic and Statistical Manual of Mental Disorders (DSM) may be applied in practices that treat psychiatric problems.

Procedural Coding

The procedural code set identified by HIPAA for use in electronic transactions by physician and other medical provider practices in the United States is HCPCS, which has two code levels. Level I codes are CPT codes copyrighted by the **American Medical Association (AMA)**. Although part of the HCPCS structure, these codes usually are referred to simply as CPT codes. CPT's alphanumeric codes traditionally have been used for Medicare Part B reimbursement and now are used by most third-party payers as well. **Evaluation and management (E/M)** codes relating to the level and complexity of an office visit are an important part of service information reported via CPT code. Data required for accurate evaluation and management assignment may require a structured entry template such as that noted in Figure 11-2. Unlike ICD, which is a classification system, CPT is a **nomenclature**. Nomenclatures are listings of terms, rather than a grouping of terms. Similar to ICD, CPT is neither detailed nor complex enough to be used as the basis for an EHR clinical vocabulary.

HCPCS Level II codes, or "national codes," are maintained by CMS and have been added to provide additional codes for medical services, equipment, and supplies not included in CPT. They are used to report such items as ambulance services and durable medical equipment provided. Modifiers that can be applied to all HCPCS codes also are included in Level II (Scott, 2007). Level II codes reflect Medicare regulations. Except for temporary Level II codes, both CPT codes and Level II codes are updated once a year in January. Updates to coding software must incorporate these changes as well as those to other systems.

classification system
A system that groups similar diagnoses or procedures together for reporting purposes.

Cooperating Parties
Representatives from four organizations that together make recommendations for ICD code modifications and additions for use in the US.

National Center for Health Statistics (NCHS)
One of the Cooperating Party organizations that participates in recommendations regarding ICD for use in the US.

American Hospital Association (AHA)
One of the Cooperating Party organizations that participates in recommendations regarding ICD for use in the US.

American Medical Association (AMA)
Organization that copyrights and coordinates CPT Level I codes.

evaluation and management codes (E/M codes)
Part of the CPT coding system that indicates the level and complexity of an office visit.

nomenclature
A listing of coding terms.

⌘ File Edit View SOAP In-Basket Tools Help

John Sample	CC: *Old MI*

E & M Advisor

Is visit primarily counseling/coordination? ❒ Yes ❒ No

What is type of patient? ❒ New ❒ Established ❒ Consultation

What was amount/complexity of data reviewed?

- ❒ Review/order clinical labs
- ❒ Review/order radiology tests
- ❒ Review/order other dx or tx interventions
- ❒ Discuss test results with other provider
- ❒ Review old records or hx from another provider
- ❒ Review and summarize old records for another provider
- ❒ Independently review dx data

What is risk of complications? ❒ Minimal ❒ Low ❒ Moderate ❒ High

This note is in compliance with CPT-99212
Code: ❒ 99211 ❒ 99212 ❒ 99213 ❒ 99214 ❒ 99215

Figure 11-2 Template for E/M determination.

Used with permission. Margret Amatayakul and Steven S. Lazarus (2005, p. 45). Electronic Health Records, MGMA.

MEDCIN, SNOMED-CT®, and Coding

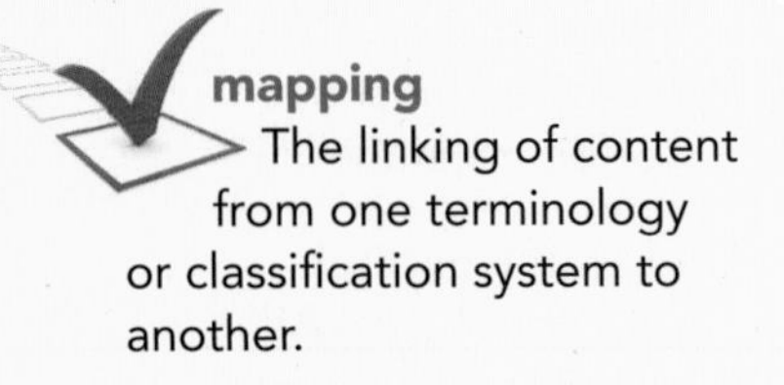

mapping The linking of content from one terminology or classification system to another.

As mentioned in Chapter 3, MEDCIN is a point-of-care terminology used to assist providers in recording patient findings, and SNOMED-CT® is an established federal information-system vocabulary standard commonly used in EHR products. These two systems have the ability to facilitate ICD and CPT coding via mapping. **Mapping** is defined as "the linking of content from one terminology or classification to another." (Foley and Garrett, 2006, p. 28.) MEDCIN has been mapped to ICD and CPT and SNOMED-CT® is mapped to MEDCIN as well as to both the ICD and CPT coding systems. As a result, if all data entered into the EHR were represented in SNOMED-CT® terms, "by using a decision support rules engine, the data could be filtered to produce CPT and ICD . . . codes automatically for billing purposes." (Amatayakul & Lazarus, 2005, p. 46.) Thus SNOMED-CT®—together with application of the current ICD and HCPCS, including CPT codes—provides the code sets and vocabulary needed for payment and most reporting requirements. Refer to Chapter 3 for more information on these vocabularies.

ENCODERS AND COMPUTER-ASSISTED CODING

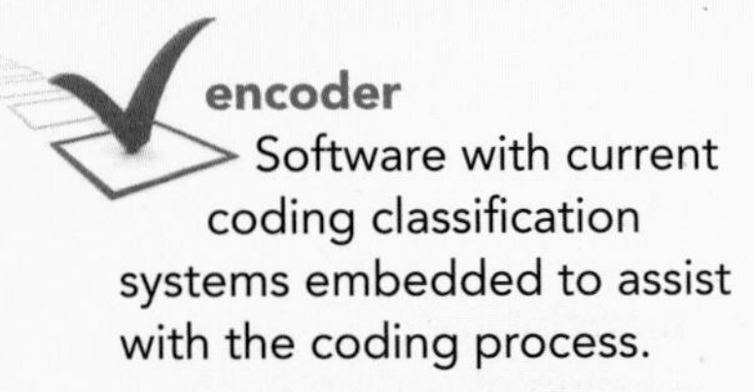

encoder Software with current coding classification systems embedded to assist with the coding process.

Encoders (software that is designed to reproduce a coding system and assist with code assignment) may be used in the coding process. Once determined by the provider, diagnoses and procedures entered into the EHR using SNOMED-CT® as the vocabulary can be transferred from those specific locations to the encoder program either by the provider or a staff member. The encoder software presents additional questions or code choices until an exact ICD, CPT, or DSM code that matches the patient situation can be identified. An example of an encoder screen is shown in Figure 11-3.

OPTUM™ EncoderPro.com Expert

All Code Sets | Search | Help with Search?

Coding ▾ Policy Lookup Reimbursement ▾

CPT® Code Section (97001-97006)

CPT ® Code Section (97001-97006)

▼To Bottom

Actions	Code	Description	References	Edits
	97001	Physical therapy evaluation	CCI LCD 100 CMS PQRS	
	97002	Physical therapy re-evaluation	CCI LCD 100 CMS PQRS	
	97003	Occupational therapy evaluation	CCI LCD 100 CMS PQRS	
	97004	Occupational therapy re-evaluation	CCI LCD 100 CMS PQRS	
	97005	Athletic training evaluation	LCD 100 CMS	
	97006	Athletic training re-evaluation	LCD 100 CMS	

Courtesy of Optum EncoderPro

Figure 11-3 Outpatient encoder screen from EncoderPro.

Claim Lines Fee Type ● Facility ○ Non-Facility

▼To Bottom

Line #	Date Of Service	Code	Mod	Mod	Primary ICD-9-CM Dx	Secondary ICD-9-CM Dx	Fee	Total RVU	Work RVU	Edit Conflicts	Delete
1	08/07/2012	58290					1169.53	34.36	20.27	CSX ICM	

▲To Top

Records 1 - 1 of 1

? Coding Questions...Click here. *Optum Coding Answers*

With ever-changing government regulations, the demands of accurately coding intricate procedures and keeping abreast of all the annual code changes, it's understandable that you may not have all the answers. Fortunately, Optum now offers *Optum Coding Answers*, a web-based solution that allows you to submit your toughest questions online and receive responses from our experts in 48 to 72 hours.

Edit Conflicts

▼To Bottom

Line #	Icon	Edit Type	Edit Conflict	Description
1	CSX	Review	Procedure Not Typical For Gender of Patient	Procedure Code 58290 is not typically performed for gender of patient (M).

Courtesy of Optum EncoderPro

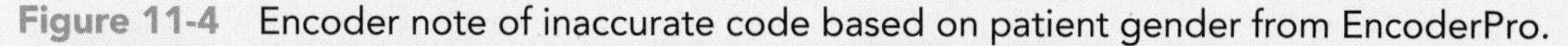

Figure 11-4 Encoder note of inaccurate code based on patient gender from EncoderPro.

The questions or alternatives presented by the encoder either assist in the choice of codes (so that they are as specific as possible) or identify related disease factors that may have an impact on code assignment. Codes for services provided and diagnoses entered on bills are required to match, which means that the services must be appropriate for the diagnoses indicated or payment will be denied. Denial also may occur if the service is determined not to be medically necessary. Encoders can perform edits to ensure that inconsistencies between codes or between codes and demographic information are evaluated for accuracy before posting final codes. For example, encoders will create an error message on the computer screen when a code for a hysterectomy is entered for a male patient (see Figure 11-4). Once an accurate code is determined, it can be transferred electronically to the appropriate location on the patient's bill by following the software interface directions.

Programs with built-in coding intelligence also can assist with E/M code selection. If visit recording is structured appropriately the system can, for example, "count" the number of items evaluated in a review-of-systems category. Prompts may assist the health care provider to document more completely. However, caution is in order. Prompts are meant to trigger documentation of services that actually were performed. Misuse of prompts such as adding a code for a diagnosis not documented or a service not performed is referred to as upcoding, a federally prohibited act. Codes submitted to payers are monitored by them for trends. Inappropriate coding patterns can be identified and can result in required payment refunds or legal action. Quality review of this portion of coding is also important to ensure that the E/M codes chosen are supported by documentation and medical necessity.

computer-assisted coding (CAC) Use of coding software that automatically generates medical codes based on documentation in the patient record.

natural-language processing Software that applies artificial intelligence to narrative text in order to extract terms and data.

Computer-assisted coding (CAC) goes a step further than an encoder in automating the coding process. The American Health Information Management Association's e-HIM Workgroup on Computer Assisted Coding (AHIMA, 2004, p. 48A) defines CAC as "the use of computer software that automatically generates a set of medical codes for review, validation, and use based upon clinical documentation provided by healthcare practitioners." There are two ways that documentation in the patient record automatically can be translated electronically into a code. The first is called **natural-language processing**. With this system, providers can document in an EHR using their standard terminology and reports and then the software, applying artificial intelligence, will extract terms and data from text and assign codes. The second model uses structured input via menus of clinical terms that have been mapped to their respective codes. A care provider chooses a menu item and its related code immediately is presented. In both models, no additional processing is required, in contrast to an encoder. An example of a CAC coding program is shown in Figure 11-5.

Advantages of CAC include increased efficiency and productivity, consistent and comprehensive code assignment, and the production of an audit trail or record of the steps taken in coming to a final choice of codes. Of course, these systems are complex and expensive. Because CAC is a relatively new technology, errors may occur. For this reason, it is important that coding professionals review or edit the assigned codes. At this time in their evolution, CAC systems also work best in specialty areas with limited vocabularies or limited source documents. (AHIMA, 2004.)

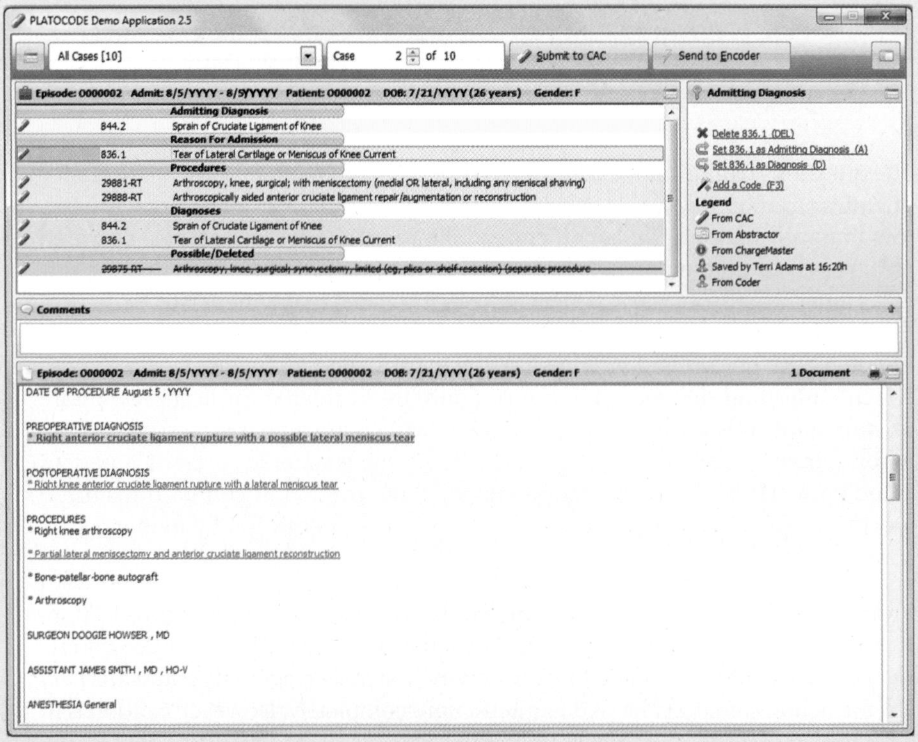

Figure 11-5 Example of a computer-assisted coding program.

ELECTRONIC BILL SUBMISSION

Through instructions within the practice's coding software, chosen codes are transferred to a bill electronically. Patient demographic information, payer information, national provider identifiers (NPIs), service location, and other required information are added either via transfer from the EHR or from data stored in the practice management software. Fees for services are obtained and transferred from the fee schedule component of the practice management system. These fees are predetermined by the practice as set by contract with the patient's particular payer. Next, the bill is reviewed by those indicated in practice policies. Billing data also can be processed through software developed to review it for errors and to check for compliance with regulatory mandates. This software commonly is referred to as a **scrubber**. Scrubbers can include general billing guidelines as well as specific payer information and guidelines. A newer development is a web-based scrubber. Bertrams (2004, p. 46) describes the unique features of web-based scrubbers in this way:

> In addition to the traditional procedural and diagnosis coding components, they factor in medical necessity mandates, quarterly updates from the National Correct Coding Initiative (CCI) and modifier specifications as well as customized edits in response to individual payer requirements. Claim files or charges are uploaded from the practice management system to the Web-based scrubber . . . It flags potential problem claims and returns them to the practice management system with an explanation of the error or omission that interferes with the claims' validity. Coding and billing staff can make corrections and submit clean claims to the payer the first time.

scrubber

Software developed to review claims for discrepancies or errors and to validate compliance with regulatory mandates prior to submission to third-party payers.

This may be a step performed within the practice, or the verification of information and scrubbing of bills may be contracted to a claims clearinghouse before forwarding to the actual insurance company or payer. When manual steps or hand-completed encounter forms are eliminated and replaced by electronic processes, bills can be forwarded more quickly. Once bills are received, third-party payers perform their own reviews of the electronically submitted information. If approved, payment (often in the form of an electronic transfer) can be made promptly. If questions develop, electronic communication via an EOB or RA shortens the inquiry and response time. Of course, quality control of the practice's entire coding and billing process is important. This requires the expertise of someone on the office staff who is well versed in coding and billing.

Steps in the accounting process that are related to billing—including the patient account ledger, the daily log, and patient statements—also can be performed by the practice management system. Letter or e-mail templates can be developed for the most frequently sent communications to patients or others as needed for the reimbursement process.

PRACTICE REPORTS

Quality service to patients, efficient provider practice patterns, and adequate practice income are important for the success of the health care provider practice. Decisions about purchasing a new piece of equipment, adding another medical assistant, accepting more patients from a managed care organization, or choosing the most effective medication for a particular diagnosis all can be aided by sound practice data. An EHR is particularly useful in this area because defined data fields can be combined in many combinations to provide the reports needed. Of course, in the past some information has been available from the scheduling and billing components of practice management software. An

EHR adds the benefit of integrating medical record data with practice management data and eliminating the need to transfer data manually from one system to the other. Standard reports that routinely pull data from both systems can be developed. Special "one time only" data requests also can be performed with the assistance of someone trained in using the system's reporting capabilities. Revenue cycle management, practice pattern evaluation, staff productivity monitoring, and quality management activities are all examples of areas where reports provide essential information to support management decision making.

As patients are seen and bills submitted, it is important for an assigned individual in the practice to monitor the claims process and its results. Revenue-cycle management reporting, typically a function of practice management systems, is enhanced with the EHR. For example, database queries can provide lists of patients receiving treatment for which no bill has been generated, and then categorize them by provider, by type of treatment, or by the length of time since the patient's visit. Lists of unpaid claims (accounts receivable) can be generated that are categorized by third-party payer, diagnosis, care provider, or days since the bill was submitted. Monitoring of payment denials—including reason for the denial, action taken, appeal status, and primary care provider—is also possible. Linkage with EHR treatment data provides opportunities to relate the claims process more closely with supporting service documentation and with the actual care received.

Practice-pattern monitoring also requires EHR data. Patients taking two alternative medications for a disease could be divided into two groups: one taking the medication usually covered by payers and the other taking a newer medication that is usually not covered. Within those patient groupings, data could be subdivided further by prescribing provider or by desired outcome measures. In this case, results may influence future prescription practices. Other practice-pattern reports may focus on patient health, such as the number of patients reported to health authorities for communicable diseases during the past year who have not been seen for follow-up treatment. In addition, some reports currently available via the scheduling or billing components of a practice-management system can be enhanced by further detail obtained from the EHR system. For example, established patients receiving prescriptions for narcotics by month over the past two years could be generated. This data could be matched against prescription data received from other care providers via a continuity of care record (CCR; see Chapter 13) in order to identify potential patterns of drug abuse by a patient moving from practice to practice or city to city.

Another type of report that can be generated from an EHR helps manage the daily functions of a practice. For example, work can be distributed by an office manager to staff or care providers via the EHR's work distribution system. The assigned task then appears on the work list for the designated individual. It can be monitored until a notation of completion is received or reassigned, if necessary. Summaries of tasks performed over a period of time (say, a week or a month) can be compiled for productivity evaluation. Tabulations also can be made of numbers of times specialized practice equipment is used. These reports support staffing levels, help justify the purchase of new equipment, and assist in the timely ordering of medical and related supplies. An example of a report using care data along with practice information is shown in Figure 11-6.

Finally, practice service patterns can be compared with established industry or practice protocols to evaluate the quality of care provided. Once again, reports can be generated "by provider" so that a provider–practice profile is created. Topics for monitoring could change according to the interest of the care providers, as mandated by third-party payers, or when directed as part of a data-reporting system such as the Health Plan Employer Data and Information Set (HEDIS). The CCHIT has recognized the importance of report functions for ambulatory care EHRs and has developed standards for them as well.

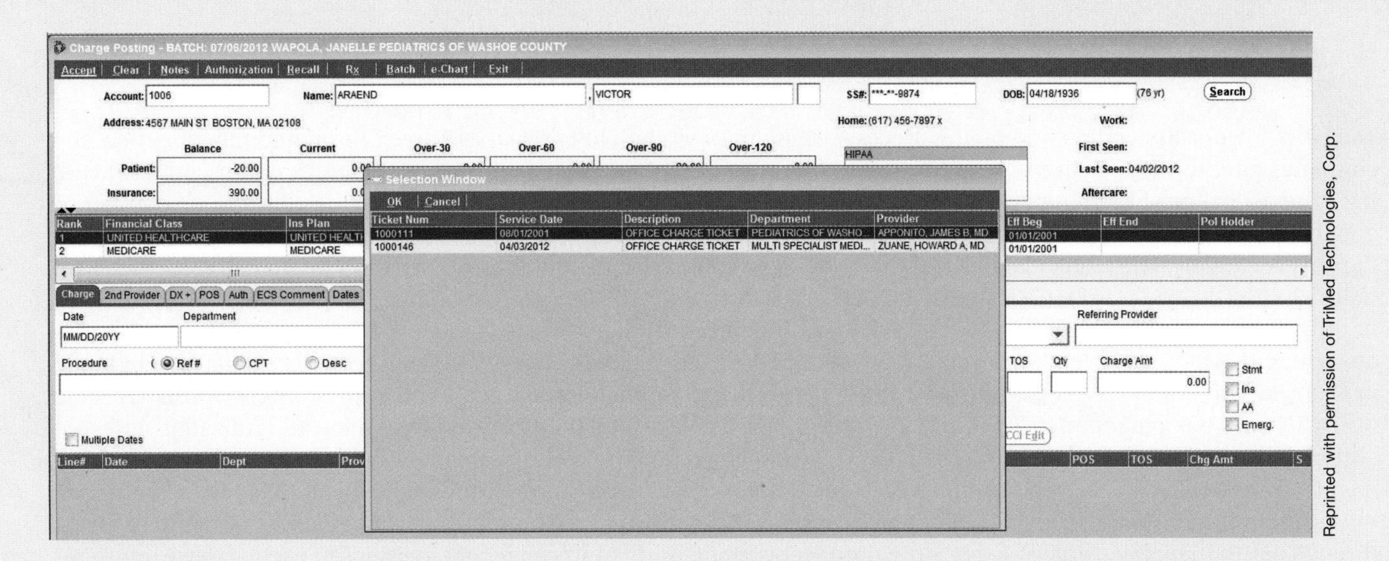

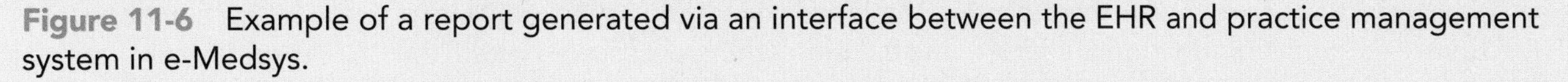

Figure 11-6 Example of a report generated via an interface between the EHR and practice management system in e-Medsys.

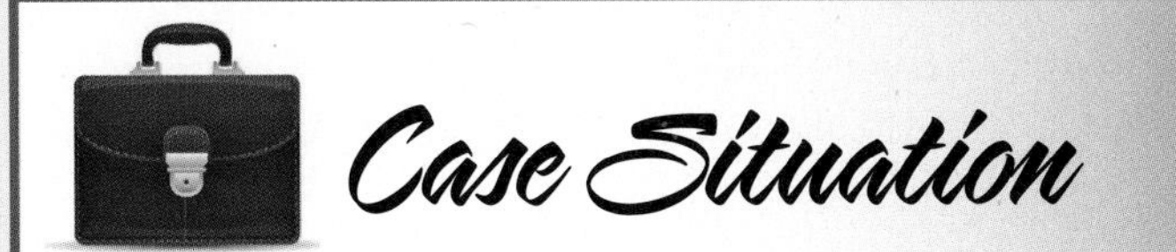

Case Situation

An established patient sees his internist for a medication check. A claim for service is initiated through linkages in data documented as part of the patient registration process, the physician and practice identifiers in both databases, the practice fee schedule, and payment information available online from the patient's third-party payer. Only diagnoses and codes need to be added. The billing coordinator next enters the patient's record number into the encoder screen. The patient's diagnoses for this visit are pulled from the visit record database (problem list) and shown on the screen. The diagnoses include hypertension and depression. The billing coordinator, who is also a trained coder, highlights the first diagnosis; then an ICD screen is presented by the encoder software with the associated diagnostic code. Since hypertension requires more specificity, the encoder presents options for more detailed codes. The correct code is selected via highlighting, and it is automatically transferred to the claim form along with the wording associated with the code. It is listed first because it was the primary reason for the visit.

The same process then occurs for the depression diagnosis. The diagnosis of depression was added at this visit, so a new code must be selected. No procedures were performed at this visit, but an E/M code must be added. Visit documentation has been programmed to support the information needed for E/M coding. Thus, a CPT E/M code is presented by the coding software. The biller/coder accesses the patient record to verify that there is documentation to support the suggested code. The code appears to describe the visit correctly, and it is highlighted. Upon selection, it too is added to the claim form.

The claim is now ready to be processed by the practice management scrubber. The scrubber indicates that there are no noticeable problems, and the claim is submitted electronically to the patient's third-party payer. Two weeks later, an EOB is generated from the payer and is sent electronically to the practice, indicating that full payment (minus the patient's $10 co–pay amount, which he paid during his visit) will be transferred to the practice's bank account. The deposit is verified by the billing specialist a few days later.

SUMMARY

The workflow for the coding and billing process begins prior to the patient visit as part of the scheduling function and continues after the visit until payment for services is received. Using defined clinical vocabularies and established coding systems, patient-treatment documentation can be linked to diagnostic and procedural codes. In turn, codes can be applied to bills for submission to third-party payers. Standards for these processes are important for sharing and interpreting data accurately. HIPAA regulations identified standard code sets for submitting information for an ambulatory service bill, including the use of ICD , CPT, and HCPCS Level II codes. The ICD is an international classification system that is used in provider practices for recording diagnoses. Recording of procedures is done with the CPT nomenclature. CPT codes are actually Level I HCPCS codes. Level II HCPCS codes are used nationally for services and equipment that are not found in CPT. The SNOMED-CT® is the primary clinical vocabulary identified for use within an EHR. Both SNOMED-CT® and MEDCIN have been mapped to ICD, CPT, and other specialized vocabularies in order to permit standardization and consistency in the use of medical terms in an EHR. Once diagnoses and procedures are identified via a problem list or other means, an encoder can assist personnel with code assignment. If computer-assisted coding is applied, then no human intervention is required except for auditing purposes. CAC software programming facilitates code assignment either through natural-language processing or structured menu input. Audit trails can record the steps in each of those processes in the event that questions about assignment develop. Assigned codes then can be transferred to the billing component of the EHR system. Additional information is added to the bill from other data sources within the EHR, scrubbers are applied to edit codes and bills for errors, and then the bill is sent electronically to the primary payer. Communication with that payer or the patient continues electronically, if possible, until service payment has been received.

The billing function in the health care provider office has long included electronic procedures. In the EHR system, interoperability among the billing system and the medical record is key to increasing the accuracy and efficiency of this important business activity. Finally, the interaction of the two systems also supports gathering data to assist practice owners and managers in monitoring activities and performance and in making sound management decisions.

Computer Exploration

Using your e-Medsys® Educational Edition 2.0 access code provided with this text, complete the e-Medsys® Computer Exploration Exercises in Appendix B.

REFERENCES

AHIMA e-HIM Work Group on Computer-Assisted Coding. (2004). Delving into computer-assisted coding. (AHIMA Practice Brief.) *Journal of AHIMA, 75(10)*, 48A–H.

Amatayakul, M., & Lazarus, S. S. (2005). *Electronic health records, Transforming your medical practice.* Englewood, CO: Medical Group Management Association.

Bertrams, C. (2004, November/December). Well scrubbed, look for quality of data, flexibility in a claims validation system. *MGMA Connexion,* pp. 46–49.

Foley, M. M., & Garrett, G. S. (2006). The code ahead, Key issues shaping clinical terminology and classification. *Journal of AHIMA, 77(7)*, 24–28, 30.

Scott, K. S. (2011). Clinical vocabularies and classification systems. In M. L. Johns (Ed.), *Health Information Management Technology, An Applied Approach* (3rd ed.), (pp. 237–262). Chicago, IL: AHIMA.

REVIEW QUESTIONS

1. Outline the major steps in the coding and billing workflow in an EHR environment.

2. What code sets have been mandated by HIPAA for use in ambulatory care interactions?

3. What is a classification system? What is a nomenclature?

4. What four groups are responsible for providing recommendations for updates of ICD in the United States?

5. How frequently is ICD updated? How frequently are CPT and HCPCS Level II codes updated?

6. What system is used to code dental disorders? What system is used to code mental disorders?

7. What group is responsible for updates to CPT? To HCPCS Level II?

8. How are the use of MEDCIN and SNOMED-CT in an EHR useful to the coding process?

9. What is an encoder and how does it work?

10. What are the two methods used to identify terms for computer-assisted coding?

____

____

____

11. What advantages does computer assisted coding have over an encoder?

____

____

____

12. How are audit trails and scrubbers used in the coding and billing process?

____

____

____

13. What additional pieces of information are required for a complete bill, and from where within the EHR can they be obtained?

____

____

____

14. List at least three distinct types of practice reports that can be generated using data gathered from a combination of the medical record and practice management components of an EHR.

____

____

____

CHAPTER 12 Research, Registries, and Reportable Events

CHAPTER OUTLINE

OBJECTIVES

Upon completion of the chapter, the learner will be able to:

1. Define terms and key concepts used in relation to the research process.
2. Name the most common type of clinical trial and its purpose.
3. Describe the steps and phases in the product research process that involve patients and consequently content of EHRs and practice-management systems.
4. Describe the impact of research participation on the patient's electronic health record (EHR) in relation to patient identification, patient-care documentation, reimbursement for care, and sharing of patient-participant information.
5. Identify organizations that provide documentation standards relating to research in the practice setting
6. Define the terms "registries" and "reportable events".
7. Describe the role of an EHR in providing information to registries, in responding to reportable event requirements, and in meeting meaningful use criteria regarding research and public health.

KEY TERMS

case report form
clinical trial (clinical study)
diagnostic trials
Institutional Review Board (IRB)
Medicare qualifying trial
placebo
prevention trials
principal investigator
Privacy Board
protocol
quality-of-life trials
reportable event
screening trials
treatment trials

INTRODUCTION

On any day in the United States, there are thousands of medical research projects underway. Some will be successful and produce new drugs, devices, vaccines, and other biologic products; some may discover unknown facts about a disease or its treatment. Others will be dropped because the results show no impact or even adverse findings. Some research projects require identification of the patient to be effective, others do not. Discovery research often can be performed entirely in a laboratory setting or via reporting of data for summarization. However, before new products can be placed on the market in the United States, they must be tested thoroughly. To ensure that products are tested appropriately, and to protect humans who volunteer as participants in the research projects, the U.S. Food and Drug Administration has developed specific guidelines for all aspects of the research process. These guidelines help limit the risks of participating in a study and ensure that volunteers have all the information needed to make an informed decision regarding participation.

From the practice perspective, many health care providers are involved in research studies. Providers may be the primary researchers and administer the project. They may be contacted by other researchers to recommend patients that fit a study's criteria, or they may have patients that volunteer themselves as research participants. Whatever the role, it is important to note that content and use of an EHR will be affected. Patient compliance with study parameters may mean that care must also be adjusted. In the long run, supporting research eventually will result in better health care, a benefit from all views.

In addition, states or the federal government may require care-provider reporting of some diseases so that they can be monitored more thoroughly. For example, providers may be required to report data when they diagnose or treat neoplasms, especially malignant neoplasms. Data is transferred to a central registry where research, statistical analysis, and disease monitoring can be performed. Another type of government-mandated reportable event relates to the discovery of injuries or death potentially resulting from a crime or foul play. Care providers must comply with the laws and provide the patient information required. The EHR often can facilitate that reporting process.

MEDICAL PRODUCT DEVELOPMENT

To be able to describe the role of an EHR in research, a basic understanding of the research process is useful. Individuals develop ideas every day for new products, or new questions about disease development and responses that need investigation. Before products can be developed to answer these questions or offered to the public, research must be performed. Research tests the products and tries to uncover answers to questions raised without creating harm to the population for which the product is intended. Before the U.S. Food and Drug Administration can approve any new product, the product must undergo extensive testing. Drugs, vaccines, treatments, devices, and diagnostic tools are all subject to the federal government's review. A sequence of steps is followed routinely by researchers. The steps start in the laboratory, gradually introduce the product to a select number of humans, and eventually expand to larger and larger groups of volunteers. The part of testing involving humans is referred to as a **clinical trial or clinical study**.

clinical trial (clinical study)
Steps in the medical research process that involve humans.

Organization for Clinical Research

The first step of a clinical trial is formation of a research team that may include scientists, physicians, nurses, and other health care professionals. One member of the team serves as its leader or **principal investigator**. The team develops a detailed plan, called a **protocol**, for the study. The protocol will include the reason for the study, safeguards planned for participants, the length and timing of the study steps, how many volunteers will be needed, eligibility for participation, and details regarding information to be gathered including volunteer testing, medications, procedures, and so forth. Everyone who participates in the study uses the same protocol.

Next the protocol goes through a process of organizational review, usually by a committee referred to as an **Institutional Review Board (IRB)**. At least five multidisciplinary IRB members, including representatives of the general public, screen the plan carefully to ensure that it is sound, that the risk for volunteers will be minimal, that its focus is both legal and ethical, and that volunteers will be safeguarded, which includes being fully informed about the study and what it involves. In fact, all volunteers will be required to review and sign an informed consent. The IRB's work does not end there, because it also determines the frequency of project reviews and conducts them as the volunteer's advocate throughout the study. Another entity, a **Privacy Board**, also may be formed with the task of reviewing the protocol for compliance with HIPAA privacy regulations. This board also is a multidisciplinary group with expertise in privacy standards. Any concerns raised here must be addressed before the research can proceed.

After approval of the protocol and informed consent, research funding from a foundation or government agency may be sought, particularly if the team is part of a university or health care setting. The IRB-approved protocol for the project will be the foundation for the funding request. Some research is sponsored by the team's employer—for example, a drug company—or by health care providers themselves.

Clinical Research Focus and Steps

There are five types of clinical trials performed in the United States today (U.S. National Institutes of Health, 2007):

1. **Treatment trials** test experimental treatments, new combinations of drugs, or new approaches to surgery or radiation therapy.
2. **Prevention trials** look for better ways to prevent disease in people who have never had the disease, or to prevent a disease from returning. These approaches may include medicines, vaccines, vitamins, minerals, or lifestyle changes.
3. **Diagnostic trials** are conducted to find better tests or procedures for diagnosing a particular disease or condition.
4. **Screening trials** test the best way to detect certain diseases or health conditions.
5. **Quality-of-life trials** (or supportive-care trials) explore ways to improve comfort and the quality of life for individuals with a chronic illness.

Traditionally, treatment trials have been the most common type, but practice patients could participate in any of these types of trials.

Whichever trial type is the focus, once research funding is in place, defined steps must be performed by the sponsoring organization or group. Each research step

principal investigator
Member of a research team who serves as its leader.

protocol
Detailed plan for a research study.

Institutional Review Board (IRB)
Multidisciplinary group that reviews research protocols for soundness, risks to participants, safeguards, and legal and ethical issues.

Privacy Board
Multidisciplinary group of individuals from a health care setting that reviews a research protocol for compliance with HIPAA privacy regulations.

treatment trials
Type of clinical trial that tests experimental treatments, new combinations of drugs, or new approaches to surgery or radiation therapy.

prevention trials
Type of clinical trial that looks for better ways to prevent a disease in people who have never had it or to prevent a disease from recurring.

diagnostic trials
Type of clinical trial conducted to find better tests or procedures for diagnosing a particular disease or condition.

screening trials
Type of clinical trial that tests the best way to detect certain diseases or health conditions.

includes the name of the trial, its sponsor and protocol number, and at least a copy of the signed informed consent for trial participation. More information may be included as needed for proper reimbursement. The design of the EHR must support gathering this information, and a special alert may need to be added to remind care providers of the patient's study participation.

Care providers also must become familiar with the study treatment protocol so that, in addition to completing routine visit documentation, they also can monitor particular responses to the research treatment. The *Accreditation Handbook for Ambulatory Health Care* published by the AAAHC (2011, p. 42) goes one step further, stating: "Any notation in a patient's clinical record indicating diagnostic or therapeutic intervention as part of clinical research is clearly contrasted with entries regarding the provision of non-research related care." The Joint Commission has similar criteria stating that clinical records must contain "[a]ny documentation of clinical research interventions distinct from entries related to regular patient care, treatment or services." (RC.02.01.01, EP 4, p. RC-7.) Thus, if a practice seeks either Joint Commission or AAAHC accreditation, documentation related to research must be easily recognized as such. Special labeling, highlighting, or a distinct location for this type of documentation can be part of the EHR software program to meet this requirement.

If the research is not performed entirely within the practice, data from research participant records will be requested routinely by the research team. The HIPAA privacy rule includes special provisions for research allowing disclosure without consent, if information has been "deidentified." However, Privacy Board review is required for approval of a waiver of patient authorization to release information. (OCR HIPAA Privacy, 2002.) Both the research team and the practice must be in compliance with these rules before any information is shared. That means that the practice must develop some approval process, perhaps via an IRB/Privacy Board, to review informational requests and to develop guidelines. Data requested must be consistent with the project's protocol. If patient identifiers are to be shared, then an authorization for release of information (signed by the patient or the patient's representative) will be needed. If the group performing the research is within the practice, those providers must develop a process to abstract data and, of course, protect patient confidentiality. EHRs provide the opportunity for efficient data exchange after appropriate safeguards have been met.

Finally, if a patient develops adverse effects that possibly could be associated with research interventions, it is a provider's obligation to contact the research team, report the findings, and document them in the EHR. The patient's situation then will be evaluated by the research team, and the patient may be pulled from the study. It is the documentation of the primary care provider that often provides evidence for or against success for the research team. If required documentation is not currently part of the practice EHR, then programming changes will be required.

Reimbursement

Reimbursement for the medical care provided in clinics or offices as part of research studies may or may not be covered by third-party payers. Treatment types of studies are covered more frequently. If the study's approach is seen as "experimental" or "investigational" the possibility of funding decreases. Some states have passed legislation that requires reimbursement for the routine costs of patient care in a study. These routine costs of care involve the visits, tests, and studies that usually would be done for patients with the particular disease even if they were not part of the study. Some payers may have other requirements, and some costs may not be paid. Such unpaid costs are often, but not always, reimbursed through the research funding. It is important that providers obtain clear information about reimbursement at the beginning of a patient's qualifying treatment, just as it is for patients seen in a practice who are not part of a research study.

In 2000, Medicare changed a long-standing policy and began reimbursing for the routine costs of care and associated costs from medical complications in Medicare-approved treatment studies, referred to as **Medicare qualifying trials**. (CMS, 2011.) This change of policy was meant to encourage patients who qualify for Medicare to participate in research. Most research studies are performed with younger age groups, but many treatments address the Medicare population. It is important to understand the impact of a new product on this population if it will be the targeted age group, and this can be done only if research studies include individuals from that group. Since then the policy has been updated several times. Updates include guidelines for what Medicare will or will not pay and which patients can be covered, among other aspects. If a practice has Medicare patients participating in qualified studies, these guidelines must be followed to receive reimbursement and the EHR will be the source document for evidence of compliance.

Medicare qualifying trial Clinical trial meeting Medicare's criteria as an approved study so that the routine costs of care and associated costs from medical complications it may produce can be reimbursed.

Medicare usually covers reasonable and necessary services that are normally covered by Medicare but are associated with a trial, as well as those costs that relate to the diagnosis and treatment of medical complications from participating in a clinical trial. The participant's medical records and the bill forwarded to Medicare must contain qualifying trial information. The EHR must be able to capture all required data.

Bills submitted to Medicare for services provided to qualifying trial research patients must meet federal guidelines. Medicare requires that a special Q1 or Q0 modifier code (QV or QA prior to January 1, 2008) be added to certain line item codes to indicate routine services or investigational items or services provided in a qualifying trial. CMS suggests that practices voluntarily report the specific eight-digit clinical trial number as well. These guidelines may be revised in the future, so it is important that care providers routinely review Medicare publications to maintain current billing practices. The CMS web site or the contracted Medicare Part B claims processor in the practice area are possible resources for this information. (See also the Computer Exploration at the end of this chapter.)

Patients who participate in non-Medicare studies may be covered for routine care as well, particularly if the practice is located in a state with mandatory coverage legislation. Providers need to be aware of state laws that may affect billing. It may be necessary to contact the research team regarding coverage for care that is not reimbursable by third-party payers. Billing to the research team requires detailed information so that claims meet funding requirements and are sent to the correct location. Meeting these requirements means that practice management software or EHR content changes occur. In an EHR environment, all claims are sent electronically via interface of the practice management program with EHR data.

STANDARDS THAT SUPPORT RESEARCH

Four national groups provide standards that impact the research process in practice settings. In addition to the standards on record documentation described previously in this chapter, the AAAHC's 2011 *Accreditation Handbook*

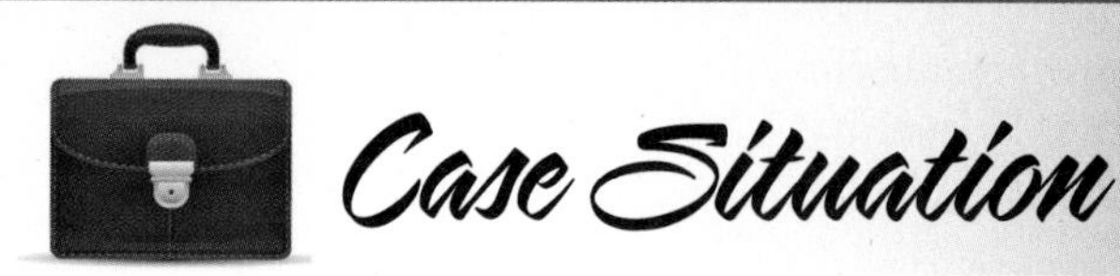

Two psychiatrists have been approached by a drug company to include in a Phase III trial several of their adult patients being treated for bipolar disorder. The psychiatrists receive comprehensive information from the drug company, including the company's internal IRB review, specific guidelines for protection of human subjects, and the results of previous human testing. Under the research protocol, the partners would continue to see and supervise their patients while on the new medication. Because the partners have been active in research studies in the past, they have written practice policies to follow. They perform their own review of the research protocol against the policy criteria and also provide their lawyer a copy for review. The study seems to have all components addressed in practice policies, including those that allow patients to opt out at any time. The lawyer for the practice also is satisfied with the study parameters.

Patients are approached regarding participation. If interested and willing, the study is explained to each in detail and a lengthy informed consent—which includes the steps in the study, the length of the study, the confidentiality provisions, the opt-out choice, and any possible adverse findings—is explained. Then the informed consent is signed and witnessed. The patient's psychiatrist closely monitors the patient's progress on the medication and documents specific notes in the patient record. Laboratory tests are performed as outlined in the protocol and practice policies. Reports to the study investigators are required periodically. According to set privacy guidelines, they are produced by sending portions of the patient record and a research report (both part of the EHR) to them electronically.

for Ambulatory Health Care and The Joint Commission's 2011 *Standards for Ambulatory Care* include entire sections related to setting up and maintaining research studies, including patient rights. If a practice decides to take this step, those standards should be reviewed.

The third set of research-related standards comes from the federal government's "meaningful use" criteria. Federal standards note simply that the EHR system must be able to "[g]enerate lists of patients by specific conditions to use for quality improvement, reduction of disparities, research or outreach." (Federal Register, 2010, p. 44373.) Two CCHIT ambulatory functionality criteria address clinical trials indirectly through guidelines for setting up patient-monitoring practices or reminder lists based on selected demographic data, and for removing patient identifiers prior to exporting data (CCHIT, 2010).

REGISTRIES AND REPORTABLE EVENTS

Registries often are sponsored by government agencies to gather health care data on specific populations. For example, a cancer registry records medical data for patients diagnosed with a malignant tumor, and a birth defects registry records data on newborns with birth defects. Registries help identify geographic areas where diseases are found, effective treatments, life spans of those with the disease, conditions under which the disease occurs, and so forth. Federal and state laws at times require providers to participate in submitting data for registries so that information gathered is comprehensive and effective preventive efforts or treatment can be identified. If built into the EHR software, required data elements for this type of reporting can be identified, automatically abstracted, and electronically sent via secure networks to the appropriate government agency. This type of routine reporting saves the practice time and money while contributing to population research on the incidence and prevalence of diseases.

State laws also may require reporting of suspected illegal activities such as child or elder abuse or injury caused by violent means (hitting, stabbing, etc.). Certain contagious diseases such as tuberculosis and sexually transmitted diseases also may require reporting. These defined situations are referred to generically as **reportable events**. Laws or regulations covering such events also will designate the specific government health agency or department to receive the report or medical information. If programmed appropriately, the EHR is particularly efficient at gathering required abstracted information from treatment data. It also can be the tool for reporting information to authorized groups without the repetition of manually transferring information to a report. Regional data then can be provided for health care planning, education, and timely interventions such as preventive or treatment activities.

reportable events Medical diagnoses or disorders that a government entity has mandated be reported for public health or safety reasons.

If at all, standards groups focus on patient rights in the reporting process, rather than on the process itself. For example, The Joint Commission section on the Rights and Responsibilities of the Individual states, "The informed consent process includes a discussion about any circumstances under which information about the patient must be disclosed or reported." A note is then added to provide examples. "Such circumstances may include requirements for disclosure of information regarding cases of HIV, tuberculosis, viral meningitis, and other diseases that are reported to organizations such as health departments or the Centers for Disease Control and Prevention." (2011, p. RI-8.) More specific to the EHR, the Federal Register Stage 1 Meaningful Use Objectives indicate that the EHR of Eligible Professionals should provide the "[c]apability to submit electronic data to immunization registries or Immunization Information Systems and actual submission in accordance with applicable law and practice . . . [and the] [c]apability to submit electronic syndromic [signs, symptoms, etc.] surveillance data to public health agencies and actual submission in accordance with applicable law and practice." (2010, pp. 44374, 44375.)

SUMMARY

Research plays an important role in the United States, accounting for many of the medical advances that have become commonplace today. Because there is potential for harm to research participants, safeguards have been put in place to protect human volunteers. These safeguards include the development of a written protocol, review and approval of the protocol by an IRB/Privacy Board, provision of an extensive participant written-informed consent, and graduated steps for involvement of humans in clinical trials. There are five basic types of trials: treatment, diagnostic, prevention, screening, and quality-of-life. Practices may become involved in research by sponsoring it, referring patients to projects, or monitoring patients while they participate in a study. Each level of participation has an impact on the practice in relation to its review processes, documentation of care in the EHR, and reimbursement. Special challenges may be discovered by practices in identification of research participants, meeting documentation guidelines, and receiving appropriate reimbursement. A fully functioning EHR can address all of these concerns, in part or in full, while meeting standards set by a number of approval bodies including the AAAHC, The Joint Commission, the CCHIT, and "meaningful use" criteria. An EHR also can facilitate mandatory reporting for reportable events and provide data for health care registries.

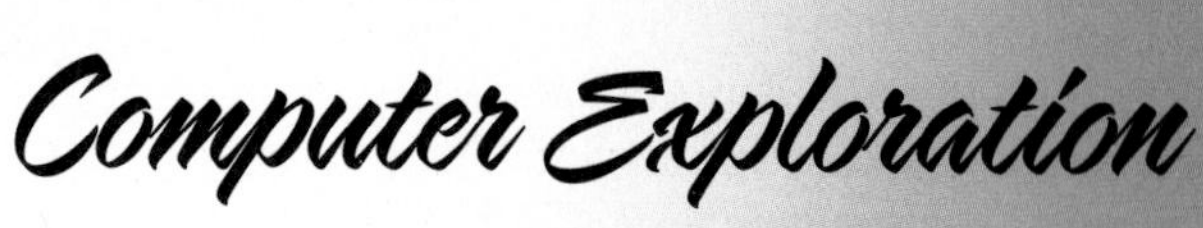

1. Visit http://www.cancer.gov/clinicaltrials/payingfor/laws and identify the states that require health plans to cover patient care costs in clinical trials. Does your state require coverage? If so, click on your state and read the information provided about coverage. If not, click on any other state and note the coverage it provides.
2. Visit https://www.cms.gov/ClinicalTrialsPolicies/ and locate the link to Chapter 32, Section 69 of the Medical Claims Processing Manual. Open that document and find Subsection 69.6 that provides the directions for coding of research-participant claims in the provider office-setting. What codes are used for reporting routine costs associated with a Clinical Trial?
3. Each state defines its own reportable communicable diseases, often in its public health laws or regulations. As an example, Arizona's list can be found at http://www.azdhs.gov/phs/oids/pdf/rptlist.pdf Access that list and find the diagnoses that must be reported electronically or by telephone within 24 hours after diagnosis, treatment, or detection. What are those diagnoses?

REFERENCES

AAAHC [American Association for Ambulatory Health Care, Inc.]. (2011). *Accreditation handbook for ambulatory health care.* Wilmette, IL.

CCHIT [Certification Commission for Healthcare Information Technology]. (2010). CCHIT Certified 2011 Ambulatory EHR Certification Criteria. Retrieved August 7, 2010, from http://www.cchit.org/.

CMS [Centers for Medicare & Medicaid Services]. (2011). Medicare clinical trial policies. Retrieved from http://www.cms.hhs.gov/ClinicalTrialsPolicies.

Crerand, W. J., Lamb, J., Rulon, V., Karal, B., & Mardekian, J. (2002). Building data quality into clinical trials. *Journal of AHIMA, 73(10)*, 44–46.

OCR HIPAA Privacy. (2002, December). Research [45 CFR 164.501, 164.508, 164.512(i)], pp. 85–98.

The Joint Commission. (2011). *Standards for ambulatory care.* Oakbrook Terrace, IL.

U.S. Department of Health and Human Services. (2010). *Federal register 42CFR parts 412, 413, 422 et al, Medicare and Medicaid programs; Electronic health record incentive program; Final rule,* 75(144)Washington, DC: National Archives and Record Administration.

U.S. National Institutes of Health. (2007, September). Understanding clinical trials. Retrieved from http://www.clinicaltrials.gov/ct2/info/understand.

REVIEW QUESTIONS

1. Define each of these terms in relation to the research process:

   a. case report form

   b. IRB

   c. placebo

   d. principal investigator

   e. Privacy Board

   f. protocol

2. What is a clinical trial? What is a Medicare-qualified clinical trial?

3. Several hundred healthy individuals are testing the use of a new drug. What clinical trial step or phase does that statement describe?

4. Two years after a new heart drug is FDA approved it is recalled and banned because evidence has developed that it has side effects that are potentially fatal. What clinical trial step does this statement describe? What data might have the participant EHRs provided to support the recall action?

5. Research can affect a care provider's practice in many ways. Describe how it might change the EHR or practice management system content in relation to:

   a. **The type of identifying information collected from the patient.**

   ____

   ____

   ____

   b. **Documentation of the health care provider regarding a patient's visit.**

   ____

   ____

   ____

   c. **Assignment of codes submitted on a bill for services.**

   ____

   ____

   ____

   d. **Requests for release of/provision of patient information.**

   ____

   ____

   ____

6. The AAAHC, Joint Commission, and CCHIT all have standards that affect the content or functioning of an EHR in relation to research. Which of these three requires that documentation relating to research monitors be separate from standard visit documentation?

   ____

   ____

   ____

7. How does an EHR assist in submission of patient information to registries or as required by the government for reportable events?

   ____

   ____

   ____

CHAPTER 13 Personal Health Records and Continuing Care Records

CHAPTER OUTLINE

Personal Health Record
Communication Among Providers for Continuing Care
Continuity of Care Record

OBJECTIVES

Upon completion of the chapter, the learner will be able to:

1. Define personal health record (PHR) and continuity of care record (CCR).
2. Describe the reasons supporting the development of both types of records.
3. Name several alternatives for maintaining/storing a PHR.
4. List a variety of data categories and elements from the American Health Information Management Association (AHIMA) and the Medicare descriptions for the content of a PHR.
5. Identify groups that provide standards or criteria that address documentation of communication between care providers.
6. Describe the American Society for Testing and Materials (ASTM) content standards for continuity of care records.
7. Identify the key to and process for accessing a CCR.
8. Describe two options for maintaining a CCR.

KEY TERMS

continuity of care record (CCR)

personal health record (PHR)

INTRODUCTION

Health care has seen many changes over the past decade, including easy access to many sources of health-related information. This information is available not only to health care providers, but also (via the Internet) to patients, the consumers of health care. Patients can perform their own research on diseases, compare the costs of one medication payment plan to another, check quality of care data provided by accrediting and licensing organizations, and learn about a new treatment, all via the Internet. Patients also can compile records of their own health information so they can communicate more accurately with, and ask informed questions of, their care providers. Personal health records (PHRs) provide a service to both the patient and the health care provider. Patient recording of health care events when and wherever they occur helps to ensure that information will not be forgotten at the next provider visit. Providers appreciate receiving more thorough information about the patient's condition to assist in treatment. This information or portions of it can be added to a practice's EHR. As a result, steps to define, develop, and encourage the use of PHRs, a patient-controlled type of EHR, have come from both consumers and health-related organizations.

Another new method of communication is used entirely by health care providers. Communication is important between providers that are currently involved in the care of a patient, or between a current provider and one who has treated the patient in the past. At times, access to health care treatment information (e.g., current medications and allergies) can prevent a life-threatening situation from developing. Emergency services can be more focused if a patient's diagnoses and health problems are known. Access to results of tests previously performed by other care providers can save both time and the cost of repeat testing. At times, information provided by the patient may not be specific enough for the needs of a health care provider, or the patient may be severely injured and unable to communicate. The EHR provides the framework for sharing of information between health care providers via what is referred to as the continuity of care record.

PERSONAL HEALTH RECORD

personal health record (PHR) Documentation system that allows consumers to gather, store, access, and coordinate their health information.

For a variety of reasons, patients may want to develop a **personal health record (PHR)**, defined as a "system (or combination of systems) that allows consumers to store, access, and coordinate their health information." (Friedman, 2005, p. 43.) Patients may have already, out of necessity, gathered records for themselves or family members who have complicated medical conditions or who are seeing multiple care providers. Putting medical information into an electronic format is more efficient than keeping copies of volumes of paper. Patients may be encouraged by their health care provider to keep a personal record. Perhaps they could not remember all the historical detail that the provider needed and began keeping records as a result. They may be receiving a variety of medications and need records to manage them, or they just may want to take a more active role in monitoring their own health status.

For whatever reason, health care consumers/patients are creating personal health records. The records may originate on paper, but more frequently are maintained electronically on a personal computer, a web-based private account, a smart card (electronically readable card similar to a credit card; see Chapter 1), a portable device such as an iPad, or some combination of these.

In the future, a computer-readable chip or a microchip implant in an arm or other accessible area of the body may become common. Smart cards and implanted chips, often sponsored by medical care-related organizations, require digital electronic readers to transfer the information to a computer for use in treatment situations. Because of this, sponsoring medical groups or health plans must make sure that practices have the proper equipment available to use them effectively.

PHRs benefit not only the patient but also care providers, payers, employers, and the health of the public in general. The National Committee on Vital and Health Statistics summarized these benefits in a special report. The benefits identified can be found in Table 13-1.

The sources for information contained in a PHR also may vary. For example, there may be times where the patient or the patient's guardian or legal representative requests information from a care provider to add to a PHR. Once the right to access has been verified, information can be shared. The practice's EHR must contain all copies of legal papers, entered via scanning, as well as a record of what actually was shared with the patient. This information becomes part of the EHR's logs of internal access and release of information. Patients can obtain other information from payers, employers, the Internet, self-monitor flow charts, or public health records. Recent federal regulations have given a qualified patient the right to receive laboratory tests directly from the labs where testing occurs. Information from all of these sources can become part of a PHR. As a result, a PHR can become a lifelong record that is owned and managed by the individual patient. Access is provided only by that individual, who maintains and protects the record.

Early national efforts outlining the content of a PHR were completed by a work group of AHIMA. These data elements are listed in Table 13-2 (see AHIMA, 2005a, for further definition of many of the elements). As evidenced by the content outline, the information maintained provides a comprehensive, lifelong view of the patient's health history and status. Of course, not all elements may be found in all PHRs, but the AHIMA guidelines serve as an excellent resource.

Medicare encourages its members to compile a PHR and provides a less extensive list of elements. The Medicare sample PHR content items can be found in Table 13-3. These basic items are a good starting place for all health care consumers when reviewing a variety of PHR products for personal use. The same Medicare web site provides additional resources including questions to use when choosing a PHR vendor.

Other efforts are under way to support and encourage development, standardization, and use of PHRs. For example, policies for electronic sharing of information between providers and patients were the focus of the "Connecting for Health" collaboration between the Markle Foundation and the Robert Wood Johnson Foundation. This group of 25 industry leaders found that:

> Widespread use will require the adoption of common data sets, methods of patient identification, and privacy and security protections. Patients must be at the center of the PHR, controlling its use and access as well as maintaining responsibility for its content. (Burrington-Brown, 2005, p. 1.)

To date, however, the work toward a standardized base of information still is being sought, although the Continuity of Care Record discussed later in this chapter, (see Table 13-4) is suggested by some as an appropriate foundation. Other standards relating to use or transfer of information between health care provider EHRs and PHRs also are being promoted.

TABLE 13-1 Key Potential Benefits of PHRs and PHR Systems

ROLE	BENEFITS
Consumers, patients, and their caregivers	Support wellness activities. Improve understanding of health issues. Increase sense of control over health. Increase control over access to personal health information. Support timely, appropriate preventive services. Support health care decisions and responsibility for care. Strengthen communication with providers. Verify accuracy of information in provider records. Support home monitoring for chronic diseases. Support understanding and appropriate use of medications. Support continuity of care across time and providers. Manage insurance benefits and claims. Avoid duplicate tests. Reduce adverse drug interactions and allergic reactions. Reduce hassle through online appointment scheduling and prescription refills. Increase access to providers via e-visits.
Health care providers	Improve access to data from other providers and the patients themselves. Increase knowledge of potential drug interactions and allergies. Avoid duplicate tests. Improve medication compliance. Provide information to patients for both health care and patient services purposes. Provide patients with convenient access to specific information or services (e.g., lab results, Rx refills, e-visits). Improve documentation of communication with patients.
Payers	Improve customer service (transactions and information). Promote portability of patient information across plan. Support wellness and preventive care. Provide information and education to beneficiaries.
Employers	Support wellness and preventive care. Provide convenient service. Improve workforce productivity. Promote empowered health care consumers. Use aggregate data to manage employee health.
Society/population health benefits	Strengthen health promotion and disease prevention. Improve the health of populations. Expand health education opportunities.

Source: National Committee on Vital and Health Statistics, "Personal Health Records and Personal Health Systems," February 2006, p. 7 (available at www.ncvhs.hhs.gov/0602nhiirpt.pdf)

TABLE 13-2 AHIMA Defined Common Data Elements in the PHR

PERSONAL INFORMATION	
Name	Address (multiple)
Contact information	Personal identification
Marital status	Employer information (multiple)
Languages spoken	School
EMERGENCY CONTACTS	
Contact type	Name
Relationship	Address
Contact information	Employer information
HEALTH CARE PROVIDERS (MULTIPLE ENTRIES ALLOWED)	
Health care provider type	Name
Group or association name	Primary care physician (yes or no)
Address	Contact information
INSURANCE PROVIDERS (MULTIPLE ENTRIES ALLOWED)	
Insurance provider type	Company name
Address	Contact or agent
Identification	Contact information
Deductible	Co–pays
Primary insured person	
LEGAL DOCUMENTS AND MEDICAL DIRECTIVES (MULTIPLE ENTRIES ALLOWED)	
Document or directive type	Document location (physical location)
Legal representative (person assigned legal authority)	Organ donation
Contact (person with access to the document)	
Date filed	
Document image (image or copy of actual legal document)	
GENERAL MEDICAL INFORMATION	
Height (feet and inches)	Weight (pounds)
Blood	Last physical or check-up
General conditions checklist	

(*continues*)

TABLE 13-2 *(continued)*

ALLERGIES AND DRUG SENSITIVITIES (MULTIPLE ENTRIES ALLOWED)	
Allergy or sensitivity type	Reaction
Severity	Date last occurred
Doctor	Treatment
Comments	
CONDITIONS (MULTIPLE ENTRIES ALLOWED)	
Condition type	Date diagnosed
Doctor	Age at onset
Treatment	Condition status
Comments	
SURGERIES (MULTIPLE ENTRIES ALLOWED)	
Procedure	Description
Date	Doctor
Hospital	Results
Comments	
MEDICATIONS—PRESCRIPTION AND NONPRESCRIPTION (MULTIPLE ENTRIES ALLOWED)	
Medication name	Dosage
Quantity number	Quantity form
Frequency	Start date
Stop date	Prescribed by
Prescription date	Prescription number
Pharmacy	Allergic reaction
Comments	
IMMUNIZATIONS (MULTIPLE ENTRIES ALLOWED)	
Immunization type	Date
Booster (yes or no)	Administered by
Reason	Comments
DOCTOR VISITS (MULTIPLE ENTRIES ALLOWED)	
Visit type	Date
Doctor	Reason
Diagnosis	Comments

TABLE 13-2 *(continued)*

HOSPITALIZATIONS (MULTIPLE ENTRIES ALLOWED)	
Hospitalization type (includes ER)	Admission date
Discharge date	Doctor
Hospital	Reason
Diagnosis	Complications
Comments	
OTHER HEALTH CARE VISITS (MULTIPLE ENTRIES ALLOWED)	
Visit type	Date
Health care professional	Reason
Diagnosis	Treatment
Comments	
PREGNANCIES (MULTIPLE ENTRIES ALLOWED)	
Pregnancy term	Due date or date of birth
Delivery type	Weeks early or late or weeks of gestation
Gender	Child's name
Doctor	Hospital
Admission date	Discharge date
Complications	Comments
MEDICAL DEVICES (MULTIPLE ENTRIES ALLOWED)	
Device type	Doctor
Hospital	Reason
Date	Comments
FAMILY MEMBER HISTORY (MULTIPLE ENTRIES ALLOWED)	
Relationship	Birthplace
Date of birth	Current health status
If deceased (age and cause)	Comments
Family general history	Social history
FOREIGN TRAVEL (MULTIPLE ENTRIES ALLOWED)	
Country (dates and comments)	

(continues)

TABLE 13-2 *(continued)*	
THERAPY (MULTIPLE ENTRIES ALLOWED)	
Therapy type	Start date
Stop date	Frequency
Therapist	Administered by
VITAL SIGNS (MULTIPLE ENTRIES ALLOWED)	
VISION (MULTIPLE ENTRIES ALLOWED)	
DENTAL (MULTIPLE ENTRIES ALLOWED)	
MISCELLANEOUS	
AUDIT LOG	

A number of health plans, health-related associations, foundations, employers, physician practices, and vendors have become involved in the funding or development of PHR products. The PHRs that they develop may be available to the general public or may be released only to members of a specific group. For example, U.S. military veterans have a PHR specifically designed for them called MyHealtheVet. Consumers have many choices available to them directly.

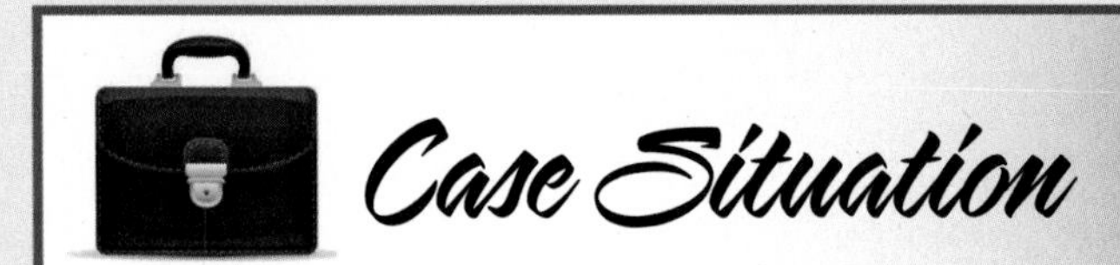

At the encouragement of her physician, a patient accessed the http://www.myPHR.com web site and located an organization that offered a free PHR template. She downloaded the template and began entering the information (personal identification, personal and family history, medications, immunization, etc.) that it required. The information was quite comprehensive, so she also made a list of the questions she wanted to ask her physician about her prior and current care the next time she had an appointment. She continued to add information over the following months until she felt she had a thorough and accurate record. Whenever she traveled out of state, she carried a copy of the electronic file with her. Her insurance company even provided her with the option of loading the information onto a smart card. She was grateful that she had the information when she was involved in an automobile accident while visiting her sister in another state. Her sister knew of the card and referred the emergency room (ER) personnel to it for her current medication and allergy information and general health status. Because they had a card reader and could access the information, the ER personnel could provide needed attention more quickly and with limited chances of an adverse reaction from medications administered.

TABLE 13-3 Elements Suggested by Medicare for a PHR

Name	Birthdate
Current Address	
Name(s) of emergency contact(s)	Telephone number(s) of emergency contact(s)
Name(s) of all doctors, specialists, dentists	Telephone number(s) and address(es) of all doctors, specialists, dentists
Name of health insurer(s) (third party payers)	Telephone number(s) for insurer(s) contacts
Current medications	Medication dosages
Allergies (food, drug, and other substances)	
Important events and hereditary conditions in family history	Dates associated with historical events
Significant illnesses	Dates of significant illnesses
Significant surgical procedures	Dates of significant surgical procedures
Results of recent doctor visits	
Important test results	
Eye records	Dental records
Immunization records	
Other information such as exercise regime, over-the-counter and herbal medicines taken, counseling received, etc.	

Source: Manage Your Health at www.medicare.gov

The web site http://www.myPHR.com, sponsored by the American Health Information Management Association, includes a listing of many private PHR vendors. Some vendors charge for access to their PHR product, some host a PHR on a web site and require online registration and password protection for use, while others provide products that are free and can be downloaded to personal computers.

COMMUNICATION AMONG PROVIDERS FOR CONTINUING CARE

Communication from one care provider in a practice to another provider outside of the practice about a patient's treatment is also important. Health care providers need to have accurate information about the patient's current diagnoses, medications, health status, and important test results in order to provide quality care. Current information is particularly important in the event of an accident, emergency, or other situation when the patient is unable to communicate. Various studies across the nation have reported a large number of adverse patient incidents that developed when care providers treated patients without necessary information, as well as the time and money wasted when repeat examinations and testing took place.

Another type of inter-provider communication occurs when a patient is referred to a specialist or therapist for consultation or is discharged from an inpatient facility. In these instances, information must be transferred to the patient's other care providers for coordination of services. As a result of these situations, federal regulations have been written to support data sharing among providers.

HIPAA guidelines specifically state that confidential patient information may be exchanged between care providers for health care purposes without patient consent. HIPAA also allows the exchange of information to public health agencies mandated by law to receive information from providers regarding communicable diseases or other health concerns. Usually consents also are not needed for these specialized releases of information. However, a notation of the information shared must be placed in the patient's record (EHR), and the patient must be given access to those notations.

Accreditation associations also recognize the importance of sharing information across providers, and include basic guidelines in their standards. The AAAHC standard is found in Section 6, Clinical Records and Health Information:

> O. The organization is responsible for ensuring a patient's continuity of care. If a patient's primary or specialty care provider(s) or health care organization is elsewhere, the organization ensures that timely summaries or pertinent records necessary for continuity of patient care are:
>
> 1. Obtained from the other (external) provider(s) or organization and incorporated into the patient's clinical record
> 2. Provided to the other (external) health care professional(s) or consultant and, as appropriate, to the organization where future care will be provided. (2011, p. 42.)

The Joint Commission standards note that clinical records need to contain "[a]ny referrals or communications made to internal or external care providers and community agencies ... [and] a copy of any information made available to the practitioner or medical organization providing follow-up care, treatment, or services" after urgent care is provided. (2011, p. RC-7.)

An EHR easily can perform these functions. In fact, the Federal Register includes two EHR criteria for sharing of information for health care purposes that "Eligible Professionals" ("EPs") must meet to be eligible for "meaningful use" Stage 1 incentive funding:

> **Improve care coordination** - Capability to exchange key clinical information (for example, problem list, medication list, medication allergies, diagnostic test results), among providers of care and patient authorized entities electronically ... The EP ... who transitions their patient to another setting of care or provider of care or refers their patient to another provider of care should provide summary of care record for each transition of care or referral. (Federal Register, July 28, 2010, p. 44372, 44374.)

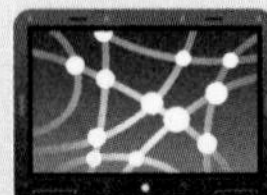

View the functional criteria used by CCHIT to certify ambulatory EHRs at the CCHIT website: www.cchit.org/.

The federal standards are further defined and supported by CCHIT's criteria for certification of ambulatory care EHR products.

Providers may share information via all the methods (e.g., paper, fax, e-mail) noted in Chapter 10 with respect to patient-focused communication. Electronic sharing of patient information has some unique characteristics. Information shared between providers via secure computer networks is presented as organized data elements instead of forms. Once the data is received, the receiving provider may use the data as a basis for current health care decisions.

Sending an entire patient record (or records of multiple encounters) from one provider to another is cumbersome and often unnecessary. Providers focus on specific information for follow-up care, so a defined summary of current treatment usually is sufficient. No clear definition has existed, however, regarding what routinely should be shared. Practices currently set their own policies regarding this process. In the EHR environment, the task can become essentially an electronic one if there is consistent identification of patients across providers involved and a common description of record components to be included in exchanges. Thus the process becomes more efficient and requires less personnel time.

CONTINUITY OF CARE RECORD

The **continuity of care record (CCR)** is a tool—designed especially for the EHR environment—for communicating important patient information among authorized providers. The CCR includes sets of information from the patient's electronic health record database contributed by any health care provider who has treated the patient. As defined by the ASTM (2005, p. 3), the continuity of care record is:

> a core data set of the most relevant administrative, demographic, and clinical information facts about a patient's healthcare, covering one or more healthcare encounters. It provides a means for one healthcare practitioner, system, or setting to aggregate all of the pertinent data about a patient and forward it to another practitioner, system, or setting to support the continuity of care.

continuity of care record (CCR)

Tool for communication between authorized health care providers from different settings; includes defined sets of information from a provider's EHR database.

Data from a provider is gathered during and after the patient visit. Upon a request for information from an authorized system user, the CCR (or a designated portion of it) is sent via a secure health network (e.g., one used by an established RHIO, HIE, SNO, ACO, or NHIN; see Chapter 1). The CCR also can be printed for delivery in paper format for providers who are not part of an established network. Care providers receiving the data online can access and update it anytime during a patient visit. Therefore, office time to locate information and then copy and perhaps mail it is reduced or eliminated, and current data is consistently available when care actually is being provided (i.e., at the point of care).

As with the EHR itself, standards for the content of a CCR are important. If standards exist, providers who share information will know exactly what data is available, and software can be developed by vendors to support the CCR dataset. Standard specifications for a CCR were developed and released by ASTM under the sponsorship of 11 technology and physician groups. The purpose of the specifications is to:

> enhance patient safety, reduce medical errors, reduce costs, enhance efficiency of health information exchange, and assure at least a minimum standard of health information transportability when a patient is referred, transferred, or is otherwise seen by another practitioner. (ASTM, 2005, p. 5.)

The ASTM specifications subdivide the CCR information into three distinct core sections: the CCR header, CCR body, and CCR footer. Table 13-4 provides specific information on the content of each of these sections. The individual patient's data is provided at the time the CCR is produced—either before, during, or after the point of care.

TABLE 13-4 ASTM Standard Content for the CCR

CCR HEADER INFORMATION	
UNIQUE IDENTIFIER	INFORMATION GENERATED BY THE ORIGINATING SYSTEM UNIQUELY IDENTIFYING THIS SPECIFIC CCR.
Language	Language used to express the CCR.
Version	Version of CCR Implementation Guide used.
Date/Time	Date and time the CCR data was produced.
Patient	Single patient identifier used in the CCR system.
From	Role and identification of originator of CCR information.
To	Role and identification of receiver of CCR information.
Purpose	Reason for CCR generation (e.g., admission, discharge, transfer, referral, consult).
CCR BODY INFORMATION	
Payers	Pertinent payers for this specific CCR, including contact and billing information and specific authorization data.
Advance directives	Existence of any advance directive and its location.
Support	Patient's support providers and contacts (e.g., family, legal guardian, clergy, caregivers).
Functional status	Status of functioning (e.g., competency, activities of daily living, ambulatory status, self-care ability).
Problems	Patient's relevant current and historical problems, conditions, diagnoses, symptoms, findings, and complaints presented in a designated sequence; coded via SNOMED-CT and ICD.
Family history	Relevant health risk factors in blood or genetic relatives.
Social history	Patient's occupation, lifestyle, social, and environmental history; health risk factors; demographic information such as race, ethnicity, religion, marital status.
Alerts	Allergies, adverse reactions, and other patient safety alerts.
Medications	Current and pertinent history of medications.
Medical equipment	Current and pertinent history of implanted and external medical devices and equipment; current durable medical equipment.
Immunizations	Current and historical immunizations.
Vital signs	Current and relevant history of vital signs (includes standard vitals plus others as appropriate including body mass index, head circumference, crown to rump length, pulse oximetry, pulmonary function tests).
Results	Most recent and pertinent laboratory, diagnostic, and therapeutic results.

TABLE 13-4 (*continued*)

Procedures	Historically pertinent interventional, surgical, diagnostic, or therapeutic procedures or treatments; coded via SNOMED-CT, LOINC, and CPT.
Encounters	Hospitalizations, office visits, home health visits, long-term care stays, or other encounters.
Plan of care	Pending orders, interventions, encounters, services, and procedures and clinical reminders.
Health care providers	Current and pertinent historical care providers.
CCR FOOTER INFORMATION	
Actors	Individuals, organizations, locations, and systems associated with data in the CCR.
References	External reference data for information in the CCR (e.g., articles, URLs, images, patient records).
Comments	Comments relating to a CCR section; cannot contain clinical or administrative data.
Signatures	Signatures associated with any CCR data.

Most of the information in the CCR body (as described in Table 13-4) will be part of standard EHR documentation maintained in a practice EHR database. Those items can be identified and transferred electronically to the shared record through mapping from one system to the other. The contents of the header and footer sections are part of the CCR system structure itself and would be added by those who maintain the CCR. A sample of a CCR is shown in Figure 13-1.

The key to sharing information through a CCR is correct patient identification so that data can be retrieved regionally, nationally, and (in the future) even internationally. To be able to do this, each care provider must use the same definitions for entering patient identifying information—including name, birth date, and other demographic data—in order to distinguish each patient uniquely. Computer programs then can match information from one provider with information from another for the same patient. If the CCR is part of a larger network of providers, a network patient identifier also may be assigned and used. This may become a national patient identifier, as advocated by HIPAA regulations, at some time in the future. When a patient arrives in a health treatment setting, or when the care provider decides that additional treatment information is needed, the patient identifier (RHIO, HIE, SNO, ACO, or NHIN) or the full CCR patient index is queried for the existence of a record for the specific patient. If the identifier or a patient index entry is found by matching the patient identifier and other patient identification data exactly, then the patient's current CCR is accessed. The CCR appearing on the provider's computer screen is a summary from care providers contributing to the CCR. The treating physician can add information to the CCR and update it with current treatment information. Thus the CCR is a dynamic or ever-changing

Continuity of Care Record

Date Created:	Sat Sep 16, 2006 at 08:03 PM UTC
From:	Dr. John Smithers (Primary Care Provider) TEPR CCR Demo Health Clinic Solventus CCR ViewPort V1.0
To:	Shirley Eichenwald Maki (Primary Care Provider)
Purpose:	Request For Consult

Patient Demographics

Name	Date of Birth	Gender	Identification Numbers	Address / Phone
Shirley Ann Demo	May 16, 1955	Female	MRN: 112233 SSN: 239-00-0000	**Home:** 3333 Maxwell Blvd Xavier, ME59988 Home: 612-455-9999

Advance Directives

Type	Date		Description	Status	Source
Resuscitation Status	Recorded Date:	Sep 16, 2006	**No Code**	Supported By Healthcare Will	Dr. John Smithers

Support Providers

Role	Name
Legal Guardian	Adam Demo

Functional Status

Type	Date	Code	Description	Status	Source
Colitis	Onset: Sep 16, 2006			Active	Dr. John Smithers

Social History

Type	Date	Code	Description	Status	Source
Marital Status			**Married**		Dr. John Smithers
Language			**English**		Dr. John Smithers
Ethnicity			**Non-Hispanic**		Dr. John Smithers
Religious Preference			**Protestant**		Dr. John Smithers
Race			**White**		Dr. John Smithers
Pregnancies			**2**		Dr. John Smithers
Term Pregnancies			**2**		Dr. John Smithers
Abortions			**0**		Dr. John Smithers
Ectopic Pregnancies			**0**		Dr. John Smithers
Pre-term Pregnancies			**0**		Dr. John Smithers
Living Children			**2**		Dr. John Smithers

Figure 13-1 Sample of a Continuing Care Record.

Additional Information About People & Organizations

People

Name	Specialty	Relation	Identification Numbers	Phone	Address/ E-mail
Shirley Ann Demo			112233 239-00-0000	Home 612-455-9999	**Home:** 3333 Maxwell Blvd Xavier, ME59988
Adam Demo					**Home:** 3499 Maxwell Blvd Xavier, ME56699
Shirley Eichenwald Maki					
Dr. John Smithers	Internal Medicine			Home 415-555-1212	**Home:** 94044 Link Road San Francisco, CA94304 jsmith@ccrdemohealthclinic.com

Organizations

Name	Specialty	Relation	Identification Numbers	Phone	Address/ E-mail
TEPR CCR Demo Health Clinic				Main 415-555-1212	**Main:** 94044 Link Road San Francisco, CA94304 jsmith@ccrdemohealthclinic.com

Information Systems

Name	Type	Version	Identification Numbers	Phone	Address/ E-mail
Solventus CCR ViewPort		V1.0			

This stylesheet is provided by the American Academy of Family Physicians and the CCR Acceleration Task Force

Powered by the ASTM E2369-05 Specification for the Continuity of Care Record (CCR) which includes:

Advance Directives	Alerts / Allergies	Encounters	Family History	Functional Status
Health Care Providers	Immunizations	Insurance	Medical Equipment	Medications
Plan Of Care	Problems	Procedures	Results	Social History
Support Providers	Vital Signs			

Figure 13-1

data set. Because of this, and given that care decisions may be based on the information obtained, data from other care providers may need to be included in the legal definition of the practice medical record. This is contrary to past policies, when information from other care providers was generally not considered part of a practice legal record. (AHIMA, 2005b.) If at all possible, the CCR should be identified as the source of the data along with the date and time it was added to the practice record. If the information later is found to be erroneous, or if the data source needs to be identified, this notation will allow tracing it to its originator.

There are two primary options for access to and retention of CCR data for sharing across the established provider-exchange network. For example, each practice may retain the information in existing databases until requests are entered into the CCR exchange network. Once a patient is identified electronically as having existing information in the network, the computer systems of the practice (or practices) that have treated the patient are notified of the request. Designated components of the patient's information in the practice's computer are identified and electronically "pulled" from the patient's health care database and from those of other participating providers who also have treated the patient. If necessary, information from multiple patient providers is summarized via the network software and then forwarded to the requesting provider as the CCR. A second option is the transfer of CCR information regarding treated patients from the practice database to a central CCR network repository (holding place) for retention. This repository actually would be the site queried for availability of patient information. Providers contribute information that has been defined as part of the repository as patients are seen. The new data is stored in the CCR, or existing information is updated. This option requires that some entity (group or organization) and site be identified as the host for the CCR database and that individuals are designated for its maintenance.

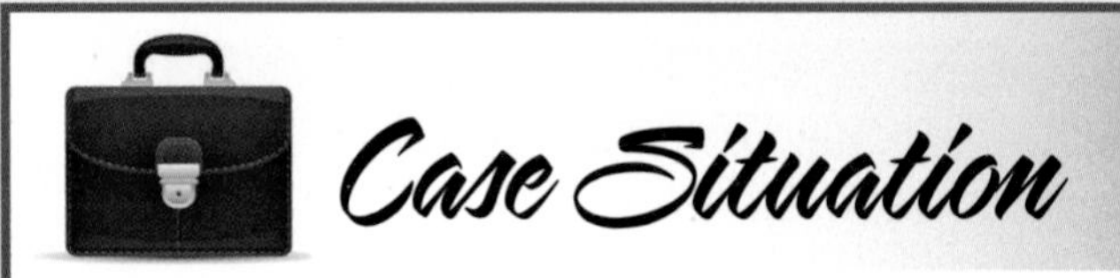

A patient is a newly diagnosed diabetic being closely monitored for compliance with the plan of care and medications ordered. The patient's employer, however, needs the patient to relocate to a city across the state for several months to work on a special project. The patient's primary physician happens to know a good physician in that city and shares this information with the patient. Both care providers participate in a state health information exchange (HIE). The HIE's patient database is shared by most physicians in the state and has defined standard components. With the patient's knowledge and encouragement, the primary physician contacts the other doctor, who agrees to supervise the patient for the months involved. To support continuity of care, the patient's primary physician makes sure that the patient's HIE CCR information is current and electronically sends it to the new provider's EHR. Upon the patient's return home, the temporary physician can do the same thing. In addition, while the patient is under care, the temporary provider can send the primary physician periodic reports via electronic transfer. Thus the primary physician receives needed information about the progress of the patient, whose care is as seamless as possible.

SUMMARY

Personal health records are gathered and maintained by patients themselves. These records may be used for a variety of purposes and may be maintained via computers, smart cards, or even computer chip implants. Although there are no specific standards for the content of a PHR, a work group of AHIMA has developed a suggested list of data items for inclusion and Medicare has provided a more streamlined option. If used, the data becomes a lifelong record of personal health treatment whose content may be shared with providers or other individuals as the need arises. A number of organizations in the United States have taken an interest in PHR development, encouraging the public to become more involved in their own health care. Efforts include a site that provides web links for products, awarding of PHR development grants by philanthropic foundations, and projects sponsored by health plans or employers.

Another tool for care communication used by a defined population of health care providers is the CCR. The CCR abstracts data elements from participating provider records to share with other providers so that current and some historical patient information is available when the patient is being treated. The ASTM has developed CCR content specifications for use in development of standards, products, and actual formation of a data repository. The key for access to a CCR is accurate patient identification. Consistent gathering of patient identification and demographic information by practices will permit sharing of patient data across multiple care providers. Two options exist for maintenance of the CCR data. The first is retaining CCR-formatted data within the practice EHR until access is requested; the second option is a network CCR repository developed under the guidance of those who participate in and contribute to it. Confidentiality and security are important considerations for whichever option is chosen.

REFERENCES

AAAHC [Accreditation Association for Ambulatory Health Care, Inc.]. (2011). *Accreditation handbook for ambulatory health care.* Wilmette, IL.

AHIMA e-HIM Personal Health Record Work Group. (2005a). The role of the personal health record in the EHR, Appendix B: Common data elements in the PHR. Retrieved from http://library.ahima.org.

AHIMA Work Group. (2005b). Update: Guidelines for defining the legal health record for disclosure purposes. *Journal of AHIMA, 76(8),* 64A–G.

ASTM [American Society for Testing and Materials]. (2005). *Designation: E 2369-05 standard specification for continuity of care record (CCR).* West Conshohocken, PA.

Burrington-Brown, J. (2005). The PHR effect. *Journal of AHIMA, 76(2),* 1–2.

Friedman, B. (2005). Health records get personal: A technology outlook for consumer access to personal health information. *Journal of AHIMA, 76(1),* 42–45.

Medicare. (2011). Manage your health. Managing your health information online. Retrieved from http://www.medicare.gov/.

National Committee on Vital and Health Statistics. (2006). Personal health records and personal health record systems. Retrieved from http://www.ncvhs.hhs.gov/0602nhiirpt.pdf.

The Joint Commission. (2011). *Standards for ambulatory care.* Oakbrook Terrace, IL.

U.S. Department of Health and Human Services. (2010). *Federal register, 42 CFR parts 412, 413, 422 et al. Medicare and Medicaid programs; Electronic health record incentive program; Final rule,* 75(144). Washington, DC: National Archives and Records Administration.

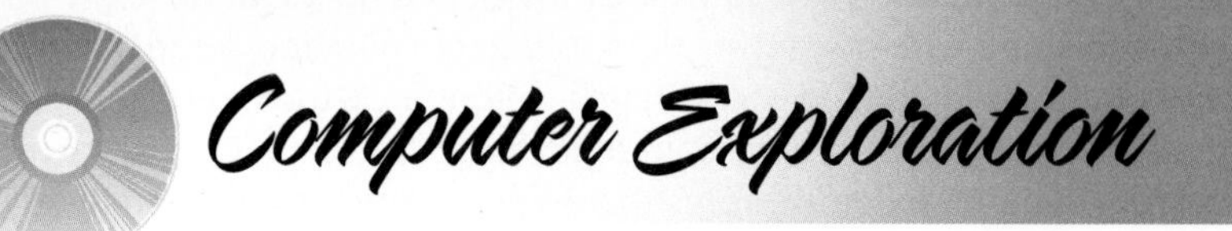

Significant amounts of information about Personal Health Records are available at this web site: http://www.myPHR.com/. Access the site and:

a. Click on "Start a PHR" at the top of the home page and then "Choose a PHR" on the drop-down menu that appears. Select "Web-based" under "Format" and "Free" under "Cost" (bottom of page) and then "Submit." Click links for at least two free products (e.g., MyMediConnect and IntuitHealthPHR—formerly iHealthRecord). Next return and select at least two products "For Purchase" under "Cost" (e.g., Mymedicalrecords.com and Lynxcare).

b. For each of the four products you select:

(1) Find the product demo, tour, or overview available via its web site and describe the product features that you find most appealing or useful as a potential customer.

(2) Review the FAQs (frequently asked questions) available via its web site or presented in videos and document at least four facts that you find most informative as a potential customer.

(3) Describe how the issue of "security" of personal health data is addressed within the content of this product's web site.

(4) Write a brief comparative analysis of the four PHR products: what was common among them, what was unique about one as compared to the others, etc.

REVIEW QUESTIONS

1. What is the definition of a PHR?

2. What purpose does the PHR serve for the patient and for health care providers?

3. In what formats might a PHR be maintained by the patient?

4. What data categories are identified by the AHIMA work group for the content of a PHR?

5. What content has Medicare suggested for a PHR?

6. According to the federal Stage 1 "meaningful use" criteria, what EHR content should be shared among providers when coordination of care is needed?

7. What is the definition of a CCR?

8. What (as determined by the ASTM) are the three major sections of a CCR? What data elements would be found in each section?

9. What is the key to accessing the CCR?

10. What is the general process for accessing a CCR?

____

____

____

11. What two alternatives might be used to retain CCR data?

____

____

____

e-Medsys® Educational Edition 2.0 Overview

ABOUT e-Medsys®

The e-Medsys® Solution Suite from TriMed Technologies is a fully integrated and fully online practice management (PM) system, electronic health records (EHR) system, and patient portal used across the country in thousands of medical offices. The e-Medsys® EHR is CHIT-certified in Ambulatory Medicine, Cardiovascular Medicine, and Child Health. For more information about TriMed Technologies, visit www.trimedtech.com.

The e-Medsys® Educational Edition 2.0 from TriMed Technologies is a custom version of this powerful product. Since e-Medsys® is completely online, it is completely portable, allowing you to work on your exercises on any computer that has e-Medsys® installed—both in the computer lab and at home—without losing any work.

e-Medsys® Educational Edition 2.0 has two interfaces—a practice management (PM) interface and an electronic health records (EHR) interface. These two interfaces work seamlessly together, forming a practical and powerful total practice management system (TPMS)—allowing all tasks in a medical office to be performed electronically. The EHR interface is accessed through a drop-down menu on the main screen of the PM interface.

- In the PM interface, you have the ability to register patients, work in the appointment schedule, add authorizations, and post patient charges and credits.
- In the EHR interface, you have the ability to work in individual patient charts; you will create new patient notes, prescriptions, and lab orders.

Your log-in information is printed on the inside front cover of this book. If you change your password, write it in the space provided on the inside front cover of this book. There is no way to retrieve your password once changed. We have also included an administrator log-in for your instructor on the inside back cover of the book. When you begin your class, you should cut off the card on the inside back cover of the book and give it to your instructor. If your instructor chooses, he or she can log in and view the entries that you have made in the program to check your work.

ABOUT THE EXERCISES

A *total practice management system* (TPMS) allows all tasks in a medical office to be done electronically. It is a term that encompasses both (1) a PM system (which performs front-office tasks such as appointment scheduling and billing) and (2) an EHR system (which performs back-office tasks such as electronic charting and e-prescribing).

The exercises in Appendix B are designed to give you practice working within a TPMS, using e-Medsys® Educational Edition 2.0. At the beginning of each exercise, step-by-step instructions are given for each task. As you gain confidence and proficiency working in the program, "Putting It into Practice" exercises require you to perform the tasks without step-by-step instructions.

The final section in Appendix B applies the tasks you have learned to two patient case studies.

It will take approximately 5–10 hours to complete all of the e-Medsys® exercises in Appendix B. The time will vary depending on your computer background.

The section titled "Getting Started with e-Medsys®" will help orient you to the software and provide some guidance on how to use it prior to starting the activities.

e-Medsys® SUPPORT AND PREMIUM WEBSITE

For technical support related to e-Medsys® Educational Edition 2.0, contact Delmar Technical Support, Monday–Friday, from 8:30 a.m. to 6:30 p.m. Eastern Standard Time:

- Telephone: 1-800-354-9706
- E-mail: delmar.help@cengage.com
- URL: www.cengage.com/support

Software support and additional resources for students and instructors can also be found on our Premium website. Follow the directions on the printed access card to log on at www.cengagebrain.com. The Premium Website includes:

- Software support: FAQ, "How To" Recorded Tutorials, Software Documentation
- Instructor resources: Instructor Notes, Answer Key Screen Shots and Printouts
- Student resources: Files to complete Exercises 8-3 and 8-4

INSTALLING e-Medsys® EDUCATIONAL EDITION 2.0

The e-Medsys® database and all of your work will be stored online on the TriMed Technologies server; however, you will need to follow the installation routine found at the end of this appendix to install the e-Medsys® PM Client in order to access the program with your specific computer. You must perform this installation on every computer on which you plan to access the program. Installation of the e-Medsys® PM Client simply allows your computer to interface with the program and the TriMed Technologies server. All data are saved online to your specific log-in account, so no work is lost between computers or locations. The e-Medsys® PM Client is self-contained within a single folder on your computer and only takes up 59.2 MB on your hard drive.

In order for e-Medsys® to work optimally on your computer, you must follow all the guidelines in the "System Requirements" section in this appendix. Since e-Medsys® is an online program and uses pop-up windows, it is critical that you follow the instructions provided for Internet settings. Some of the e-Medsys® features require third-party programs like Microsoft Word and Acrobat Reader, and these are also outlined in the "System Requirements" section.

Instructions for uninstalling e-Medsys® Educational Edition 2.0 are found at the back of this appendix, following the installation instructions.

> **Important Note:** e-Medsys® log-ins will expire 12 months after initial log-in. Three months prior to expiration, a notification message will display each time you log in.

> **Important Note:** When you are using the e-Medsys® program, a DOS window will always be present and minimized on your taskbar. Do not close that DOS window or you will close the program.

Using e-Medsys® in Multiple Locations: User Scenarios

Scenario #1: Students Use e-Medsys® in the School Computer Lab

The e-Medsys® program should be installed by following the installation instructions at the back of this appendix. The program must be installed on every computer on which students will work in order for them to access the program. Once the e-Medsys® PM Client is installed, students double click on the e-Medsys® icon and then log in to e-Medsys® with the information provided on the inside front cover of this book.

Students can work on any computer in the lab on which e-Medsys® is installed, and all work will be saved to their log-in account. No work is lost between computers.

The installation time is very quick for the e-Medsys® PM Client program once the install program is downloaded. The e-Medsys® PM Client program is self-contained within a single folder. Some of the e-Medsys® PM features require third-party programs like Microsoft Word and Acrobat Reader.

Because the e-Medsys® program is self-contained, it is fairly easy for systems administrators to automate an e-Medsys® PM Client program install. If a school re-images workstations or restores workstations to a "clean" state, it is recommended that e-Medsys® be included as part of the image or "clean" state so that the e-Medsys® PM Client program does not have to be reinstalled.

In order for e-Medsys® to work optimally on any computer, the guidelines in the "System Requirements" section found at the back of this appendix must be followed. Since e-Medsys® is an online program and uses pop-up windows, it is critical that systems administrators follow the instructions provided for Internet settings.

Scenario #2: Students Use e-Medsys® on their Personal Computers

Students must follow the installation routine at the back of this appendix, installing the e-Medsys® PM Client on their individual computers. Once the e-Medsys® PM Client is installed, students double click on the e-Medsys® icon and then log in to e-Medsys® with the information provided on the inside front cover of this book.

Again, in order for e-Medsys® to work optimally on any computer, students must follow the guidelines in the "System Requirements" section found at the back of this appendix. Since e-Medsys® is an online program and uses pop-up windows, it is critical that students follow the instructions provided for Internet settings.

Scenario #3: Students Use e-Medsys® in the School Computer Lab and on their Personal Computers

It is easy and seamless for students to use e-Medsys® in the school computer lab and on their own computers at home. However, e-Medsys® must first be installed in the computer lab and on their own computers.

Students log in to e-Medsys® at school with the information provided on the inside front cover of this book. Students log in to e-Medsys® on their own computers with the same log-in information.

All work students complete at the computer lab and on their own computers is saved to their log-in account. No work is lost between locations.

GETTING STARTED WITH e-Medsys®

Setting Up the Configuration Tool

Prior to opening the program and logging in, you must set up the Configuration Tool to configure your unique enterprise number on the computer.

1. Go to: START > ALL PROGRAMS > E-MEDSYS > E-MEDSYS CONFIGURATION.

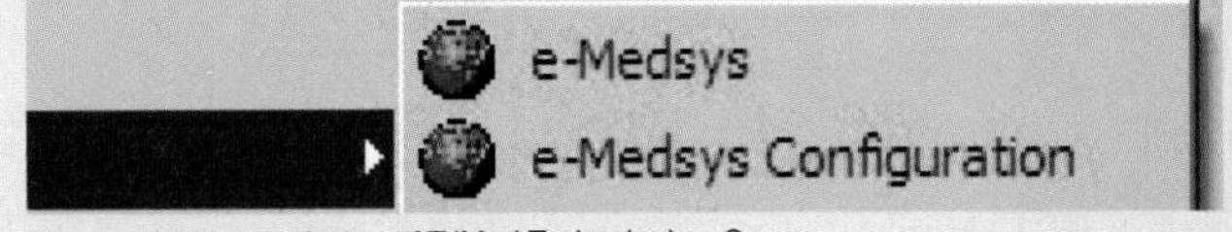

Reprinted with permission of TriMed Technologies, Corp.

2. You may receive a prompt asking whether you are an e-Medsys® customer. If you do, click Yes through the prompt.
3. Type your Enterprise Number (printed on the inside front cover of your book), and click OK.

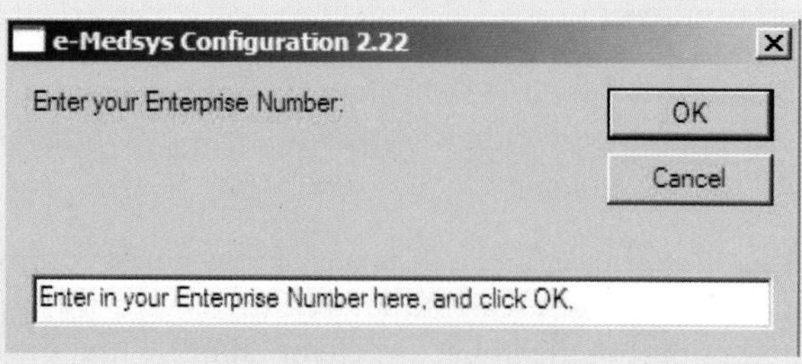

Reprinted with permission of TriMed Technologies, Corp.

4. You may receive several prompts; click Yes and OK through the prompts until you have confirmed that the program has been configured.
5. Now, continue using the directions under "Logging In to e-Medsys®" (step 2).

Logging In, Changing Your Password, and Logging Out

Logging In to e-Medsys®

1. Set up the Configuration Tool by following the preceding instructions.
2. Double click the e-Medsys® icon on your desktop.
3. Enter the enterprise number, user name, and password found on the inside front cover of your book, and click the Login button.

Reprinted with permission of TriMed Technologies, Corp.

4. Now you are at the e-Medsys® home page and can begin working. *Note:* In addition to the e-Medsys® home page, there will be another window open. *This window must be kept open on your desktop.* This will sometimes be referred to as "the black screen." It will always be running in the background when a user is logged in to the program.

Changing Your Password

> **Please be Advised:** If you lose your password, there is no way to recover your data. If you change your password, write it in the space provided on the inside front cover of your book.

1. On the Main Screen Menu Bar, click File. From the drop-down menu, click Change Password.

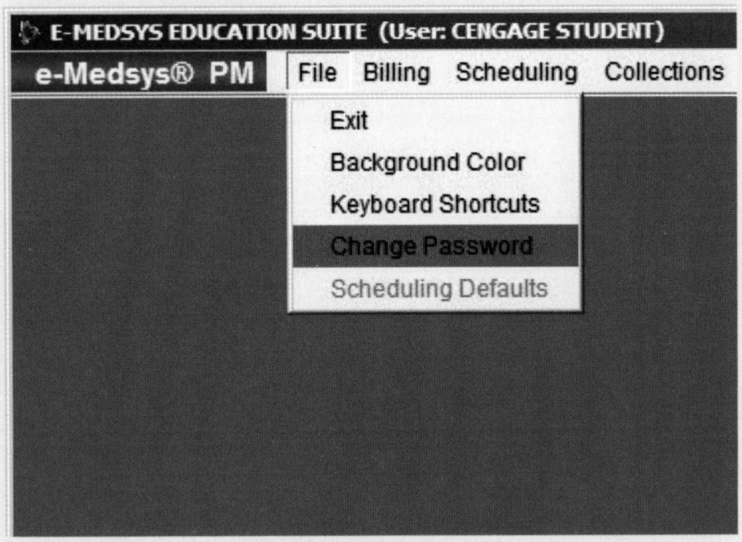

E-MEDSYS EDUCATION SUITE (User: CENGAGE STUDENT)
e-Medsys® PM | File | Billing | Scheduling | Collections
Exit
Background Color
Keyboard Shortcuts
Change Password
Scheduling Defaults

2. A Change Password Utility window will open. Click the button for Change Now.
3. Enter your current password and then your new password (the password you would like to change to). When you have finished, click the Accept button.

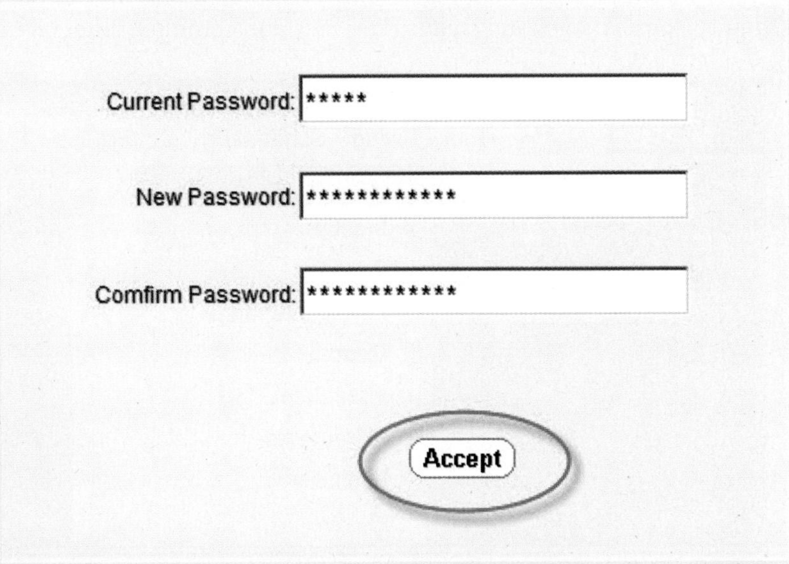

Current Password: *****
New Password: ************
Comfirm Password: ************
Accept

4. Your password has been changed, and you will use your new password the next time you log in to the program.

Logging Out of e-Medsys®

Log out by closing the software application. This is done by going to File > Exit within the application. *Note:* A warning will pop up if you close the application by using the X in the upper right corner.

Practice Management Interface: Main Screen Menu Bar

Clicking on the menu bar in the Practice Management interface produces a drop-down menu listing all of the functions in that module. The modules that we will use in Appendix B include File, Billing, Scheduling, and EHR (Electronic Health Records).

E-MEDSYS EDUCATION SUITE (User: CENGAGE STUDENT)
e-Medsys® PM File Billing Scheduling Collections Recall RX EDI EHR Dashboard Admin E-Comm Windows Help Messages: 0

Reprinted with permission of TriMed Technologies, Corp.

File Menu

The file menu allows you to log out of the program (Exit), review the keyboard shortcuts, and change your password.

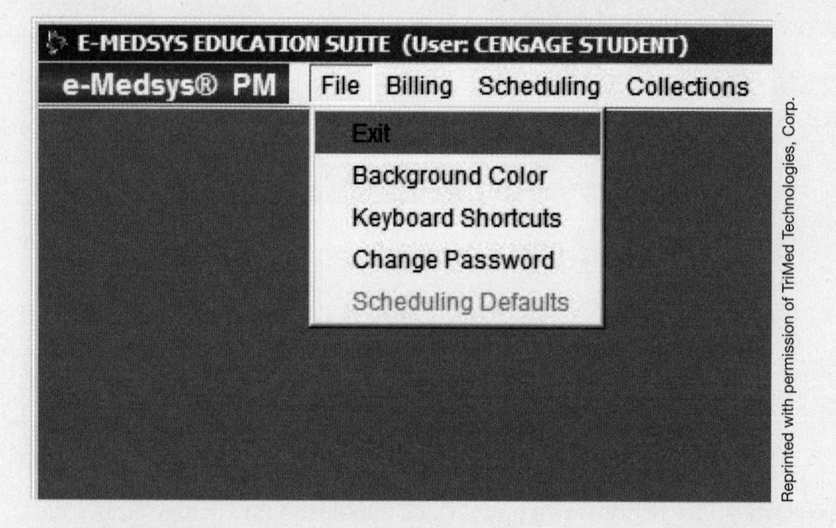

Reprinted with permission of TriMed Technologies, Corp.

Billing Menu

The billing menu allows you to work in the patient registration area to add and update patient information, add and modify authorizations (Inquiry), post charges and credits (Posting), and complete other billing-related tasks.

E-MEDSYS EDUCATION SUITE (User: CENGAGE STUDENT)
e-Medsys® PM File Billing Scheduling Collections Rec
Patient Registration Ctrl+P
Inquiry Ctrl+I
Posting
File Maintenance
Reports
Insurance
Statements
Eligibility
EDI Manager

Reprinted with permission of TriMed Technologies, Corp.

Scheduling Menu

The scheduling menu allows you to work in the PM appointment schedule (Appointment Schedule).

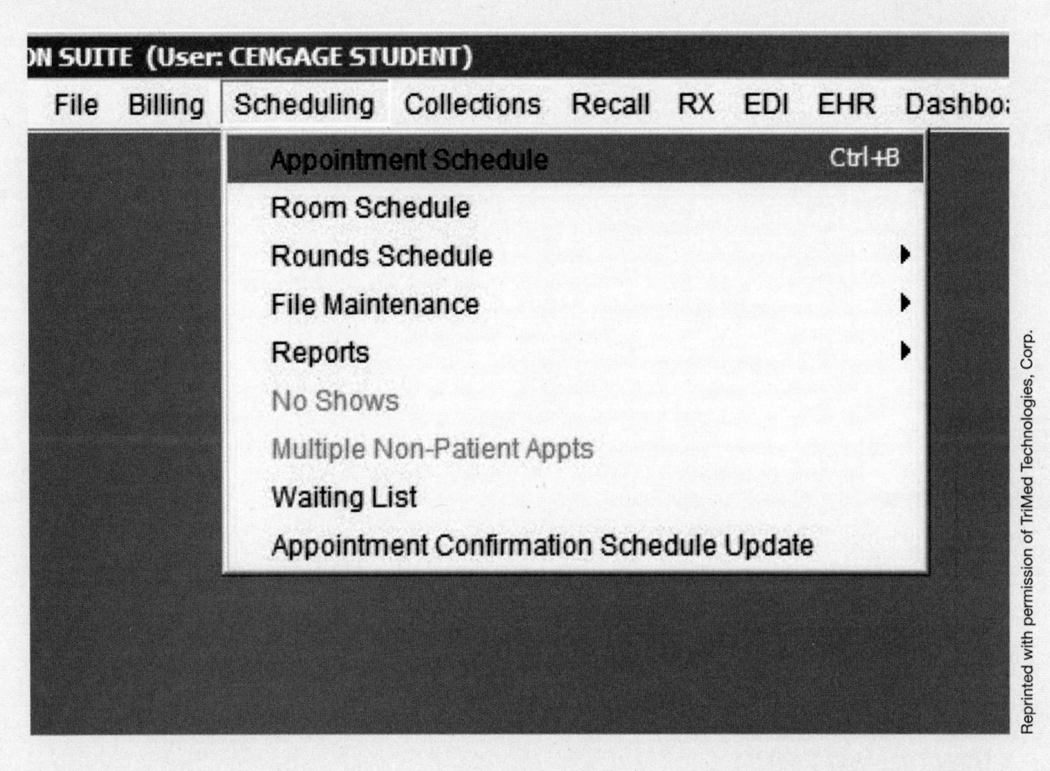

Reprinted with permission of TriMed Technologies, Corp.

EHR Menu

The EHR menu provides access to the EHR interface, where you can add new patient notes, prescriptions, orders, and lab results to individual patient charts.

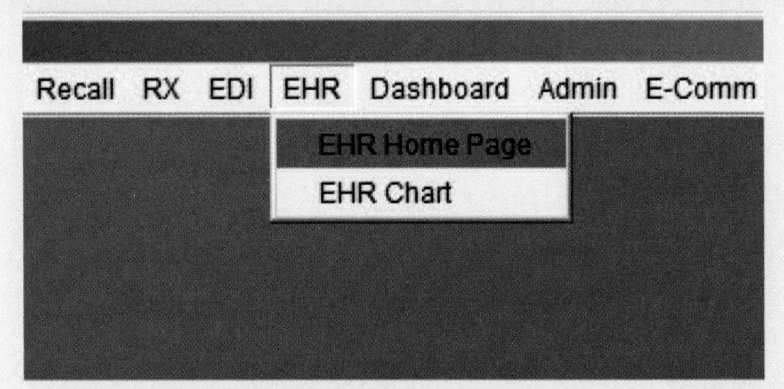

Reprinted with permission of TriMed Technologies, Corp.

Keyboard Shortcuts

Throughout the system there are default "shortcut keys" that can be used to select items from the Main Screen Menu Bar. For example, Ctrl + E is a shortcut for Exiting or Logging Out of the program. These default keys have been set up by the system:

- Ctrl + P = Patient Registration
- Ctrl + I = Inquiry
- Ctrl + B = Appointment Schedule
- Ctrl + H = Charge Posting
- Ctrl + R = Credit Posting

EHR Interface: Menu Bar

Home

The home page for the EHR is the provider schedule page. All appointments made in the PM interface (Scheduling > Appointment Schedule) will also appear in this schedule.

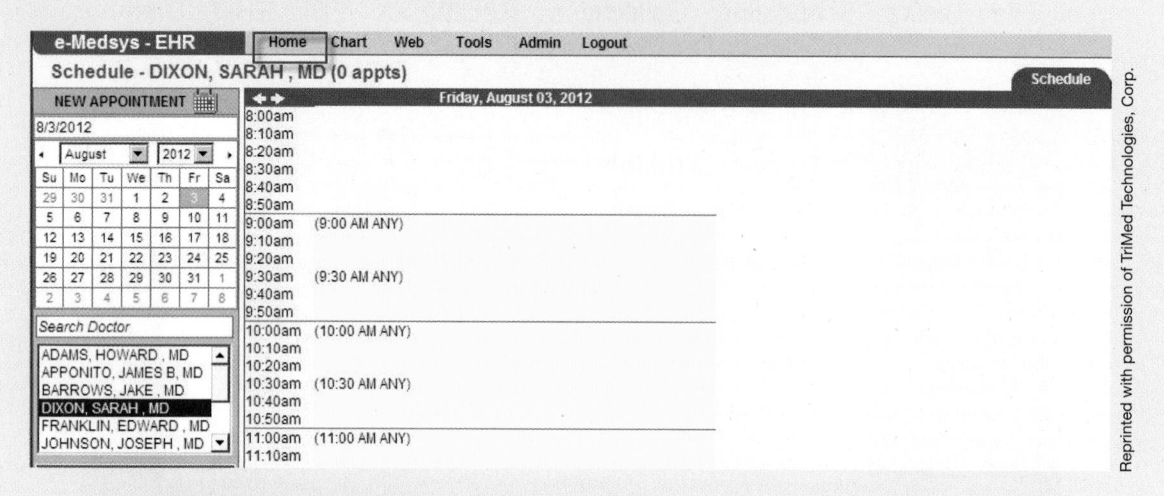

Reprinted with permission of TriMed Technologies, Corp.

Chart

Use the Chart button (at the top of the screen) to look up individual patient charts.

e-Medsys - EHR | Home | Chart | Web | Tools | Admin | Logout

PATIENT/CHART FIND

Pat. Name: | SSN: | MRN:

Provider: ALL | DOB: | ID:

Search | Clear | 0 records found. | Open in New Window

Patient	Pat ID	SSN	DOB	Address

A
B
C

Reprinted with permission of TriMed Technologies, Corp.

Features of the e-Medsys® Program

Enter Key or Tab Key

Using the Enter key or the Tab key on your keyboard allows you to move from field to field in the system.

Search for Items by Name

You can search many fields in the software by name, including Patient, Insurance Company, Procedure, and Code. To search a field for an item by its name, enter the first few letters (or numbers, in the instance of a code), and press Enter on your keyboard. For example, suppose you want to search for patient Ashley Mansfield:

1. Enter "MAN" in the Last Name field, and press Enter on your keyboard.
2. The software will bring up a selection window showing all patients in the system whose last name starts with those letters.

Patient	Pat ID	SSN	DOB	Address
MANNING, LINDA	1031	987-52-1234	10/10/1968	8787 WANDERING WAY
MANSFIELD, ASHLEY	1036	774-55-6222	3/17/1983	85523 CYNTHIA ST

Reprinted with permission of TriMed Technologies, Corp.

3. Highlight the selection by clicking on it with the mouse. Once the correct item is highlighted, you can select it in a number of ways. You can click the OK button, double click on the highlighted row, or press the Enter key on your keyboard.

Search for Items Using Table Look-Up

You can also search many fields in the software using Table Look-Up. Some of these fields include Patient, Procedure, Diagnosis, Insurance Plan, and Referring Physician.

As an example, we will search for a patient on the Patient Tab of the patient registration screen. To bring up a list of *all* items in the program associated with a particular field:

1. Type "%" in the Patient field, and click the Search button.
2. The software will bring up a selection window showing all patients in the system.

Patient Search

OK | Exit

Patient | Guarantor | Show Members | Phonetic Name Search | Include Historical Records | Include Inactive Accts

Account No: | Last Name: % | First Name: | Search | Clear

Home | Work | Cell

Birth Date: MM/DD/19YY | SSN: ***-**-**** | Phone: (***) ***-**** x | Policy#:

Last Name	First Name	M	Number	MRN	DEPT	FC	Birth Date	SS Num	HomePhone	Guar Last	Guar First
ADAMS	LILY		1051		SMG	BLUE CROSS	10/31/1960	495127435	(310) 784-7212	ADAMS	LILY
ALMOND	BARRY		1005		BFH	MEDICARE	12/15/1936	665478974	(815) 447-9797	ALMOND	BARRY
ARAEND	VICTOR		1006		IMB	UNITED HEALTHCARE	04/18/1936	654789874	(617) 456-7897	ARAEND	VICTOR
AUGUST	ROSEMARY		1007		SMG	MEDICARE	07/12/1936	332547897	(805) 654-8974	AUGUST	ROSEMARY
AUGUSTINE	JENNIFER		1027		PEDS	PRIVATE INS	06/10/1998	444669999	(805) 465-4652	AUGUSTINE	TINA
BAGLEY	VIRGINIA		1082		BFH	AETNA PPO	11/01/1940	633984295	(312) 982-6168	BAGLEY	VIRGINIA
BARR	DONALD		1008		SMG	MEDICARE	12/15/1936	333665478	(805) 456-7897	BARR	DONALD
BARTEL	DELORES		1054		SMG	CIGNA PPO	07/18/1952	987766677	(805) 678-9098	BARTEL	DELORES
BATES	ANTHONY		1049		SMG	PRIVATE INS	07/28/1965	599784326	(818) 899-4848	BATES	ANTHONY
BECKER	ETHEL		1009		SMG	MEDICARE	09/16/1936	326547897	(805) 987-4567	BECKER	ETHEL
BEST	DIANE		1010		SMG	MEDICARE	01/15/1936	326457874	(805) 547-8974	BEST	DIANE

Reprinted with permission of TriMed Technologies, Corp.

3. Highlight the correct selection, and click OK (or press Enter or double click).

If you want to narrow your search down, you can type "%" and then the first few letters of what you are looking for. For example, if you are looking for Donald Barr:

1. Type "%BA," and click the Search button.

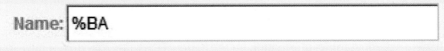

Reprinted with permission of TriMed Technologies, Corp.

2. The software will bring up a selection window showing all patients with "BA" in their name that are in the system.

Patient Search

OK | Exit

Patient | Guarantor | Show Members | Phonetic Name Search | Include Historical Records | Include Inactive Accts

Account No: | Last Name: %BA | First Name: | Search | Clear

Home | Work | Cell

Birth Date: MM/DD/19YY | SSN: ***-**-**** | Phone: (***) ***-**** x | Policy#:

Last Name	First Name	M	Number	MRN	DEPT	FC	Birth Date	SS Num	HomePhone	Guar Last	Guar First
BAGLEY	VIRGINIA		1082		BFH	AETNA PPO	11/01/1940	633984295	(312) 982-6168	BAGLEY	VIRGINIA
BARR	DONALD		1008		SMG	MEDICARE	12/15/1936	333665478	(805) 456-7897	BARR	DONALD
BARTEL	DELORES		1054		SMG	CIGNA PPO	07/18/1952	987766677	(805) 678-9098	BARTEL	DELORES
BATES	ANTHONY		1049		SMG	PRIVATE INS	07/28/1965	599784326	(818) 899-4848	BATES	ANTHONY

Reprinted with permission of TriMed Technologies, Corp.

3. Then highlight the correct selection, and click OK (or press Enter or double click).

Entering Dates

Dates are entered in a six-digit date format (DD/MM/20YY). For the Date of Birth fields, the system defaults to DD/MM/19YY. There are several shortcuts for entering dates that can be used.

When the cursor is in the Date field:

1. Type "t" to populate the field with today's date.
2. Typing "3M" will populate the field with the date three months from today, "6W" will populate with the date six weeks from today, "5D" will populate with the date five days from today, and so on.

Selecting Items from a Window

As mentioned previously, items can be selected in a number of ways. First, highlight the selection by clicking on it once with the mouse, and then:

1. Click the OK button, or
2. Double click on the item, or
3. Press the Enter key on the keyboard, or
4. Press Alt + O on the keyboard.

WORKING IN THE e-Medsys® PROGRAM

Patient Registration

From the Main Menu: *Billing > Patient Registration*

Exercises and step-by-step procedures covering this material are found in Appendix B.

Creating a New Patient

1. Select Billing > Patient Registration from the main menu. The patient registration screen appears.
2. Click the New Patient button.
3. Enter the patient's demographic information on the Patient (Pat) Tab. You do not have to fill in every field with information; however, at a minimum, you must complete the fields colored in *red*.
4. Click the Accept + Ins button if you plan to enter the patient's insurance information immediately; otherwise, click the Accept button to save the information.

Updating Patient Information

1. Select Billing > Patient Registration from the main menu. The patient registration screen appears.
2. Search for a patient by typing his or her last name in the Last Name field and clicking Search. (You can also search by date of birth, social security number, or home telephone number.)
3. If there are no other patients in the database with that last name, the patient's account will populate the screen. If there are multiple patients with that last name, highlight the patient's name on the pop-up window, and click OK.
4. Update the screen with the new patient information by typing over previous information.
5. Click the Accept button to save the updated information.

Description of Fields on the Patient (Pat) Tab

- **Account Number:** When the New Patient button is clicked, the next chronological number is assigned automatically. The user can also key in an existing patient's account number and click the Enter key to pull up the patient's information.
- **Last Name:** Enter the patient's last name with no punctuation. The system will default to capital letters.
- **First Name:** Enter the patient's first name with no punctuation. The system will default to capital letters.
- **Address 1/Address 2:** Enter the patient's address with no punctuation. Users may want to input data in all capital letters for uniformity throughout the system and for any merge documents or reports.
- **May Phone?:** The default is Yes. The drop-down options are Yes, No, and Special. If No or Special is selected, the Phone Number fields become color-coded: No = red; Special = yellow.
- **Marital Status:** The drop-down list includes Single, Married, and Other. An option can be selected by typing in the first letter of the desired option. Other selections can be added to this default list through Billing > File Maintenance > General Codes. Select Marital Status from the drop-down menu, and add more options.
- **Verify Address:** When this box is checked, a Verify Address Alert window is created when the patient's account is pulled up in the system.
- **Verify Phone:** When this box is checked, a Verify Phone Alert window is created when the patient's account is pulled up in the system.
- **Relationship to Guar:** The drop-down options are Self, Spouse, Child, and Other.
- **User:** This field will populate based on the user's log-in name.

Buttons on the Patient (Pat) Tab

- **Accept Button:** This button saves or updates all patient demographic information added.
- **Accept +Ins Button:** This button not only saves or updates all patient demographic information added but also automatically takes the user into the Insurance Tab to add the patient's insurance information.
- **History Button:** Any information changed and accepted (saved) in a patient's account is kept in the history. The user can view not only the historical information but also the effective dates of the information, the fields that were changed, and the person who made the changes.

Using the History Button

To view a patient's historical information in the system:

1. You must be in a patient's account, on the Pat Tab.
2. Click the History button.
3. Highlight the selection you wish to view.

4. Click OK.
5. You will then be viewing the historical data. To get back to the active information, click the Active button. When you are in the historical record, the Accept buttons are unavailable for you. Also the only option is to click back on the Active button to return to the active record.

Adding an Insurance Plan to a Patient's Account

1. If you are registering a new patient and have clicked the Accept + Ins button on the Pat Tab screen, the system will take you to the Insurance (Ins) Tab automatically.
2. Otherwise, select Billing > Patient Registration, and search for a patient. (Type in the patient's last name, and click Search. Select the correct patient from the pop-up window if applicable; otherwise, patient information will appear on screen automatically.)
3. Click the Ins Tab.
4. Click the ADD INS button on the right side of the screen.
5. Enter the plan name in the Insurance Plan field. (Table Look-Up is available.)
6. Select the patient's relation to the policyholder. Policyholder information fields will open up if the policyholder is someone other than Self. Enter the policyholder information if applicable.
7. Enter the effective date and all group, policy, co-payment, and deductible information.
8. Click the Accept button to save changes.

Modifying an Insurance Plan

1. Select Billing > Patient Registration, and search for a patient. (Type in the patient's last name, and click Search. Select the correct patient from the pop-up window if applicable; otherwise, patient information will appear on screen automatically.)
2. Click the Ins Tab.
3. Begin by highlighting the insurance plan you wish to modify, and click on the Modify Ins button on the right side of the screen. This will populate the insurance screen with the current information regarding the plan.
4. The plan information can now be changed. Once the correct information is entered, click Accept to save the changes made.

Note: If the insurance plan address is incorrect, the plan must be inactivated and the correct plan added.

Inactivating an Insurance Plan

1. Select Billing > Patient Registration, and search for a patient. (Type in the patient's last name, and click Search. Select the correct patient from the pop-up window if applicable; otherwise, patient information will appear on screen automatically.)
2. Click the Ins Tab.
3. Begin by highlighting the insurance plan you wish to inactivate, and click on the Modify Ins button on the right side of the screen. The system will pull forward all of the current information for the plan. This will populate the insurance screen with the current insurance information plan.
4. Uncheck the Active box in the center of the screen, and enter a valid ending date.
5. Once these changes have been made, click the Accept button to save the changes.
6. The system will create an alert prompt, asking the user whether the charges should be updated. If you answer Yes to this prompt, the system will make the necessary changes to the transactions posted with a date of service that falls within the effective dates of this change.

Changing the Order of an Insurance Plan

1. Select Billing > Patient Registration, and search for a patient. (Type in the patient's last name, and click Search. Select the correct patient from the pop-up window if applicable; otherwise, patient information will appear on screen automatically.)
2. Click the Ins Tab.
3. Begin by clicking on the Change Order button on the right side of the screen. The system will then bring up an instruction window.
4. Double click on the insurance plan that should be the primary; the system will hold the new rank in the Pending Rank field on the left side of the screen.
5. Then double click on the insurance plan that should be the secondary.
6. The system will then rebuild the table in the new order.
7. The system will then prompt the user to update the charges with the new ranking. Click Yes or press the Enter key to update the charges, as appropriate.

Description of Fields on the Insurance (Ins) Tab

- **Insurance Plan:** Table Look-Up is available. Choose the correct plan from the list.
- **Patient's Relation to Policy Holder:** The drop-down options are Self, Spouse, Child, and Other. Select an option by typing in the first letter of the desired option.
- **Policy Holder Information:** Fields will open up if the relation to the policyholder is something other than Self.
- **Effective Beginning Date:** Enter the date the insurance plan became effective for the charges that will be posted to this patient's account.
- **Effective Ending Date:** Enter the date the insurance plan ended for this patient in your office. This is completed when the plan is inactivated.
- **Co-Pay Amount:** Enter the patient's co-pay. This field prints on charge tickets and will be displayed in the insurance grid throughout the system.
- **Deductible:** This is an informational field. It will be displayed in the insurance grid throughout the system.

Working in the Guarantor Information Tab

The guarantor screen controls where the patient's statement will be sent and who is ultimately responsible for the payment on the account. The system will populate the guarantor information fields with the data that were entered in Patient Registration, Pat Tab. Click on the Guarantor (Guar) Tab in the patient registration screen *if* the patient and the guarantor are different.

To add a new guarantor:

1. Select Billing > Patient Registration, and search for a patient. (Type in the patient's last name, and click Search. Select the correct patient from the pop-up window if applicable; otherwise, patient information will appear on screen automatically.)
2. Click the Guar Tab.
3. Click on the Change Patient's Guar button.
4. Click on Add New Guar.

5. Enter the information for the guarantor. If the guarantor lives at the same address as the patient or shares other information, you can click the buttons for Copy Patient Address and Copy Patient Data.
6. Click Accept to save any changes made to the guarantor screen.

Description of Fields on the Guarantor (Guar) Tab

- **Guarantor Number:** The system will automatically assign the next available guarantor number. *Note:* This number may not match the patient account number.
- **Copy Patient Address:** Click on the Copy Patient Address button. The system will keep the patient address information and clear out only the First Name field.
- **Copy Patient Data:** Click on the Copy Patient Data button. The system will keep the patient information.
- **Employment Status:** The options in the drop-down menu are Full Time, Part Time, Unemployed, Retired, and Student. The default is Full Time.
- **Send Mail:** The drop-down options are Yes, No, and Special. The default is Yes.
- **Dunning Message?:** If this field is checked, the patient will receive statement messages. The default is Yes.
- **Credit Card Button:** Clicking the Credit Card button will pop up the credit card information screen, which allows the user to add, change, or clear credit card data.
- **Verify Address:** When the box is checked, a Verify Address Alert window is created when the patient's account is pulled up in the system.
- **Verify Phone:** When the box is checked, a Verify Phone Alert window is created when the patient's account is pulled up in the system.

Patient Appointments

From the Main Menu: *Scheduling > Appointment Schedule*

Exercises and step-by-step procedures covering this material are found in Appendix B.

1. Select Scheduling > Appointment Schedule from the main menu. The scheduling screen appears.
2. Click on the Provider button. Choose the patient's provider from the Select a Resource pop-up window by highlighting the provider name and clicking OK.
3. Back on the scheduling screen, enter the patient's last name, and press Search to bring up the patient's account. If more than one patient with that last name exists in the database, highlight the patient's name, and click OK.
4. The patient's information screen is brought up; this is a snapshot of the patient's account. Click Exit to return to the scheduling screen.
5. Use the Calendar icon to select the date on which the appointment should be scheduled.
6. Use the drop-down menu to select the correct visit type.
7. Click Book.
8. On the supplemental information screen, type any notes or comments about the appointment.
9. Click Clear to book another appointment. Click Exit to return to the main menu.

Patient Authorizations

From the Main Menu: *Billing > Inquiry*

Exercises and step-by-step procedures covering this material are found in Appendix B.

Creating a New Authorization

1. Select Billing > Inquiry from the main menu. Search for and select the patient's name for which you wish to create a new authorization.
2. Click Authorization.
3. Click Add.
4. Fill in the type, status, request date, primary care provider and specialty provider, and diagnosis code(s).
5. Fill in the procedure code(s) on the Authorized Visits/Procedures Tab.
6. Click on the Accept button to save the authorization. (If you click on the Cancel button, all information will be lost.)

Modifying an Existing Authorization

1. Select Billing > Inquiry from the main menu. Search for and select the patient's name for which you wish to modify an authorization.
2. Click Authorization.
3. Highlight the authorization to be modified.
4. Click on the Modify button on the top button bar. This action will pull you into the authorization and allow any changes to be made.
5. Once all modifications are made, click the Accept button.

Description of Fields on the General Information Tab

- **Referral Type:** Enter the referral type; the options are Referral In and Referral Out.
- **Authorization Number:** Enter the authorization number; this is an alphanumeric field. When the authorized procedures are posted, this number will print in box 23 on the Standard CMS-1500 form.
- **Status:** This is a drop-down field. The options are Approved, Modified, Denied, Deferred, Expired, Cancelled, and Requested.
- **Request Date:** Enter the date when the authorization was requested from the insurance company.
- **Authorization Date:** Enter the date when the authorization was approved by the insurance company.
- **Expiration Date:** Enter the date when the authorization expires as directed by the insurance company. This is not a required field.
- **Primary Care Provider:** Enter the name of the primary care physician.
- **Specialty Provider:** Enter the name of the specialty physician.
- **Diagnosis:** Enter the diagnosis using either an ICD-9 code or a description.
- **Contact:** Enter the first and last names of the contact at the insurance company. This is an informational field.

Description of Fields on the Authorized Visits/Procedures Tab

- **Specific Procedures Tab:** Enter the specific procedure(s) for the authorization. Click the appropriate radio button to enter using a CPT code or a description.
- **Quantity:** Enter the number of times for which use of this CPT code is authorized.
- **Used:** This field will populate when the specific procedure listed on the authorization is posted through charge posting. If a specific authorized procedure is posted, the system will show the user the authorization number and count it as *used.*
- **Non-Specific Procedures:** Enter the number of times a patient can come in for nonspecific procedures. This method increments the Used column based on any CPT codes posted before the expiration date on the authorization.
- **Number of Visits—Office:** Enter the number of office visits authorized. The Used column increments based on dates of service posted with office visit codes before the expiration date on the authorization.
- **Number of Visits—Hospital:** Enter the number of hospital visits authorized. The Used column increments based on dates of service posted with hospital visit codes before the expiration date on the authorization.

Patient Reception

From the Main Menu: *Scheduling > Appointment Schedule*

Exercises and step-by-step procedures covering this material are found in Appendix B.

Indicating "Arrived" and "Registered" on the Schedule

1. Select Scheduling > Appointment Schedule from the main menu. The scheduling screen appears.
2. Use the Provider button and Calendar icon to navigate to the correct date.
3. Right click on the patient's name on the schedule, roll the mouse over the patient's name, and select Arrived.
4. The patient appointment information screen is now shown. This is a snapshot of the patient's account and can be used to confirm whether registration updates need to be made.
5. If registration updates are needed, select Billing > Patient Registration. Make the necessary updates, and click Accept.
6. Back on the scheduling screen, right click on the patient's name on the schedule, roll the mouse over the patient's name, and select Registered.
7. When you have finished, click the Clear button to prepare the calendar for the next entry or patient.

Printing Charge Slips

1. Select Scheduling > Appointment Schedule from the main menu. The scheduling screen appears.
2. Use the Provider button and Calendar icon to navigate to the correct date.
3. Right click on the patient's name on the schedule, and then select Patient Appt Info.
4. This brings up Patient Appointment Information for the patient.

5. Click the Charge Ticket button.
6. The charge ticket will print to your local printer.

Working in the Patient Electronic Medical Record

From the Main Menu: *EHR > EHR Home Page*

Exercises and step-by-step procedures covering this material are found in Appendix B.

Admitting Patients Using the EHR Schedule

1. Select EHR > EHR Home Page from the main menu.
2. A new browser window opens, opening the EHR interface.
3. On the left side of the screen, highlight the provider associated with a particular patient.
4. Also on the left side of the screen, navigate to the date of the patient's appointment.
5. Now, the provider's schedule should appear in the center of the screen, and you should see the patient's appointment on the screen if you have selected the correct date.
6. Right click on the patient's name on the schedule.
7. Roll your mouse over Status and then select Admitted.

Linking a New Patient Note to an Appointment

1. Still on the provider schedule page, again right click on the patient's name on the schedule.
2. Select Add New (Linked) and then Patient Note. Now, you are in the patient's individual medical record, and a new patient note has opened on the bottom right side of the screen.
3. Fill in the date, and select the appropriate template for the patient visit. Click Save.
4. Fill in the requested information on the template. The information will depend on the template chosen but typically includes vital signs, basic health history, and chief complaint.
5. Click Save when you have finished.
6. You may print the patient note by clicking Print > PDF Form.

Using the Tree View to View the Patient's Chart

The Tree View shows items as they are connected with one another. The Tree View will automatically build when additional items are added and linked to the patient's chart during each appointment.

1. You must be in a patient's chart to use Tree View.
2. On the lower left side of the screen, you should see a group of horizontal tabs. This is your left navigation bar within a patient's chart.
3. Click on APPTS. This will show all of the appointments that have been scheduled for the patient at the medical office. Make sure the box next to Tree is selected.
4. Make sure the box next to Appts: Inc. Canc is *not* selected (this suppresses appointments that were cancelled).

Locating a Patient Chart Without Using the EHR Schedule

1. From the menu along the top of the page, click on Chart.
2. This will bring up a search screen you can use to find a patient chart. You can either:
   - Type in the patient's last name and click Enter on your keyboard or
   - Click the first letter of the patient's last name along the left side of the screen. All patients whose last name begins with that letter will appear on your screen.

3. Double click the patient's name to open the patient's chart.
4. Once in the patient's chart, on the left menu, click on APPTS to prepare to link your new item to a patient appointment.

Creating Prescriptions for Provider Authorization

From the Main Menu: *EHR > EHR Home Page*

Exercises and step-by-step procedures covering this material are found in Appendix B.

Creating a Prescription

1. When working in the EHR interface in an individual patient record, you should always *first* indicate on the EHR schedule that you have "Admitted" the patient.
2. Still on the EHR schedule page, again right click on the patient's name on the schedule.
3. Select Add New (Linked), and then select Prescription. Now, you are in the patient's individual medical record, and a new prescription has opened on the bottom right side of the screen.
4. Within this tab, the provider name and the location will autopopulate based on the patient selected. Leave the Template field blank. The Folder field is autopopulated with Meds.
5. To the right of the ICD field, click on the binoculars to search for the diagnosis related to the medication being prescribed.
6. Beneath the Drug Tab, in the field next to Drug, enter the first three letters of the drug to be prescribed, and then click on the binoculars to the right of the field. Make sure that the box to the left of Search All has a checkmark in it.
7. Scroll through the resulting list until you find the prescribed drug and dosage. Click on it. The frequency, the form, and the route of administration will autopopulate based on your selection. The category of the drug will also autopopulate.
8. Fill in the date, the quantity, and the refills of the prescription. Make sure the checkbox to the left of Current is selected.
9. Click on Save. Note that the new prescription now appears in the Tree View, beneath today's appointment date.

Send a Prescription for Provider Sign-Off

1. With the prescription saved and the screen still open on it, click on the open envelope in the top right corner of the template. This allows you to send a message informing the provider that the prescription is ready for sign-off.
2. A new window will open. On the left side of the screen, beneath Select Individual Staff, highlight "Cengage Instructor." (In a medical office setting, you would select the patient's provider in this list.)
3. With the "Cengage Instructor" entry highlighted, click on the > button.
4. This action moves the admin name into the Route To list. Click on this entry in the Route To list to select it.
5. Click on the radio button for Send Indiv. Action Items.
6. The Route Date and Time fields will autopopulate with the current date and time.
7. In the Action Type field, use the drop-down menu to select Sign Off.
8. Leave the priority as Normal.
9. The Attachment/Routed Item field is autopopulated with the prescription information.
10. Click Send.

Recording Therapeutic Injections and Immunizations

From the Main Menu: *EHR > EHR Home Page*

Exercises and step-by-step procedures covering this material are found in Appendix B.

Documenting Injections and Immunizations

1. When working in the EHR interface in an individual patient record, you should always *first* indicate on the EHR schedule that you have Admitted the patient.
2. Still on the EHR schedule page, again right click on the patient's name on the schedule.
3. Select Add New (Linked), and then select Patient Note. The new note appears on the bottom right side of the screen.
4. The Provider, Department, Template Type, and Folder fields are autopopulated. Be sure that None is selected in the Template field.
5. Fill in the ICD field with the provider's diagnosis, and enter the date of administration.
6. In the Comments section, document the injection given.
7. Click Save.
8. When you are certain that the information documented is accurate, you will sign off on this note. Click Sign.
9. A new window opens. Enter your password (the one that you used to log into e-Medsys®), and click Save.

Completing a Charge Ticket

1. Once you have saved and signed off on the patient note, you can create a charge ticket.
2. In the patient's chart, on the left side of the screen, click on the current appointment, highlighting it.
3. When you do this, the right side of the screen brings up more information regarding the appointment. From the right-hand corner of this screen, select the Superbill Tab. The electronic superbill appears.
4. Enter the provider name and the date. The Insurance field is autopopulated based on the patient's insurance.
5. Below the Comments section, there is a section with three tabs (Ticket, Chart, and Find). The Ticket Tab is populated with some of the most common charges. If the charge is not on the Ticket Tab, select the Find Tab to look up a CPT code and add it to the charge ticket.
6. Type the code, and then press Enter on your keyboard. Now, the procedure code appears below the search field, with a box next to it. Click on the box to select it. When you do, a row at the bottom opens that indicates your selection.
7. Move your mouse into the Diag1 field. When you do, an icon of binoculars appears. Click on the binoculars. Now, the cursor moves back up to the Code field. Type the first few letters of the diagnosis in the Description field, and press Enter on your keyboard. Now, the diagnosis code appears below the search field, with a box next to it. Click on the box to select it. When you do, note that the diagnosis code now appears in the Diag1 box at the bottom.
8. Click Save. Now, you are back on the Ticket Tab.
9. Enter additional CPT codes and ICD-9 codes in the same manner.
10. When you are certain that the information documented is accurate, you will sign off on these charges. Click Sign.
11. A new window opens. Your sign-off password is your user password (the one you used to log into e-Medsys®). Enter your user password, and click Save.
12. You can click Print to print a copy of the superbill.

Ordering Laboratory Tests and Entering Results

From the Main Menu: ***EHR > EHR Home Page***

Exercises and step-by-step procedures covering this material are found in Appendix B.

Ordering Lab Tests

1. When working in the EHR interface in an individual patient record, you should always *first* indicate on the EHR schedule that you have Admitted the patient.
2. Still on the EHR schedule page, again right click on the patient's name on the schedule.
3. Select Add New (Linked), and then select Order. The new order appears on the right side of the screen.
4. The Provider, Department, Folder, and Insurance fields are autopopulated.
5. Enter the date of the order.
6. The order will be billed to the patient's insurance company, so in the Bill To option, make sure the button to the left of Insurance is selected. The Priority field has various drop-down options; select Routine. The remaining fields should be left blank.
7. Click Save.
8. Now, click on the Tests Tab.
9. In the Company field, select LabCorp from the drop-down menu. The Order Set field should be autopopulated with LabCorp Test Set.
10. From the Set Tests Tab, scroll down, and click in the box to the left of the test that the provider is ordering.
11. Note that when you select the test, a row appears at the bottom of the screen that indicates your selection.
12. Now click the ICDs Tab.
13. Type the first few letters of the diagnosis in the Desc field, and press Enter on your keyboard. This searches for all diagnosis codes in e-Medsys® that start with these letters. Click in the box to the left of the correct diagnosis code to select it.
14. Click on Save. Now, the order is ready for provider sign-off.

Uploading Laboratory Results into the Patient Chart

1. Click on EHR home page.
2. From the menu along the top of the page, click on Chart.
3. Search for the patient (either by typing the patient's last name and clicking Enter or by clicking the first letter of the patient's last name along the left side of the screen). Double click on the patient's name to open his or her chart.
4. From the left navigational tab, click on APPTS.
5. Find the correct appointment and the linked order for lab testing.
6. Right click on the correct order. Select Add New (Linked), and then select Upload File. The document upload appears on the right side of the screen.
7. Folder: Select Results from the drop-down menu.
8. Doc. Type: Select Lab Result Report from the drop-down menu.
9. In the ICD field, click the binoculars, and search for the provider's diagnosis. (*Hint:* Type the first few letters of the diagnosis in the Description field, and press Enter.)
10. Enter the date.
11. In the Name field, enter Lab Result Report if not already populated.
12. Next to the Document to Upload field, click Browse. Locate and select the laboratory results file on your computer.

13. Click Upload to Chart.
14. Now, on the left side of the screen, the lab result should appear in Tree View, as a submenu item beneath the corresponding order.

Posting Charges and Payments at the Time of Service

From the Main Menu: *Billing > Posting > Charge Posting*

Exercises and step-by-step procedures covering this material are found in Appendix B.

What Does Batch Posting Mean?

Batch posting allows you to have multiple open posting batches available at one time. This is a tool for organizing the transactions posted in the practice. For example, you could have one batch for posting a large Blue Cross EOB, another batch for patient payments, and yet another batch for charges for a specific doctor or a specific day.

Creating a New Batch Posting

1. When you select Billing > Posting > Charge Posting, a Batch Posting window opens. This window shows all open batches and gives you a chance to open a new batch or post to an existing batch.
2. To open a new batch, click on the New Batch button.
3. Populate the Open Date (the date the batch was opened; the system will default to the current date), the Batch Description, and the Department (the *physical location* of the department the user is posting from).
4. Click OK. Now, you are on the charge posting screen and can enter account charges.

Posting Charges to an Existing Batch

1. When you select Billing > Posting > Charge Posting, a Batch window opens. This window shows all open batches and gives you a chance to open a new batch or post to an existing batch.
2. To post new charges to an existing batch, highlight the batch that you wish to post charges to, and click OK.
3. Now, you are on the charge posting screen and can enter account charges.

Posting Charges

1. Search for (type in the patient's last name, and click Search) and select the patient for which you wish to post charges.
2. Press OK to accept the charge ticket number if correct, or press Cancel if there is no charge ticket number. If a charge ticket was created, the system will populate the Date, Department, and Provider fields.
3. Now, your cursor appears in the Charge Tab in the Date field. Enter the date of service, department, and provider for the charge (if not already populated).
4. Enter the first procedure code from the patient's visit. You can search for a CPT code using Table Look-Up (%).
5. Enter the diagnosis code from the patient's visit. You can search for an ICD-9 code using Table Look-Up (%). Once the primary diagnosis is entered, the Additional Diagnosis Tab will allow for the entering of up to three additional diagnoses. Enter additional diagnosis codes if appropriate.
6. Click OK to record the charges. The charges now appear in the Charge Accumulation box, which holds the charges (and allows you to enter additional procedures) until you are ready to post the entire visit's charges to the patient's account.
7. At the bottom of the screen, there are four boxes:
   - Check the box next to Credits to inform the system a payment needs to be posted after charges have been posted. Once the charges have been accepted, the system will automatically open the credit posting

screen using the same batch. When the payment is entered and accepted, the system will take the user back to the charge posting screen.

- Check the box next to Prt Stmt to indicate that a statement should be produced for this patient after charges and payments have been posted.
- Check the box next to Prt Receipt to indicate that a receipt should be produced for this patient only for those charges and payments posted today.
- Check the box next to Prt Claim if you would like to print a CMS-1500 form of the patient's visit after posting the charges and payments.

8. When you have recorded all charges and are ready to post them to the patient's account, click the Accept button. If you have checked the box next to Credits, the system will take you to the credit posting screen.

Correcting Charges Prior to Posting

1. If an incorrect charge was entered in the Charge Accumulation box, double click on the transaction in question, and click on the Clear Line button. This action will clear the transaction from the Charge Accumulation box.
2. Follow the steps for posting charges, and enter the correct values. Click OK to record the charges back to the Charge Accumulation box.
3. When you have recorded all charges and are ready to post them to the patient's account, click the Accept button.

Description of Fields on the Charge Tab

- **Date:** Enter the date of service for the charge.
- **Department, Provider, Primary Ins Plan, Referring Provider:** These fields default to the entries from patient registration.
- **Procedure:** Search by CPT code by typing "%,"the first digit of the code, or the first few digits of the code, if known.
- **Dx1:** Search for an ICD code by typing "%," the first digit of the code, or the first few digits of the code, if known.
- **Charge Amount:** The system will automatically populate with the correct fee.
- **Multiple Dates:** Check this box if the cursor should be positioned in the Date field after each charge line is posted. This box would be checked if posting multiple services done on different dates—for example, hospital charges.
- **Update Dx:** Click on the Update Dx button to indicate the primary diagnosis as the default diagnosis for that patient.
- **Credits:** Check this box to inform the system that a payment needs to be posted after charges have been posted. Once the charges have been accepted, the system will automatically open the credit posting screen using the same batch. When the payment is entered and accepted, the system will take the user back to the charge posting screen.
- **Prt Stmt:** Check this box to inform the system that a demand statement should be produced for this patient after charges and payments have been posted.
- **Prt Receipt:** Check this box to inform the system that a receipt should be produced for this patient only for those charges and payments posted today.
- **Prt Claim:** Check this box to inform the system that a demand claim form should be produced for this patient after charges and payments have been posted.

Posting Payments at the Time of Service

1. When you accept the charges on the charge posting screen, the system will automatically bring the patient from charge posting forward into the credit posting screen (since you checked the box next to Credits). The system will automatically default to the same batch and the same date of service; it will also default the credit type to a patient type payment.
2. Enter the credit type (Cash, Check, Credit Card).
3. Enter check information (check number and ABA number) if check is the method of payment.
4. Enter the amount of the payment.
5. Patient payments are posted to the patient's outstanding transactions using the Patient, Today, All Open, or All radio button.
   - To apply payments to today's charges, click the radio button next to Today.
   - To apply payments to other outstanding charges, select the radio button next to All Open.
6. When you select a radio button, an itemized list will appear below with open patient charges (either today's charges or all open charges, depending on what you selected).
7. In the Applied column, enter the amount that is to be applied to each charge.
8. Click Accept to save the payment to the patient's account.

Description of Fields on the Credits Tab

- **S:** Enter the default to Yes to have transactions appear on the patient's statement.
- **Patient Radio Button:** This button displays all charges with a remaining balance for which the patient is responsible.
- **Today's Radio Button:** This button displays all of today's charges with a remaining balance.
- **All Open Radio Button:** This button displays all outstanding charges with a remaining balance (patient responsible and insurance responsible). This radio button is normally used for posting patient payments.
- **All:** This button displays all charges—even charges with a zero remaining balance.
- **Apply:** Enter charges to the line item or items. Be sure to press the Enter key to apply the payment to the last transaction.
- **Auto Payment:** After you enter the amount and choose the All Open radio button, you can click on the Auto Payment button, which will automatically apply the payment to the oldest outstanding charge.

INSTALLATION INSTRUCTIONS FOR e-Medsys® EDUCATIONS EDITION 2.0

1. Open Internet Explorer, and enter http://www.trimedtech.com/v2delmar/ in the address bar.
2. Click the Download e-Medsys® button to start downloading the e-Medsys® client application.
3. A window will pop up, asking "Do you want to run or save this file?" Click Run.
4. After e-MedsysPM.exe is downloaded, it will ask, "Are you sure you want to run this software?" Click Run.
5. The e-Medsys® Educational Edition Setup Wizard will appear. Click Next.
6. Specify the location of the e-Medsys® directory (c:\e-Medsys). Click Next.

7. On the Ready to Install screen, click Install.
8. Type your Enterprise Number (printed on the inside cover of your book), and click OK.
9. Click Yes through the prompt concerning your enterprise number.
10. Click Finish to complete the e-Medsys® Setup Wizard.
11. Follow the directions on page 213 for using the Configuration Tool and logging in to the program.
12. *Note:* When you are using the e-Medsys® program, a DOS Window will always be present and minimized on your taskbar. Do not close that DOS Window or you will close the program.

UNINSTALLING e-Medsys®

Vista

1. Click Start > Control Panel, and then click Programs and Features.
2. Scroll to and click e-Medsys® Client for Delmar/Cengage Learning.
3. Click Uninstall at the top.

Windows XP

1. Click Start > Control Panel, and then click Add or Remove Programs.
2. Scroll to and click e-Medsys® Client for Delmar/Cengage Learning.
3. Click Remove.

SYSTEM REQUIREMENTS FOR e-Medsys® EDUCATIONAL EDITION 2.0

Minimum Requirements

- Intel Pentium 4 2.0 GHz, 1 GB of available local disk space
- 2 GB memory RAM with Microsoft Windows Vista or later
- Microsoft Internet Explorer 8 or 9
- Microsoft Word 2003 or later
- Acrobat Reader
- 1024 × 768 × 24 bit display

Third-Party Software

Third-party software (such as Yahoo! and Google toolbars, Norton, and McAfee) does not follow the rules setup in Internet Options; therefore, it tends to block e-Medsys® EHR functionality with respect to pop-ups. If this does happen, then you need to add http://ehr.elearning.emedsys.trimedtech.com to the allowed or safe sites lists of those programs. Follow the instructions in the next section, "Internet Settings (Add as Safe Site)."

Internet Settings (Add as Safe Site)

1. Open Internet Explorer, and go to the Tools Menu Bar. Select Pop-up Blocker, and set it to Turn Off Pop-up Blocker.
2. Go to Tools, and select Internet Options.
3. Select the second tab, Security; select Trusted Sites, and click on the Sites button.

4. Keep the "Require server verification (https:) for all sites in this zone" checked.
5. Add the URL http://ehr.elearning.emedsys.trimedtech.com as a trusted site, and then click Close.
6. While in the Trusted Sites location, click on Custom Level. Select Reset To: and select the Low setting; then hit the Reset button. A message will pop up, asking "Are you sure you want to change the settings for this zone?" Click Yes. Then click the Ok button and then click Ok once more to close out of Internet Options.

Installation Location

It is recommended that you install e-Medsys® PM Client in "C:\e-Medsys®." The regular installation routine will automatically designate this installation location.

Bandwidth Recommendations

It is recommended that you have a minimum Internet bandwidth of 384 kbps for upload and download. If there are multiple workstations utilizing e-Medsys®, then each active workstation will require a minimum of 64 kbps of bandwidth.

Recommended Screen Resolution

The recommended screen resolution is 1024 × 768 or higher.

Supported Browser

e-Medsys® EHR does not support browsers other than Internet Explorer 8 or 9. Mozilla Firefox and Netscape are not supported.

APPENDIX B

e-Medsys® Educational Edition 2.0 Computer Exploration Exercises

TASK 1—PATIENT REGISTRATION

Exercise 1.1: Registering a Patient

Today is August 6, 2012. Michael Minn, a friend of yours, has been looking for a new provider. You suggest that he make an appointment with your provider, Sarah Dixon, M.D., Sierra Medical Group, 231 Mountain Avenue in Truckee, CA, telephone (530) 886-8740.

Michael decides to contact the office today to set up an appointment with Dr. Dixon. Table 1-1 lists registration information that was provided by Michael.

1. Log in to e-Medsys®.
2. At the top of the screen, click on Billing.
3. Click on Patient Registration from the drop-down box.

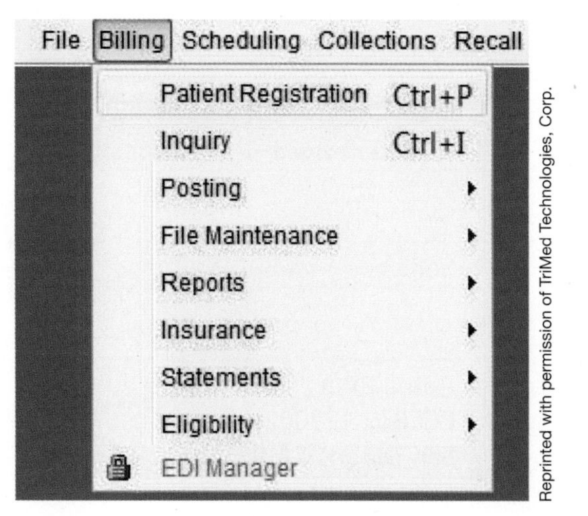

Reprinted with permission of TriMed Technologies, Corp.

4. The patient registration screen will appear.
5. Click the New Patient button. Use the information found in Table 1-1 to complete the following steps. In the e-Medsys® program, the field names in *red* indicate required fields. The other fields are additional information that can be added.
6. To maintain continuity, we recommend turning the CAPS LOCK button on.
7. Enter the patient's last name, first name, and middle initial.
8. Enter the patient's address with no punctuation.
9. Enter the patient's zip code. Once entered, the city and state will automatically populate in those fields.
10. Enter the patient's e-mail address.

TABLE 1-1 Registration Information for Michael Minn

PATIENT INFORMATION	
Patient Name	Michael B. Minn
SSN	011-65-9859
DOB	12/8/1936
Sex	Male
Home Address	2321 Sparrow Lane Calabasas, CA 91303
E-mail Address	mminn@hotmail.com
Employer	Hospitals and Clinics of America
Phone Numbers	Home: (818) 555-2323 Work: (818) 666-4545 x25 Cell Phone: (818) 555-9988 The patient said that it is OK to call him at any of these numbers.
Marital Status	Married
DLNumber	*Leave blank*
Language	English
Race	N/A
Ethnicity	Caucasian
EMERGENCY CONTACT INFORMATION	
Name	Jane Minn
Phone	(818) 555-2323
GUARANTOR INFORMATION	
Name	Self
INSURANCE INFORMATION	
Insurance Plan	Aetna PPO PO Box 129002 San Diego, CA 92112
Effective Date of Plan	1/1/2000
Subscriber	Self
Group Number	EP6589
Policy Number	MM58952525
Co-Pay Amount	$20
Deductible Amount	None

11. Enter the name of the patient's employer.
12. Enter the patient's home phone, area code first, with no spaces or dashes. Continue to add the patient's work and cell phone numbers in the same manner.
13. Enter the patient's emergency contact name and phone number.
14. The patient has indicated that he may be contacted by phone, so check YES in this field, if not already selected. If the patient had not agreed to be contacted by phone, be sure NO is selected in this field.
15. Select the patient's marital status from the drop-down box.
16. Leave the field for the patient's driver's license number blank. This is sometimes required as it could be helpful information in tracking down patients through the Department of Motor Vehicles (DMV) if they become delinquent in their payments or cannot otherwise be located.
17. From the Language drop-down menu, select English.
18. The Race field can remain blank.
19. From the Ethnicity drop-down menu, select Caucasian.
20. Enter the patient's social security number with no spaces or dashes.
21. Enter the patient's date of birth. Press the Enter key, which calculates the patient's age automatically.
22. Select Male for the patient's sex.
23. From the Department drop-down, select Sierra Medical Group, since that is where the patient will be seen.
24. From the Provider drop-down, select Dr. Sarah Dixon.
25. Leave the Referred By field blank. If there was a referring provider, you would enter the appropriate name in this field.
26. Leave the First Seen, Misc and Aftercare fields blank. The patient has not been seen yet.
27. Uncheck the boxes next to Verify Address and Verify Phone if checked. When these are selected, a pop-up alert window will appear each time the patient's account is pulled up. Keeping current with both the address and the phone number is important because the office may have to contact the patient either via telephone or through the mail. Each practice will have a preference as to whether to verify contact information each time the patient's account is accessed to make sure the information is up-to-date.
28. From the Relation to Guar drop-down, select Self.
29. Check your work with the following screen shot.

History
Active
Search
Account No: 1086
Active Account
MRN:
Name: MINN , MICHAEL B
Nickname:
SSNum: 011-65-9859
Date of Birth: 12/08/1936 75 yrs
Sex: Male Female
Address1: 2321 SPARROW LANE
Address2:
City: CALABASAS
State: CA Zipcode: 91303
Email Address: MMINN@HOTMAIL.COM
Employer: HOSPITALS AND CLINICS OF AMERI
Department: SIERRA MEDICAL GROUP
Provider: DIXON, SARAH , MD
Referred By:
Home Phone: (818) 555-2323 x
Work Phone: (818) 666-4545 x25
Cell Phone: (818) 555-9988 x
Emergency Phone: (818) 555-2323 x
May Phone? YES
Emergency Contact JANE MINN
First Seen: MM/DD/20YY
Misc: MM/DD/20YY
Aftercare: MM/DD/20YY
Deceased
MM/DD/20YY
Codes
Verify Addr
Verify Phone
Marital Status: MARRIED
DL-Num:
Relation to Guar SELF
Language: ENGLISH
Race:
Ethnicity: CAUCASIAN
Pharmacy
Accept + Ins
Accept
User: lwhalen

30. When you are finished, click on the Accept + Ins button at the bottom of the screen. This action saves all of your entries on the Patient Tab and then opens the Insurance Tab so you can continue registering the patient. Proceed directly to the next exercise.

Exercise 1.2: Entering Insurance Plan Information

Now that you have created a new record for the patient Michael Minn and have entered his demographic information, you can add his insurance plan information. Continue to use the information given in Table 1-1.

1. Click on the ADD INS button on the right side of the screen.

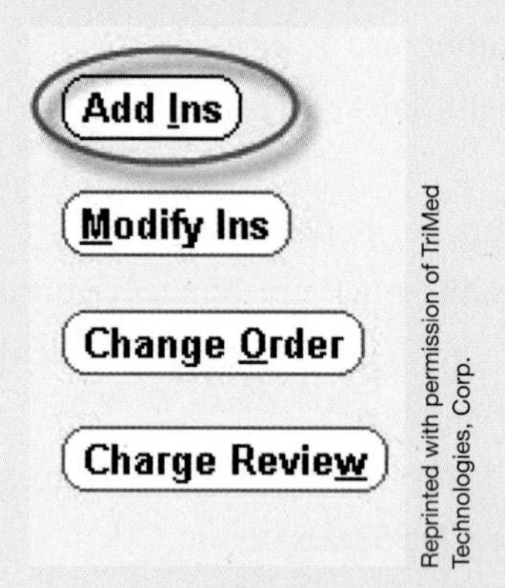

2. In the Insurance Plan field, type "AETNA," and then press the Enter key. An Insurance Plan Selection pop-up window will appear. Highlight and double click on Aetna PPO in San Diego.
3. In the Patient's relation to Policy Holder field, select Self from the drop-down menu. The policyholder information boxes will remain grayed out, as the patient is the policyholder and the system already has his information. If the policy holder was the spouse, then the policyholder information boxes would need to be filled out.
4. Tab over to the Effective Date field, and enter "1/1/2000" in the first field. This is the date the insurance plan became effective for the charges that will be posted to the patient's account. Leave the second field blank, as the plan is still effective. This will be completed when the plan is inactivated in the system.
5. Enter the group number and policy number in the appropriate fields.
6. Enter the patient's co-pay amount in the appropriate field. The co-pay amount will print on charge tickets.
7. Leave the boxes next to Accept Assign. and Sig. on File checked. Check your work with the following screen shot.

Effective: 01/01/2000 MM/DD/20YY
Group No: EP6589
Policy No: MM58952525
Policy No 2:
Special 1:
Special 2:
Copay Amt: 20.00 Copay %: 0.00
Deductible: 0.00 Family Ded.: 0.00
MSP Type: 12 Working Aged/Spouse EGHP

☑ Accept Assign.
☑ Sig. on File
☐ Outside Lab
☐ Sim. Symptoms
☐ Employ. Rel.
☐ EPSDT
☐ Accident
☐ Auto Accident
Accident State
Fam. Planning

Accept Cancel Authorization

8. Click Accept. Now, the insurance plan is listed in the top table for the patient. Also note that the box next to "No Insurance is to be billed" is now unchecked, as there is now an insurance plan in the system.

Patient: 1086 MINN, MICHAEL B   Guarantor: MINN, MICHAEL B

it | Insurance | Guarantor | Contacts | Messages | Web

☐ No insurance is to be billed   No Ins Fin Class: Update No Ins

Rank	Financial Class	Ins Plan	Policy	Grp	Copay Amt	Copay %
1	AETNA PPO	AETNA	MM58952525	EP6589	20.00	0.00

Active

9. Click Exit at the top of the screen.

PUTTING IT INTO PRACTICE

Exercise 1.3: Registering a New Patient

This exercise requires you to register a patient without step-by-step instructions, as given in previous exercises. Use the information in Table 1-2 to register Jordyn Anderson.

Today is August 23, 2012. Jordyn Anderson has been referred by her aunt, Marge Grey, to the office of Howard Zuane, M.D., of the Sierra Medical Group. Jordyn has been experiencing some abdominal pain for the past few weeks. Table 1-2 lists registration information that was provided by Jordyn.

TABLE 1-2 Registration Information for Jordyn Anderson

PATIENT INFORMATION	
Patient Name	Jordyn Ann Anderson
SSN	956-11-7812
DOB	07/01/1991
Sex	Female
Home Address	631 Flood Drive Ventura, CA 93001
E-mail Address	jaanderson@zero.net
Employer	Student
Phone Numbers	Home: (805) 544-6798 Work: N/A Cell Phone: (805) 555-6453 The patient said that it is OK to call and leave a message at any of these numbers.
Marital Status	Single
DLNumber	*Leave blank*
Language	English
Race	N/A
Ethnicity	Caucasian

(Continued)

TABLE 1-2 Registration Information for Jordyn Anderson (*Continued*)	
EMERGENCY CONTACT INFORMATION	
Name	Jessica Anderson
Phone	(805) 544-6798
GUARANTOR INFORMATION	
Patient Relation to Guar	Child
Name	Craig Anderson
Home Address	Same as Patient
DOB	2/5/1966
SSN	695-88-1803
Employer	MAT, Inc.
Sex	Male
INSURANCE INFORMATION	
Insurance Plan	Blue Shield of CA PO Box 1505 Red Bluff, CA 96080
Effective Date of Plan	10/01/2010
Subscriber	Craig Anderson
Group Number	EP659815
Policy Number	CA880323776
Co-Pay Amount	$10
Deductible Amount	None

TASK 2—PATIENT SCHEDULING

Exercise 2.1: Scheduling an Appointment for a New Patient

Today is August 6, 2012. Michael Minn is a new patient of Dr. Dixon and would like to schedule an annual exam. He would prefer an appointment at 10:00 a.m. on Thursday, August 20, 2012.

1. Log in to e-Medsys®.
2. At the top of the screen, click on Scheduling.
3. Click on Appointment Schedule from the drop-down box. (You can also get to this screen by pressing Ctrl + B [the shortcut command] on the keyboard.)

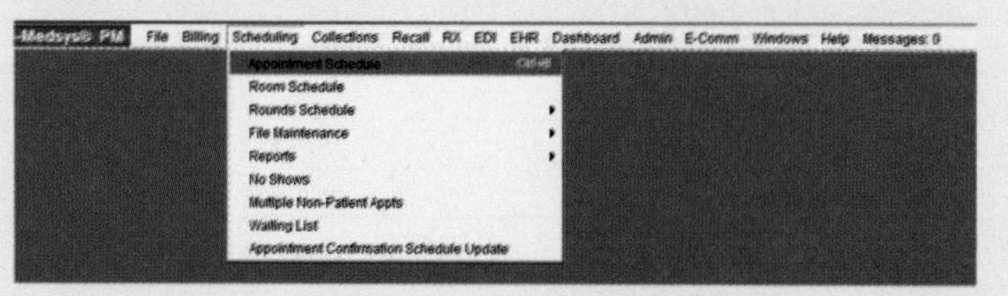

Reprinted with permission of TriMed Technologies, Corp.

4. The Appointment Scheduling screen will now appear. Click on the Provider button that appears in the left-hand corner of the screen. This will allow you to change to another provider's schedule.
5. A pop-up screen, Select a Resource(s), will appear. Highlight Dr. Sarah Dixon from the Physicians column.

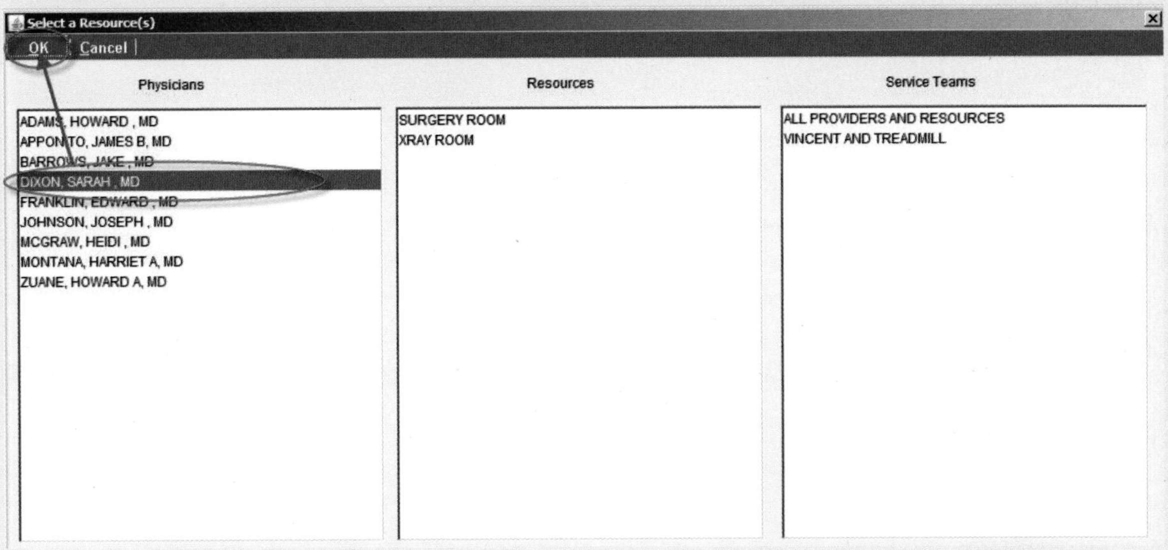

Reprinted with permission of TriMed Technologies, Corp.

6. Once the provider's name is highlighted, click OK. Now the Appointment Scheduling screen shows Dr. Dixon's schedule.
7. In the Name field, enter "MINN." Now, click on the Search button on the right side of the screen.

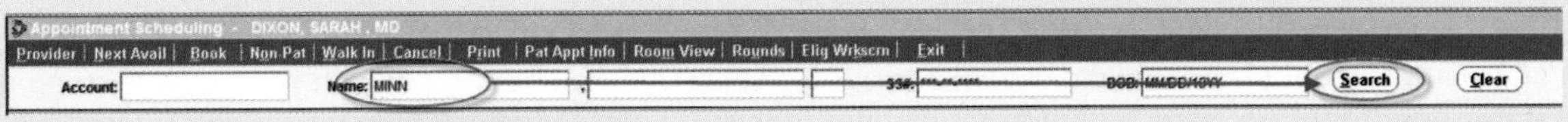

Reprinted with permission of TriMed Technologies, Corp.

8. Now the Patient Appointment Information is brought up. This screen is a snapshot of the patient's account. Click Exit to return to the Calendar screen. Note that now Michael's information is populated at the top of the screen.
9. In the top middle of the screen, there is a drop-down field for Visit Type. The default visit type is Annual (Annual exam), which is what Michael's appointment is, so this can be left as is.
10. Click the Date field in the upper left corner beneath the Provider button. (This field automatically defaults to today's date.)

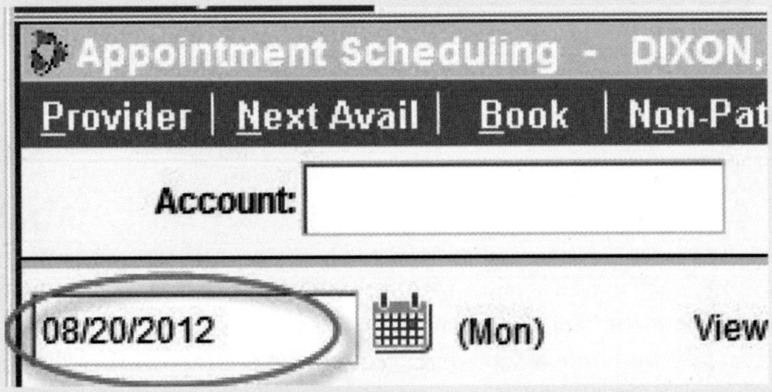

Reprinted with permission of TriMed Technologies, Corp.

11. Type "08/20/12", and press Enter on the keyboard.
12. The week of the chosen date now appears on the screen.
13. Dr. Dixon may be scheduled for any type of appointment on August 20, 2012, which is indicated by ANY in the appointment slots. On the weekly appointment calendar, highlight the requested time slot, 10:00 a.m., by clicking on it.

14. Click Book from the menu at the top of the screen.
15. A Supplemental Information screen will appear. Type "ANNUAL EXAM" in the Reason for Visit field. Note at the bottom of the screen that the system has instructions that should be given to the patient for this type of appointment.

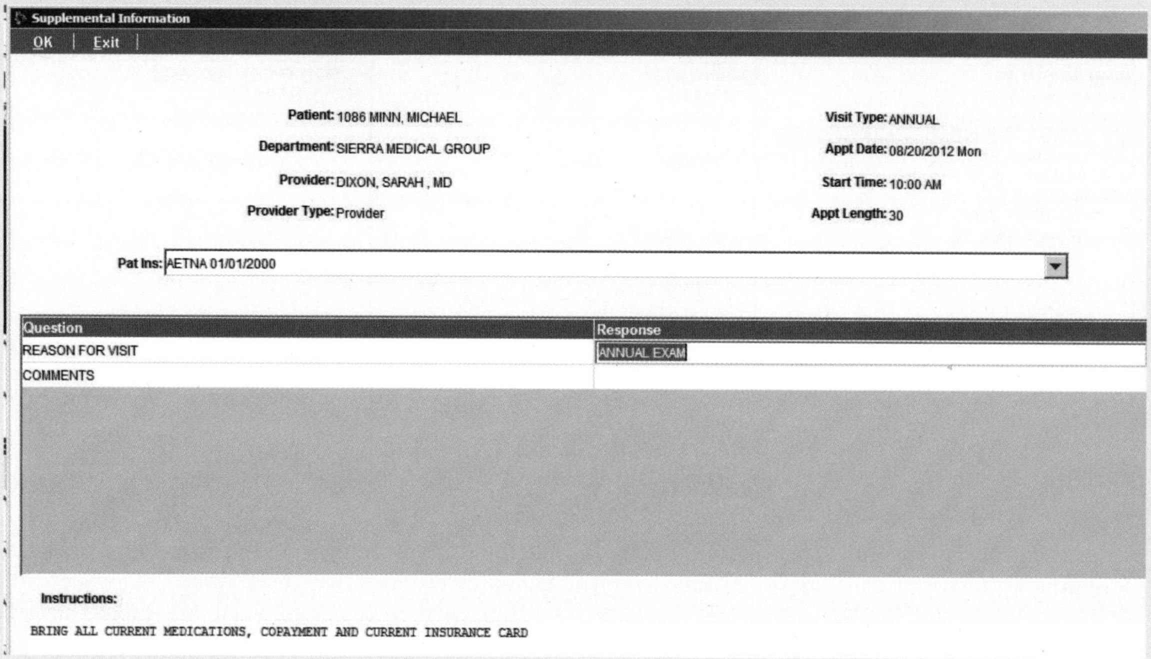

Supplemental Information
OK | Exit |

Patient: 1086 MINN, MICHAEL
Department: SIERRA MEDICAL GROUP
Provider: DIXON, SARAH , MD
Provider Type: Provider
Visit Type: ANNUAL
Appt Date: 08/20/2012 Mon
Start Time: 10:00 AM
Appt Length: 30

Pat Ins: AETNA 01/01/2000

Question	Response
REASON FOR VISIT	ANNUAL EXAM
COMMENTS	

Instructions:
BRING ALL CURRENT MEDICATIONS, COPAYMENT AND CURRENT INSURANCE CARD

Reprinted with permission of TriMed Technologies, Corp.

16. Click OK. The appointment is now booked on the weekly calendar for Dr. Dixon. If you hover your mouse over the appointment slot, detailed information about the appointment will appear.

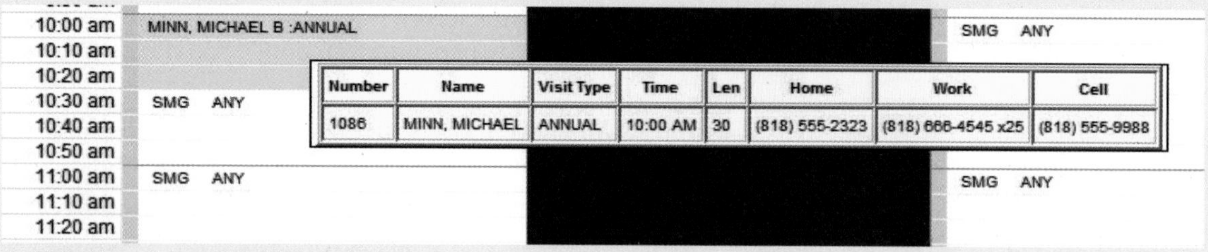

10:00 am MINN, MICHAEL B :ANNUAL — SMG ANY
10:10 am
10:20 am
10:30 am SMG ANY
10:40 am
10:50 am
11:00 am SMG ANY — SMG ANY
11:10 am
11:20 am

Number	Name	Visit Type	Time	Len	Home	Work	Cell
1086	MINN, MICHAEL	ANNUAL	10:00 AM	30	(818) 555-2323	(818) 666-4545 x25	(818) 555-9988

Reprinted with permission of TriMed Technologies, Corp.

17. Now that the appointment is booked, click the Clear button at the top right side of the screen to be prepared to book another appointment.
18. Click Exit at the top of the screen to return to the main menu.

Exercise 2.2: Scheduling an Appointment for an Established Patient

Today is August 16, 2012. Sally Jones, a patient of Dr. Heidi McGraw, calls the office this morning to request an appointment for this afternoon because she is experiencing painful urination along with back and right lower quadrant abdominal pain. She states her urine has a foul odor and she has a slight fever of 100.1°F (37°C). Looking at Dr. McGraw's schedule, you see that she has reserved time at 2:00 p.m. for any type of office visit. Sally agrees that this time will work for her. Schedule a return office visit appointment for her today at 2:00 p.m.

1. Log in to e-Medsys®, if not already logged in.
2. At the top of the screen, click on Scheduling. Click on Appointment Schedule from the drop-down box.
3. View Dr. McGraw's weekly appointment schedule by clicking the Provider button at the top left corner and then selecting Dr. McGraw.

4. Select today's date by clicking in the Date field. Type "08/16/2012", and press Enter on the keyboard. The week of the chosen date now appears on the screen.
5. Now search for Sally Jones. In the Name field, enter "JONES," and click Search.
6. Since the last name "JONES" was the only item put into the search engine, the database produced all matches. Double click Sally Jones' name, and her information is now populated across the top of the schedule.

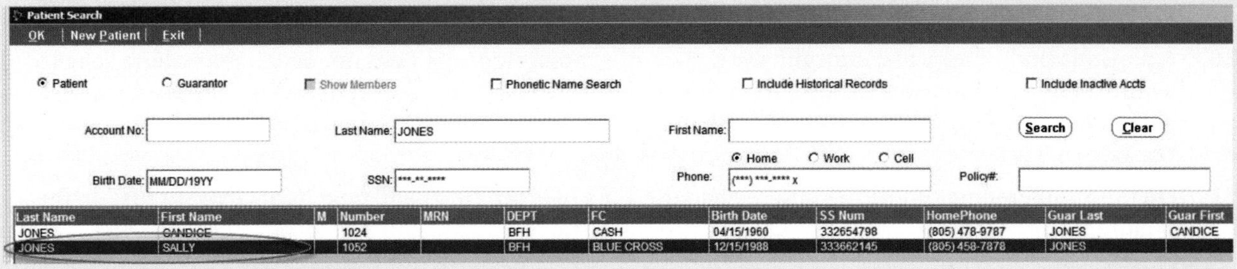

Patient Search
OK | New Patient | Exit |

Patient   Guarantor   Show Members   Phonetic Name Search   Include Historical Records   Include Inactive Accts

Account No: Last Name: JONES   First Name: Search   Clear

Home   Work   Cell

Birth Date: MM/DD/19YY   SSN: ***-**-****   Phone: (***) ***-**** x   Policy#:

Last Name	First Name	M	Number	MRN	DEPT	FC	Birth Date	SS Num	HomePhone	Guar Last	Guar First
JONES	CANDICE		1024		BFH	CASH	04/15/1960	332654798	(805) 478-9787	JONES	CANDICE
JONES	SALLY		1052		BFH	BLUE CROSS	12/15/1988	333662145	(805) 458-7878	JONES	

Reprinted with permission of TriMed Technologies, Corp.

7. From the Visit Type drop-down, select Return Office Visit (Ret OV).
8. Click on the 2:00 p.m. slot on the calendar for August 16, and click the Book button.
9. You may get a pop-up window indicating that the appointment does not use the whole time slot selected. If so, choose "Create New Slot" and click "OK."
10. On the Supplemental Information screen, in the Reason for Visit field, type "PAINFUL URINATION; BACK AND ABDOMINAL PAIN."
11. In the Comments field, type "PATIENT STATES URINE HAS FOUL ODOR; TEMP IS 100.1F."

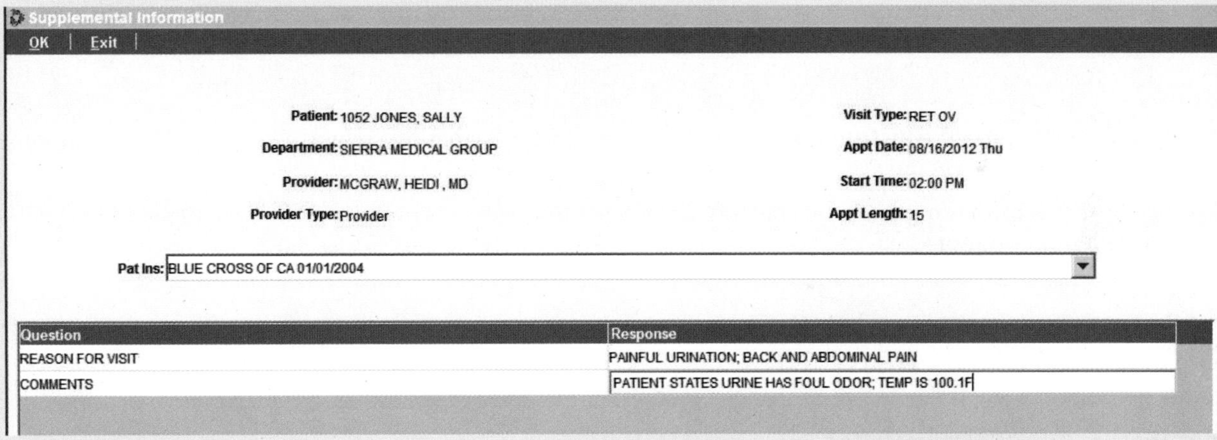

Supplemental Information
OK | Exit |

Patient: 1052 JONES, SALLY   Visit Type: RET OV
Department: SIERRA MEDICAL GROUP   Appt Date: 08/16/2012 Thu
Provider: MCGRAW, HEIDI , MD   Start Time: 02:00 PM
Provider Type: Provider   Appt Length: 15

Pat Ins: BLUE CROSS OF CA 01/01/2004

Question	Response
REASON FOR VISIT	PAINFUL URINATION; BACK AND ABDOMINAL PAIN
COMMENTS	PATIENT STATES URINE HAS FOUL ODOR; TEMP IS 100.1F

Reprinted with permission of TriMed Technologies, Corp.

12. After giving Sally the instructions on the Supplemental Information screen, click OK. Sally's appointment now appears on the schedule.
13. Now that the appointment is booked, click Clear at the top right side of the screen to be prepared to book another appointment.

Exercise 2.3: Scheduling a Procedure for an Established Patient

Valerie Violet, a patient of Dr. Zuane, has been experiencing abdominal pain for the past several days. After a consultation with Dr. Zuane, she was instructed to make an appointment for a colonoscopy. Schedule an appointment (Visit Type: PROC) for Monday, August 27, 2012, at 11:00 a.m. for the 30-minute procedure.

1. Log in to e-Medsys®, if not already logged in.
2. At the top of the screen, click on Scheduling. Click on Appointment Schedule from the drop-down box.
3. View Dr. Zuane's weekly appointment schedule by clicking the Provider button at the top left corner and then selecting Dr. Zuane.

4. Select the date by using the Calendar icon.
5. Now search for Valerie Violet. In the Name field, enter "VIOLET," and click Search.
6. Valerie has a Collections Alert in the system; click OK to close the reminder.
7. Valerie's information is now populated across the top of the schedule.
8. From the Visit Type drop-down, select PROC (procedure).
9. Click on the 11:00 a.m. slot on the calendar for August 27, and click the Book button.
10. A pop-up window appears, informing you that the appointment slot does not match the criteria selected. This feature helps remind users to book appointment visit types as indicated on the scheduler to ensure a smooth patient flow. However, this particular appointment slot indicates that a procedure appointment type may be booked, so it is all right to go ahead and book the slot.
11. On the Supplemental Information screen, in the Type of Procedure field, type "COLONOSCOPY." In the Inpatient or Outpatient field, type "OUTPATIENT." In the Need Assistant field, type "YES."

Supplemental Information
OK | Exit |

Patient: 1037 VIOLET, VALERIE
Department: SIERRA MEDICAL GROUP
Provider: ZUANE, HOWARD A, MD
Provider Type: Provider
Visit Type: PROC
Appt Date: 08/27/2012 Mon
Start Time: 11:00 AM
Appt Length: 30

Pat Ins: BLUE CROSS 02/01/2002

Question	Response
TYPE OF PROCEDURE	COLONOSCOPY
IN PATIENT OR OUT PATIENT	OUTPATIENT
NEED ASSISTANT?	YES
COMMENTS	

12. After giving Valerie the instructions on the Supplemental Information screen, click OK. Valerie's appointment now appears on the schedule.
13. Now that the appointment is booked, click Clear at the top right side of the screen to be prepared to book another appointment.

PUTTING IT INTO PRACTICE

Exercise 2.4: Scheduling Appointments

This exercise requires you to schedule appointments for the following patients without using step-by-step instructions, as given in the previous exercises. *Remember to click OK through any Collections Alerts or other reminder notes in e-Medsys® for the purposes of these exercises.*

1. Dr. Zuane has asked Scott McGuire to make an appointment to have his cholesterol levels checked. Schedule a return office visit appointment for Scott on August 8, 2012, at 2:00 p.m.
2. Bruce Sawtelle, a patient of Dr. Edward Franklin, has a history of diverticulosis. At his last visit, he was instructed to make an appointment for a sigmoidoscopy, which he does before leaving the office. Schedule an appointment (Visit Type: SIG) for Bruce on August 8, 2012, at 10:00 a.m. for the 30-minute procedure.
3. Diane Best, a patient of Dr. Howard Adams, has a family history of diabetes and would like to schedule an appointment for a blood glucose check. Schedule a follow-up visit for August 22, 2012, at 2:30 p.m.
4. Lily Adams, a patient of Dr. Dixon, needs an appointment for a B-12 shot, which was ordered by Dr. Dixon. Schedule a follow-up appointment for Lily on July 16, 2012, at 11:00 a.m.
5. Anthony Bates needs to make an appointment to receive a tetanus shot, which was ordered by Dr. Zuane. Schedule a follow-up appointment for Anthony on July 3, 2012, at 9:00 a.m.
6. Cory Haines would like to schedule an annual exam for August 6, 2012, at 10:00 a.m. with Dr. Heidi McGraw.

7. Wilma Flint, a patient of Dr. Dixon, has been experiencing extreme fatigue and dizziness for the last several weeks. She would like to schedule an appointment for her lunch hour. Schedule a return office visit appointment for Wilma on June 20, 2012, at 1:00 p.m.
8. Debbie Huston, a patient of Dr. McGraw, needs to schedule a return office visit on July 25, 2012, at 10:00 a.m. for hypothyroidism.

Exercise 2.5: Cancelling and Rescheduling an Appointment

Today is August 20, 2012. Diane Best, a patient of Dr. Adams, has potential diabetes and at her last appointment scheduled a follow-up visit for a blood glucose check for Wednesday, August 22, 2012. Because her cell phone was out of battery, she did not have her calendar with her at the time she made the appointment. Later in the day, she realized she will be out of town on that date. Diane contacts Dr. Adams' office to cancel the appointment and reschedule her follow-up at a later date. The new appointment date is Friday, August 31, 2012, at 9:30 a.m.

1. Log in to e-Medsys®, if not already logged in.
2. At the top of the screen, click on Scheduling. Click on Appointment Schedule from the drop-down box.
3. Search for Diane Best (in the Name field, enter "BEST, DIANE," and click Search). Diane Best's appointment history now appears on the Patient Appointment Information screen.
4. In the center of the screen, highlight Diane's appointment for August 22, 2012, and then click the Cancel button.

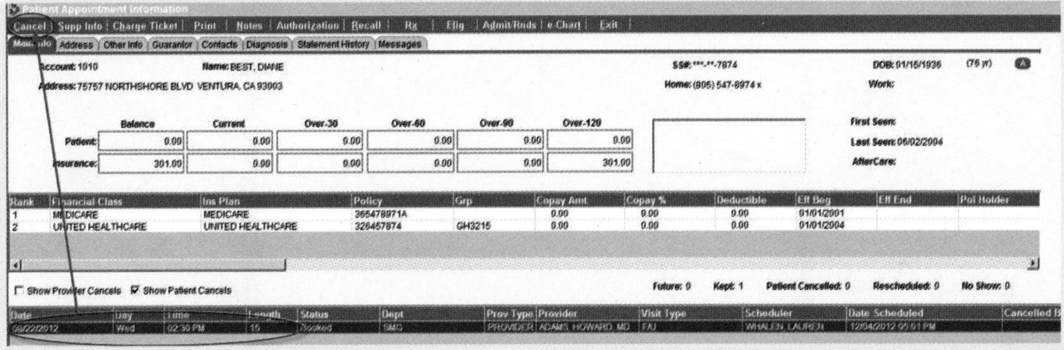

Reprinted with permission of TriMed Technologies, Corp.

5. In the Reason for Cancellation field, type "PATIENT NEEDS DIFFERENT DATE," and click the Patient Cancel button.

Cancellation Reason

Reason for Cancellation?

PATIENT NEEDS DIFFERENT DATE

Provider Cancel | Patient Cancel | Do Not Cancel

Reprinted with permission of TriMed Technologies, Corp.

6. Click Yes at the prompt for "Do You Wish to Reschedule this Appointment?"
7. This brings you to the main scheduling calendar screen. Select Diane's provider, Dr. Howard Adams, if not already selected. (*Hint:* Click on the Provider button, select Dr. Adams, and click OK.)
8. Using the Calendar icon, select August 31, 2012, the date for which Diane wishes to reschedule the appointment.
9. Be sure the Visit Type drop-down is F/U. Click on the 9:30 a.m. appointment row to highlight the slot.
10. Click Book. If you get a pop-up window, accept the information by saying Yes/OK.

11. Now the rescheduled appointment appears on the calendar.

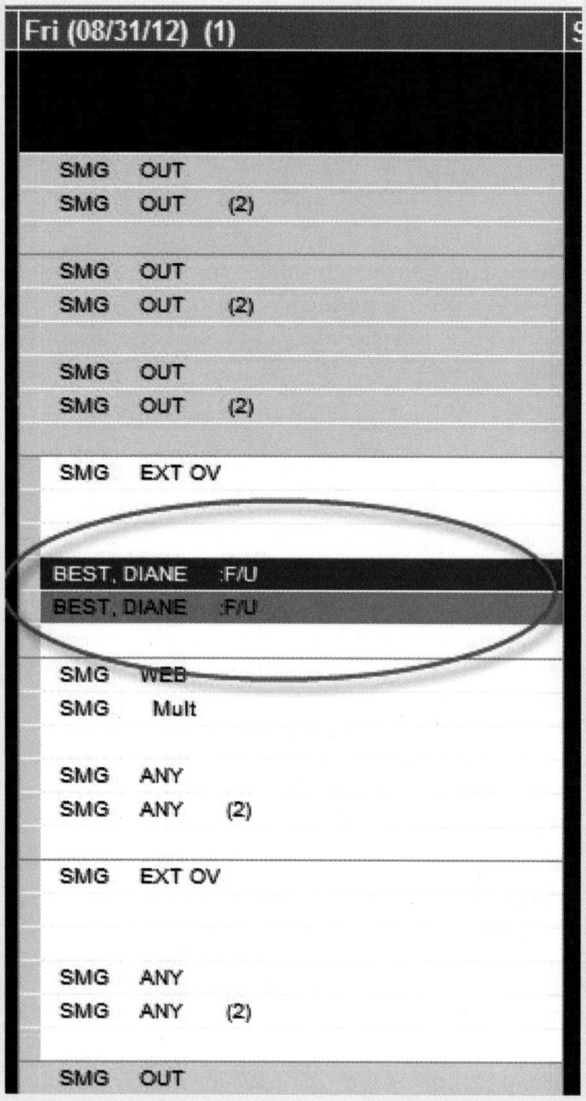

Fri (08/31/12) (1)

SMG OUT
SMG OUT (2)
SMG OUT
SMG OUT (2)
SMG OUT
SMG OUT (2)
SMG EXT OV
BEST, DIANE :F/U
BEST, DIANE :F/U
SMG WEB
SMG Mult
SMG ANY
SMG ANY (2)
SMG EXT OV
SMG ANY
SMG ANY (2)
SMG OUT

12. Now that the appointment is booked, click Clear at the top right side of the screen to be prepared to book another appointment.

PUTTING IT INTO PRACTICE

Exercise 2.6: Cancelling and Rescheduling Appointments

This exercise requires you to cancel and reschedule appointments for the following patients without using step-by-step instructions, as given in the previous exercises.

1. Scott McGuire, a patient of Dr. Zuane, has seen an increase in his weight and is concerned about developing heart issues. He would like to have his cholesterol levels checked. He had made an appointment for a return office visit for August 8, 2012, at 2:00 p.m. but realized after booking the appointment that he has family coming in from out of town that afternoon. Scott would like to reschedule his appointment to the preceding day. Schedule the new appointment for August 7, 2012, at 10:00 a.m.
2. Valerie Violet, a patient of Dr. Zuane, has been experiencing abdominal pain for the past several days. She previously scheduled a colonoscopy for August 27, 2012, at 11:00 a.m. but would like to get in sooner, due to her symptoms. She calls the office to cancel that appointment and reschedule for August 13, 2012, at the same time.

TASK 3—PATIENT AUTHORIZATIONS

Exercise 3.1: Requesting a Patient Authorization

Today is August 10, 2012. Curtis Russell is a patient of Dr. Zuane. He is being treated for constipation. Dr. Zuane refers him to Dr. Apponito for an office consultation. You call Motion Picture Industry (phone number 818-569-1234) today to request this authorization and speak with Alex Bailey. The insurance company's fax number is 818-569-5698.

1. Log in to e-Medsys®.
2. At the top of the screen, click on Billing.
3. Click on Inquiry from the drop-down box. (You can also get to this screen by pressing Ctrl + I [the shortcut command] on the keyboard.)

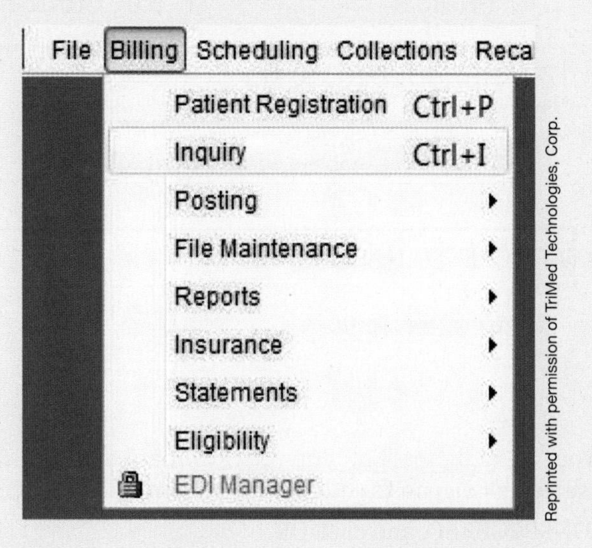

Reprinted with permission of TriMed Technologies, Corp.

4. An Inquiry screen appears.
5. Search for Curtis Russell by typing "RUSSELL" in the Name field and clicking the Search button.
6. Curtis has a Collections Alert in the system, which will appear as a pop-up. Click OK.

> **Note:** The e-Medsys® program includes built-in reminders such as this one. For the purposes of these exercises, we will click through the system reminders.

7. Now Curtis's information appears in the Inquiry screen.
8. At the top of the screen, click the Authorization button.

Inquiry
Clear | Print | Notes+ | Appt Info | Authorization | Flig | Recall | Rx | Admit/Rnds | e-Chart | Exit
Account: 1033 Name: RUSSELL, CURTIS SS#: ***-**-6677 DOB: 07/25/1975 (37 yr) Search
Main Info | Address | Other Info | Guarantor | Contacts | Diagnosis | Statement History | Messages | Totals

Reprinted with permission of TriMed Technologies, Corp.

9. The Patient Authorization File Maintenance screen appears. Click the Add button.

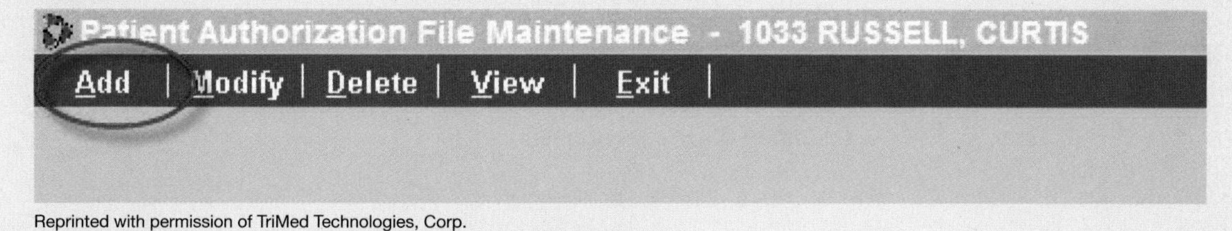

Reprinted with permission of TriMed Technologies, Corp.

10. A new screen appears. In the Type field, select Referral Out from the drop-down list, since Dr. Apponito works for another practice. (Referral In would be used to refer a patient to a provider at the same facility.)
11. In the Status field, select Requested from the drop-down list.
12. In the Request Date field, type today's date, 08/10/2012.
13. In the Primary Care Provider field, type "ZUA"—the first few letters of Dr. Howard Zuane's last name.
14. Press the Enter key on your keyboard. Dr. Zuane's name is now populated in this field. In the Specialty Provider field, type "APPO" (to search for Dr. Apponito), and press Enter on the keyboard. Dr. Apponito's name is now populated in this field.

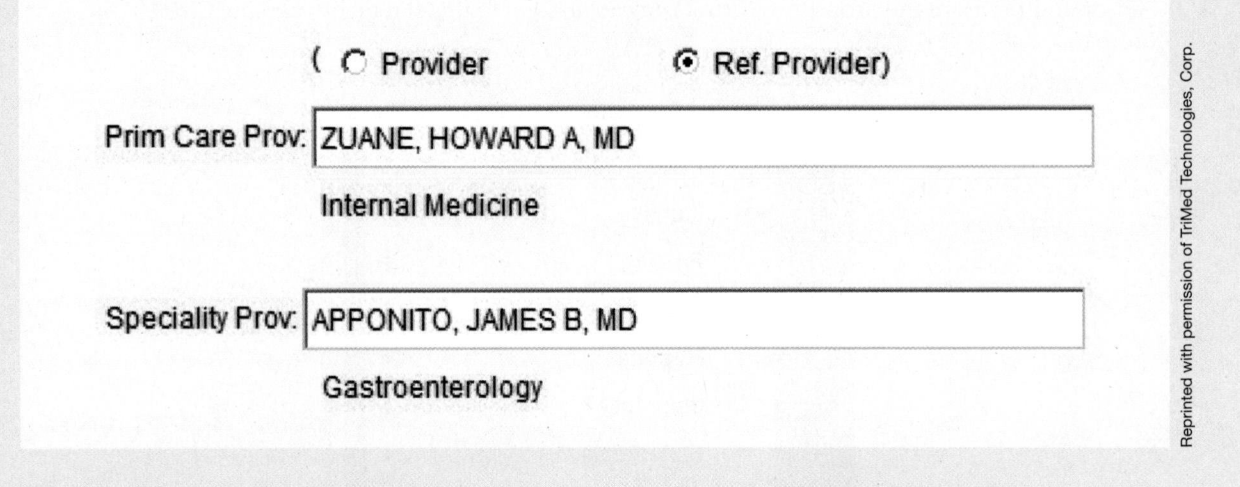

15. In the Diagnosis field, type "%," and press Enter on your keyboard to search for the diagnosis code. Using the % symbol allows you to search all diagnosis codes in the system.
16. Select CONSTIPATION UNSPECIFIED, and click OK.

Diagnosis Selection

OK | Cancel

Number	ICD9	Desc
30	592.0	CALCULUS OF KIDNEY
61	427.5	CARDIAC ARREST
5	427.9	CARDIAC DYSRHYTHMIA NOS
60	425.8	CARDIOMYOPATH IN OTH DIS
53	366.34	CATARACT IN DEGEN DIS
52	366.9	CATARACT NOS
50	682.9	CELLULITIS NOS
51	682.7	CELLULITIS OF FOOT
73	669.71	CESAREAN DELIVERY UNSPEC
11	786.50	CHEST PAIN NOS
13	496	CHR AIRWAY OBSTRUCT NEC
4	280.0	CHR BLOOD LOSS ANEMIA
12	428.0	CONGESTIVE HEART FAILURE
124	564.00	CONSTIPATION UNSPECIFIED
72	V25.9	CONTRACEPTIVE MGT UNSPEC
14	786.2	COUGH
135	626.8	D/O MENSTRUATION & OTHER ABNORMAL BLEED FE GNT
103	715.96	DEGENERATE JT LOWER LEG SPEC
120	315.8	DELAY IN DEVELOPMENT, OTHER SPECIFIED
105	692.9	DEMATITIS ECZEMA UNSPEC CAUSE
95	250.02	DIAB UNCOMP TYPE II UNCONTRD
106	V06.1	DIPTHERIA-TET-PERTIS COMBINED
76	621.9	DISORDER OF UTERUS UNSPEC

17. Type the contact person's name (Bailey, Alex), phone number (818-569-1234), and fax number (818-569-5698). Check your work with the following screen shot.

General Info | Authorized Visits / Procedures

Type: REFERRAL OUT | Auth number: | Status: REQUESTED

(C Provider ⊙ Ref. Provider) (⊙ Ref# C ICD9 C Desc)

Request Date: 08/10/2012 | Prim Care Prov: ZUANE, HOWARD A, MD | DX (1): 564.00 CONSTIPATION UNSPECIFIED

Internal Medicine

Auth Date: MM/DD/20YY | (2):

Expire Date: MM/DD/20YY | Speciality Prov: APPONITO, JAMES B, MD | (3):

Gastroenterology

Misc Date: MM/DD/20YY | (4):

Comments

Contact: BAILEY , ALEX

Phone#: 818-569-1234 fax#: 818-569-5698

E-Mail:

Reprinted with permission of TriMed Technologies, Corp.

18. Now, click on the Authorized Visits/Procedures Tab. Select the radio button next to CPT. In field 1, type "%," and press the Enter key on your keyboard to search and select the appropriate procedure code.
19. Find CPT 99243 "Office Consultation," and click OK. (*Tip:* If you click on the header labeled "Desc," the system will alphabetize the list.) Now Office Consultation is populated in field 1. Type "1" in the Qty column. Check your work with this screen.

(C Ref# ⊙ CPT C Desc) Qty Used

1. 99243 OFFICE CONSULTATION 1 0

Reprinted with permission of TriMed Technologies, Corp.

20. Click the Accept button. Click OK on the Patient Authorization pop-up that tells you the authorization has been added.
21. Click Exit to get out of the Authorizations screen. Click the Clear button to get out of the patient's account. To exit the Inquiry screen and return to the main menu, click Exit again.

Exercise 3.2: Updating a Patient Authorization

Today is August 20, 2012. Motion Picture Industry has approved the patient authorization request (from August 10, 2012) for an office consultation for Curtis Russell, a patient of Dr. Zuane. The authorization number is AP1789, and the authorization is valid until September 30, 2012.

1. Log in to e-Medsys®.
2. At the top of the screen, click on Billing.
3. Click on Inquiry from the drop-down box. (You can also get to this screen by pressing Ctrl + I [the shortcut command] on the keyboard.)
4. An Inquiry screen appears. Search for Curtis Russell by typing "RUS" in the Name field and clicking the Search button.
5. Click OK through the Collections Alert pop-up.
6. Now Curtis's information appears in the Inquiry screen.
7. At the top of the screen, click the Authorization button. The Patient Authorization File Maintenance screen appears.
8. Highlight the request from August 10, 2012, and click the Modify button.

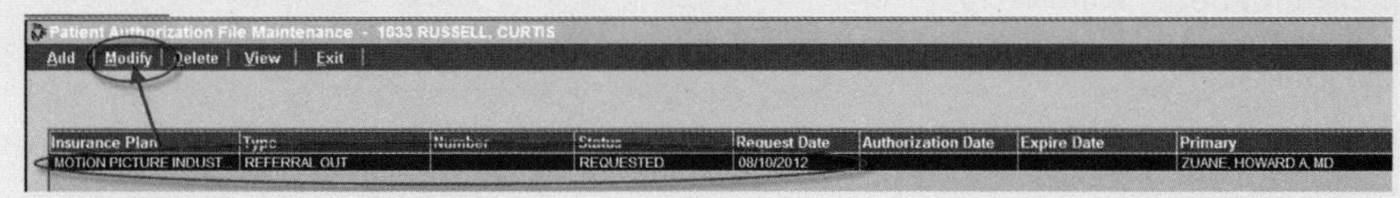
Patient Authorization File Maintenance - 1033 RUSSELL, CURTIS

Add | Modify | Delete | View | Exit

Insurance Plan	Type	Number	Status	Request Date	Authorization Date	Expire Date	Primary
MOTION PICTURE INDUST	REFERRAL OUT		REQUESTED	08/10/2012			ZUANE, HOWARD A, MD

Reprinted with permission of TriMed Technologies, Corp.

9. Type the authorization number, AP1789, in the Auth Number field.
10. Use the drop-down menu to change the status to Approved.
11. Type today's date, 08/20/2012, in the Auth Date field.
12. In the Expire Date field, type the expiration date for the authorization designated by the insurance company, 09/30/2012. Check your work with the following screen shot.

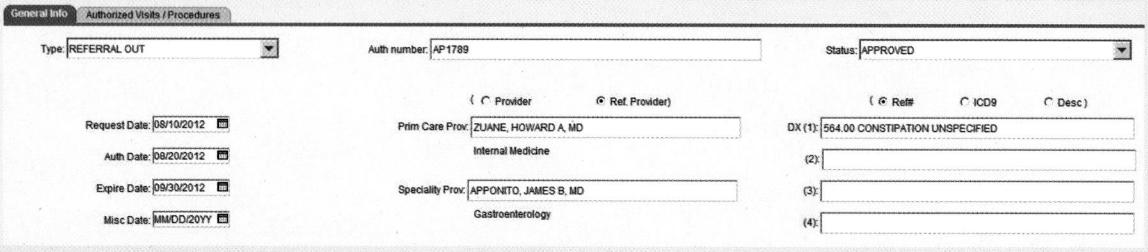

General Info | Authorized Visits / Procedures

Type: REFERRAL OUT | Auth number: AP1789 | Status: APPROVED

(Provider • Ref. Provider) | (• Ref# ICD9 Desc)

Request Date: 08/10/2012 | Prim Care Prov: ZUANE, HOWARD A, MD | DX (1): 564.00 CONSTIPATION UNSPECIFIED

Internal Medicine

Auth Date: 08/20/2012 | (2):

Expire Date: 09/30/2012 | Speciality Prov: APPONITO, JAMES B, MD | (3):

Gastroenterology

Misc Date: MM/DD/20YY | (4):

13. Click the Accept button.
14. Click Exit on the Patient Authorization File Maintenance screen. Click the Clear button to get out of the patient's account. To exit the Inquiry screen and return to the main menu, click Exit again.

PUTTING IT INTO PRACTICE

Exercise 3.3: Requesting and Updating a Patient Authorization

This exercise requires you to track an authorization for a patient without using step-by-step instructions, as given in the previous exercises.

Today is August 13, 2012. Rosemary August, a patient of Dr. Howard Adams, is experiencing some problems with atrial fibrillation and has an appointment with him to express her concerns. After examining Rosemary and discussing her symptoms, Dr. Adams would like her to make an office consultation appointment (CPT 99243) with Dr. Howard Zuane (a fellow Sierra Medical Group provider).

1. The insurance company contact is Jessica Ryan; phone 781-816-0093; fax 781-816-9300.
2. Medicare approves the authorization on September 3, 2012. The Authorization number is 7AS9887, and the authorization expires October 15, 2012.

TASK 4—PATIENT RECEPTION

Exercise 4.1: Checking in a Patient Upon Arrival—Registration Updates

Today is July 16, 2012. Lily Adams, a patient of Dr. Dixon, has scheduled an appointment to receive a B-12 shot. Lily recently moved to a new home, so her registration information will need to be updated. She would also like to add her husband as an emergency contact:

- New home address: 2626 Netherland Road, Truckee, CA 96160
- New home phone number: 310-884-3369
- Emergency Contact: Philip Adams
- Emergency Phone: 310-899-3445

1. Log in to e-Medsys®.
2. At the top of the screen, click on Scheduling. Click on Appointment Schedule from the drop-down box, or press Ctrl + B on the keyboard. The Appointment Scheduling screen will now appear.
3. Click on the Calendar icon, and use the arrows to find today's date (remember it is 07/16/12).

4. Now click on the Provider button that appears in the upper left-hand corner of the screen. Highlight Dr. Dixon to bring up her schedule for the day. Click OK.
5. Now find Lily's appointment on the schedule. Right click on the appointment slot.
6. Roll the mouse over the patient's name, ADAMS, LILY ►, and select Arrived.

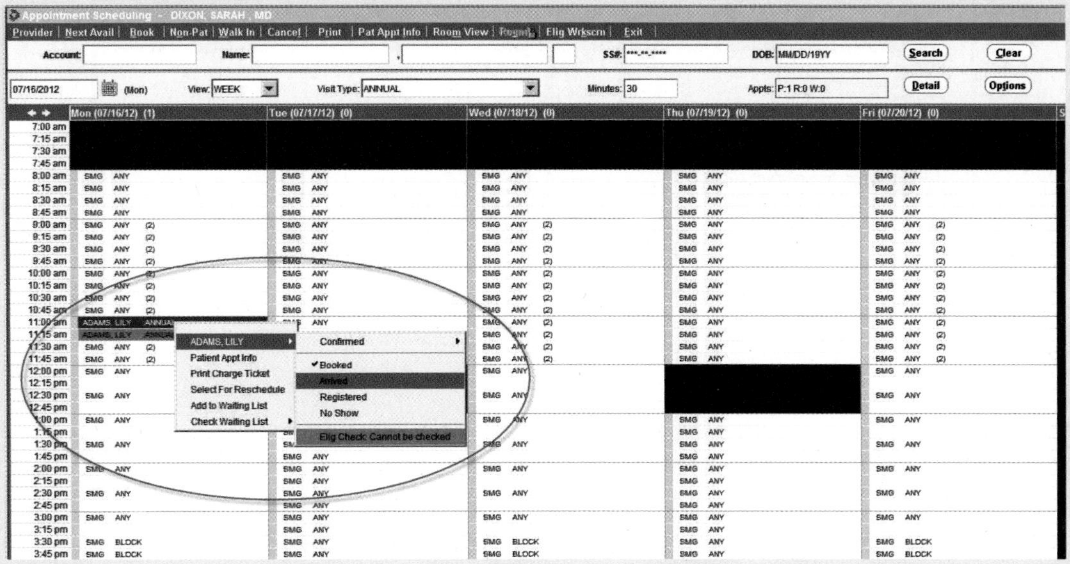

Appointment Scheduling - DIXON, SARAH , MD

Provider | Next Avail | Book | Non-Pat | Walk In | Cancel | Print | Pat Appt Info | Room View | Rounds | Elig Wrkscrn | Exit |

Account: Name: , SS#: ***-**-**** DOB: MM/DD/19YY Search Clear

07/16/2012 (Mon) View: WEEK Visit Type: ANNUAL Minutes: 30 Appts: P:1 R:0 W:0 Detail Options

	Mon (07/16/12) (1)	Tue (07/17/12) (0)	Wed (07/18/12) (0)	Thu (07/19/12) (0)	Fri (07/20/12) (0)
7:00 am					
7:15 am					
7:30 am					
7:45 am					
8:00 am	SMG ANY	SMG ANY	SMG ANY	SMG ANY	SMG ANY
8:15 am	SMG ANY	SMG ANY	SMG ANY	SMG ANY	SMG ANY
8:30 am	SMG ANY	SMG ANY	SMG ANY	SMG ANY	SMG ANY
8:45 am	SMG ANY	SMG ANY	SMG ANY	SMG ANY	SMG ANY
9:00 am	SMG ANY (2)	SMG ANY	SMG ANY (2)	SMG ANY	SMG ANY (2)
9:15 am	SMG ANY (2)	SMG ANY	SMG ANY (2)	SMG ANY	SMG ANY (2)
9:30 am	SMG ANY (2)	SMG ANY	SMG ANY (2)	SMG ANY	SMG ANY (2)
9:45 am	SMG ANY (2)	SMG ANY	SMG ANY (2)	SMG ANY	SMG ANY (2)
10:00 am	SMG ANY (2)	SMG ANY	SMG ANY (2)	SMG ANY	SMG ANY (2)
10:15 am	SMG ANY (2)	SMG ANY	SMG ANY (2)	SMG ANY	SMG ANY (2)
10:30 am	SMG ANY (2)	SMG ANY	SMG ANY (2)	SMG ANY	SMG ANY (2)
10:45 am	SMG ANY (2)	SMG ANY	SMG ANY (2)	SMG ANY	SMG ANY (2)
11:00 am	ADAMS, LILY ANNUAL	SMG ANY	SMG ANY (2)	SMG ANY	SMG ANY (2)
11:15 am	ADAMS, LILY ANNUAL		SMG ANY (2)	SMG ANY	SMG ANY (2)
11:30 am	SMG ANY (2)		SMG ANY (2)	SMG ANY	SMG ANY (2)
11:45 am	SMG ANY (2)		SMG ANY (2)	SMG ANY	SMG ANY (2)
12:00 pm	SMG ANY		SMG ANY		SMG ANY
12:15 pm					
12:30 pm	SMG ANY		SMG ANY		SMG ANY
12:45 pm					
1:00 pm	SMG ANY		SMG ANY	SMG ANY	SMG ANY
1:15 pm				SMG ANY	
1:30 pm	SMG ANY		SMG ANY	SMG ANY	SMG ANY
1:45 pm		SMG ANY		SMG ANY	
2:00 pm	SMG ANY	SMG ANY	SMG ANY	SMG ANY	SMG ANY
2:15 pm		SMG ANY		SMG ANY	
2:30 pm	SMG ANY	SMG ANY	SMG ANY	SMG ANY	SMG ANY
2:45 pm		SMG ANY		SMG ANY	
3:00 pm	SMG ANY	SMG ANY	SMG ANY	SMG ANY	SMG ANY
3:15 pm		SMG ANY		SMG ANY	
3:30 pm	SMG BLOCK	SMG ANY	SMG BLOCK	SMG ANY	SMG BLOCK
3:45 pm	SMG BLOCK	SMG ANY	SMG BLOCK	SMG ANY	SMG BLOCK

ADAMS, LILY ►
Patient Appt Info
Print Charge Ticket
Select For Reschedule
Add to Waiting List
Check Waiting List ►

Confirmed ►
✔Booked
Arrived
Registered
No Show
Elig Check: Cannot be checked

7. At the top of the screen, click on Billing. Click on Patient Registration from the drop-down box.
8. The Patient Registration screen will appear. Search for Lily Adams' account by typing "ADAMS" in the Last Name field and clicking the Search button.
9. Lily's information appears in the Patient Registration screen. Stay on the Patient Tab.
10. Update the following fields, and check your work with the following screen shot.
    - New home address: 2626 Netherland Road, Truckee, CA 96160
    - New home phone number: 310-884-3369
    - Emergency Contact: Philip Adams
    - Emergency Phone: 310-899-3445

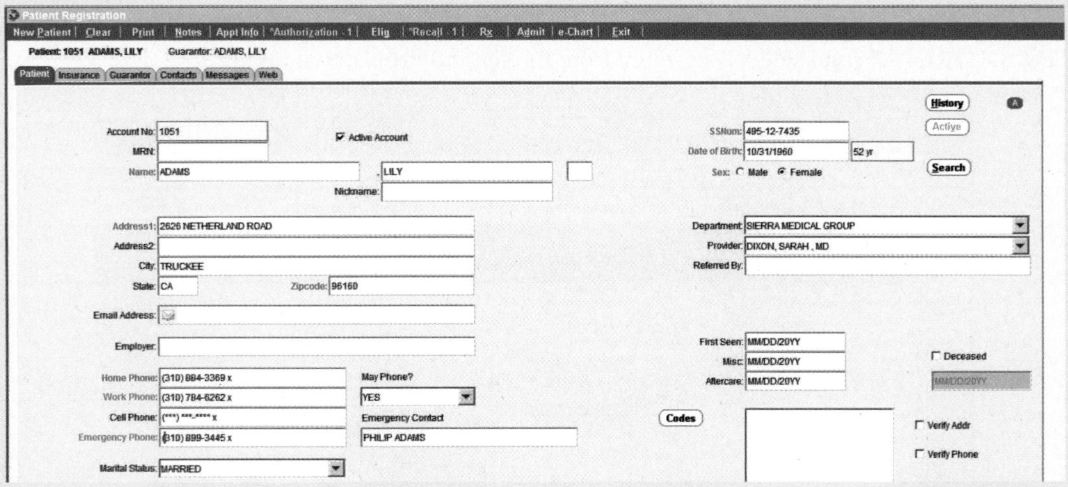

Patient Registration

New Patient | Clear | Print | Notes | Appt Info | *Authorization - 1 | Elig | *Recall - 1 | Rx | Admit | e-Chart | Exit |

Patient: 1051 ADAMS, LILY Guarantor: ADAMS, LILY

Patient | Insurance | Guarantor | Contacts | Messages | Web

History Active Search

Account No: 1051
☑ Active Account
MRN:
Name: ADAMS , LILY
Nickname:
SSNum: 495-12-7435
Date of Birth: 10/31/1960 52 yr
Sex: ○ Male ● Female

Address1: 2626 NETHERLAND ROAD
Address2:
City: TRUCKEE
State: CA Zipcode: 96160
Department: SIERRA MEDICAL GROUP
Provider: DIXON, SARAH , MD
Referred By:

Email Address:
Employer:
First Seen: MM/DD/20YY
Misc: MM/DD/20YY
Aftercare: MM/DD/20YY
☐ Deceased MM/DD/20YY

Home Phone: (310) 884-3369 x
Work Phone: (310) 784-6262 x
Cell Phone: (***) ***-**** x
Emergency Phone: (310) 899-3445 x
May Phone? YES
Emergency Contact: PHILIP ADAMS
Codes
☐ Verify Addr
☐ Verify Phone
Marital Status: MARRIED

12. Click the Accept button to save the changes.
13. Click Clear to exit out of Lily's account, and then click Exit to exit out of the patient registration area and return to the Appointment Scheduling screen.

14. Now, right click Lily's appointment slot, roll the mouse over the patient's name, and select Registered, as you have already updated her information. The program adds a time stamp after Registered.

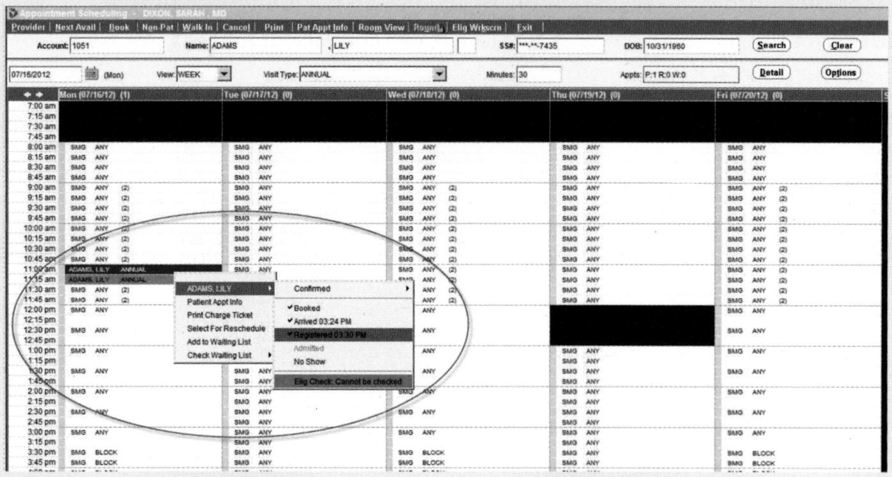

Appointment Scheduling - DIXON, SARAH , MD

Provider | Next Avail | Book | Non-Pat | Walk In | Cancel | Print | Pat Appt Info | Room View | Rounds | Elig Wrkscrn | Exit

Account: 1051 Name: ADAMS , LILY SS#: ***-**-7435 DOB: 10/31/1960 Search Clear

07/16/2012 (Mon) View: WEEK Visit Type: ANNUAL Minutes: 30 Appts: P:1 R:0 W:0 Detail Options

	Mon (07/16/12) (1)	Tue (07/17/12) (0)	Wed (07/18/12) (0)	Thu (07/19/12) (0)	Fri (07/20/12) (0)
7:00 am					
7:15 am					
7:30 am					
7:45 am					
8:00 am	SMG ANY	SMG ANY	SMG ANY	SMG ANY	SMG ANY
8:15 am	SMG ANY	SMG ANY	SMG ANY	SMG ANY	SMG ANY
8:30 am	SMG ANY	SMG ANY	SMG ANY	SMG ANY	SMG ANY
8:45 am	SMG ANY	SMG ANY	SMG ANY	SMG ANY	SMG ANY
9:00 am	SMG ANY (2)	SMG ANY	SMG ANY (2)	SMG ANY	SMG ANY (2)
9:15 am	SMG ANY (2)	SMG ANY	SMG ANY (2)	SMG ANY	SMG ANY (2)
9:30 am	SMG ANY (2)	SMG ANY	SMG ANY (2)	SMG ANY	SMG ANY (2)
9:45 am	SMG ANY (2)	SMG ANY	SMG ANY (2)	SMG ANY	SMG ANY (2)
10:00 am	SMG ANY (2)	SMG ANY	SMG ANY (2)	SMG ANY	SMG ANY (2)
10:15 am	SMG ANY (2)	SMG ANY	SMG ANY (2)	SMG ANY	SMG ANY (2)
10:30 am	SMG ANY (2)	SMG ANY	SMG ANY (2)	SMG ANY	SMG ANY (2)
10:45 am	SMG ANY (2)	SMG ANY	SMG ANY (2)	SMG ANY	SMG ANY (2)
11:00 am	ADAMS, LILY ANNUAL	SMG ANY	SMG ANY (2)	SMG ANY	SMG ANY (2)
11:15 am	ADAMS, LILY ANNUAL		ANY (2)	SMG ANY	SMG ANY (2)
11:30 am	SMG ANY (2)		ANY (2)	SMG ANY	SMG ANY (2)
11:45 am	SMG ANY (2)		ANY (2)	SMG ANY	SMG ANY (2)
12:00 pm	SMG ANY		ANY		SMG ANY
12:15 pm					
12:30 pm	SMG ANY		ANY		SMG ANY
12:45 pm					
1:00 pm	SMG ANY		ANY	SMG ANY	SMG ANY
1:15 pm				SMG ANY	
1:30 pm	SMG ANY	SMG ANY	ANY	SMG ANY	SMG ANY
1:45 pm		SMG ANY		SMG ANY	
2:00 pm	SMG ANY	SMG ANY	SMG ANY	SMG ANY	SMG ANY
2:15 pm		SMG ANY		SMG ANY	
2:30 pm	SMG ANY	SMG ANY	SMG ANY	SMG ANY	SMG ANY
2:45 pm		SMG ANY		SMG ANY	
3:00 pm	SMG ANY	SMG ANY	SMG ANY	SMG ANY	SMG ANY
3:15 pm		SMG ANY		SMG ANY	
3:30 pm	SMG BLOCK	SMG ANY	SMG BLOCK	SMG ANY	SMG BLOCK
3:45 pm	SMG BLOCK	SMG ANY	SMG BLOCK	SMG ANY	SMG BLOCK

ADAMS, LILY ►
Patient Appt Info
Print Charge Ticket
Select For Reschedule
Add to Waiting List
Check Waiting List ►

Confirmed ►
✔Booked
✔Arrived 03:24 PM
✔Registered 03:30 PM
Admitted
No Show
Elig Check: Cannot be checked

15. The patient is ready to be seen at this point. Click the Clear button to prepare the calendar for the next entry. Click the Exit button to return to the main menu.

Exercise 4.2: Checking in a Patient Upon Arrival—No Registration Updates

Today is July 3, 2012. Anthony Bates, a patient of Dr. Zuane, has arrived at the medical office at 9:00 a.m. for his appointment: administration of a tetanus shot. You go over Anthony's registration information and insurance information with him and find there are no updates to be made.

1. Log in to e-Medsys®.
2. At the top of the screen, click on Scheduling. Click on Appointment Schedule from the drop-down box, or press Ctrl + B on the keyboard. The Appointment Scheduling screen will now appear.
3. Click on the Calendar icon, and use the arrows to find the correct month (July 2012) and then to select the date, July 3.
4. Now click on the Provider button that appears in the upper left-hand corner of the screen. Highlight Dr. Zuane, and click OK to bring up Dr. Zuane's schedule on this day.
5. Now find Anthony's appointment, at 9:00 a.m., and right click on the appointment slot. Roll the mouse over BATES, ANTHONY ►, and select Registered from the second drop-down menu.

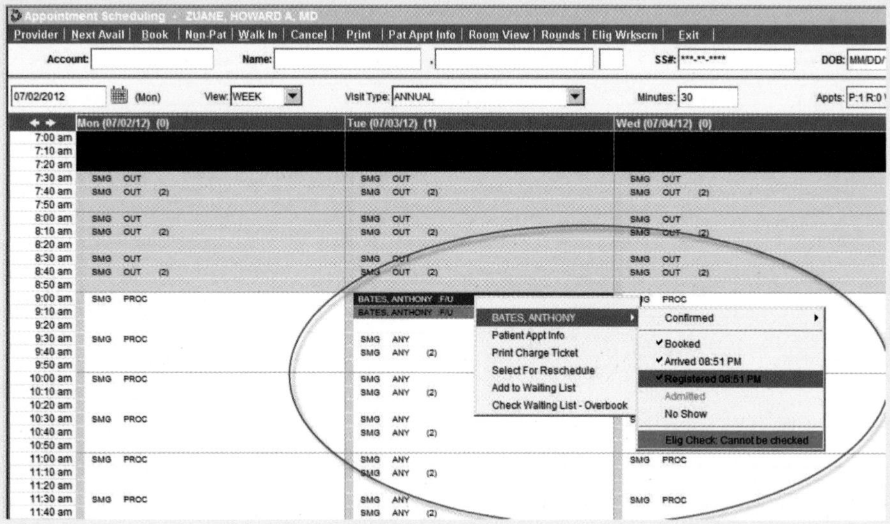

Appointment Scheduling - ZUANE, HOWARD A, MD

Provider | Next Avail | Book | Non-Pat | Walk In | Cancel | Print | Pat Appt Info | Room View | Rounds | Elig Wrkscrn | Exit

Account: Name: , SS#: ***-**-**** DOB: MM/DD/

07/02/2012 (Mon) View: WEEK Visit Type: ANNUAL Minutes: 30 Appts: P:1 R:0

	Mon (07/02/12) (0)	Tue (07/03/12) (1)	Wed (07/04/12) (0)
7:00 am			
7:10 am			
7:20 am			
7:30 am	SMG OUT	SMG OUT	SMG OUT
7:40 am	SMG OUT (2)	SMG OUT (2)	SMG OUT (2)
7:50 am			
8:00 am	SMG OUT	SMG OUT	SMG OUT
8:10 am	SMG OUT (2)	SMG OUT (2)	SMG OUT (2)
8:20 am			
8:30 am	SMG OUT	SMG OUT	SMG OUT
8:40 am	SMG OUT (2)	SMG OUT (2)	SMG OUT (2)
8:50 am			
9:00 am	SMG PROC	BATES, ANTHONY F/U	PROC
9:10 am		BATES, ANTHONY F/U	
9:20 am			
9:30 am	SMG PROC	SMG ANY	
9:40 am		SMG ANY (2)	
9:50 am			
10:00 am	SMG PROC	SMG ANY	
10:10 am		SMG ANY (2)	
10:20 am			
10:30 am	SMG PROC	SMG ANY	
10:40 am		SMG ANY (2)	
10:50 am			
11:00 am	SMG PROC	SMG ANY	SMG PROC
11:10 am		SMG ANY (2)	
11:20 am			
11:30 am	SMG PROC	SMG ANY	SMG PROC
11:40 am		SMG ANY (2)	

BATES, ANTHONY ►
Patient Appt Info
Print Charge Ticket
Select For Reschedule
Add to Waiting List
Check Waiting List - Overbook

Confirmed ►
✔Booked
✔Arrived 08:51 PM
✔Registered 08:51 PM
Admitted
No Show
Elig Check: Cannot be checked

6. The program brings up Anthony's Patient Appointment Information. This screen is a snapshot of the patient's account and can be used to confirm whether registration changes need to be made. There are no updates needed for this patient, so click Exit to return to the schedule.
7. The patient is ready to be seen at this point. When you have finished, click the Clear button to prepare the calendar for the next entry. Click the Exit button to return to the main menu.

Exercise 4.3: Printing a Patient Charge Ticket

Now that Anthony is checked in, print a charge ticket for his appointment. This allows the provider to mark services performed during a patient visit.

> **Note:** In a medical office with a total practice management system (both front-office functions and back-office electronic charting capabilities), printing charge tickets may not be required, as charges will automatically be entered into the system during the provider's examination. This exercise is included to instruct in the instance that an office has a practice management system (for front-office tasks) and still uses paper charts.

1. Log in to e-Medsys®.
2. At the top of the screen, click on Scheduling. Click on Appointment Schedule from the drop-down box, or press Ctrl + B on the keyboard. The Appointment Scheduling screen will now appear.
3. Type "BATES, ANTHONY" in the Name field, and click the Search button.
4. Once the patient's name appears at the top of the screen, click on the Pat Appt Info button. This action brings up Patient Appointment Information for Anthony. (This information may come up automatically without having to click the Pat Appt Info button.)

Reprinted with permission of TriMed Technologies, Corp.

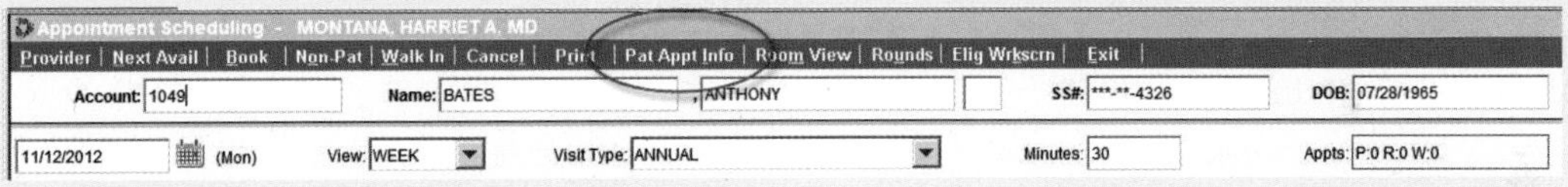

5. Make sure that the 07/03/12 appointment for Anthony is highlighted in the center of the screen, and click the Charge Ticket button.

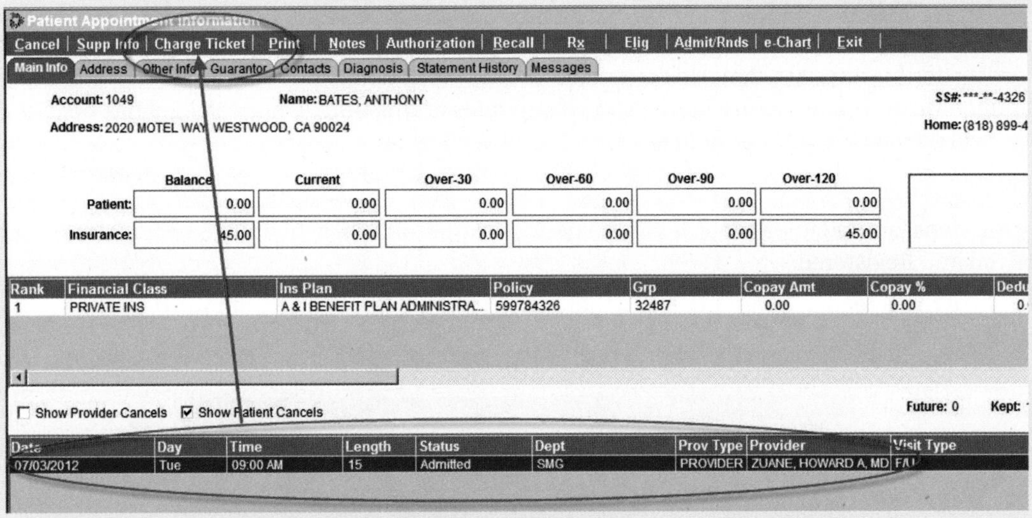

Reprinted with permission of TriMed Technologies, Corp.

6. The charge ticket will print to your local printer. Click Exit when you are finished, and click Exit again to close the scheduling area.

PUTTING IT INTO PRACTICE

Exercise 4.4: Checking in Patients Upon Arrival—(with Registration Updates)

This exercise requires you to check in patients (indicating "Arrived" on the schedule) and update their registration information (then indicating "Registered" on the schedule) without using step-by-step instructions, as given in the previous exercises.

1. Michael Minn arrives at the medical office on August 20, 2012, for his appointment with Dr. Dixon. He currently has an Aetna plan. There will now be a $25 co-payment and a deductible of $250.
2. Diane Best arrives at the medical office on August 31, 2012, for her appointment with Dr. Adams. She informs you that she has a new cell phone number, (805) 348-7665.
3. Valerie Violet arrives at the medical office on August 13, 2012, for her appointment with Zuane. She currently has a Blue Cross plan. There will now be a $40 co-payment.
4. Bruce Sawtelle arrives at the medical office on August 8, 2012, for his appointment with Dr. Franklin. Bruce currently has a United Healthcare plan. There will now be a $20 co-payment.

PUTTING IT INTO PRACTICE

Exercise 4.5: Checking in Patients Upon Arrival—No Registration Updates

This exercise requires you to check in the following patients upon their arrival to the medical office and then print charge tickets without step-by-step instructions, as given in the previous exercises.

1. Sally Jones arrives at the medical office on August 16, 2012, for her appointment with Dr. McGraw. Print a charge ticket, and label it Task 4.5A.
2. Scott McGuire arrives at the medical office on August 7, 2012, for his appointment with Dr. Zuane. Print a charge ticket, and label it Task 4.5B.

TASK 5—WORKING IN THE PATIENT ELECTRONIC MEDICAL RECORD

Exercise 5.1: Admitting a Patient using the EHR Schedule

Today is August 20, 2012. You are working with Dr. Dixon today as a clinical medical assistant. Michael Minn, a patient of Dr. Dixon, arrives for his annual exam. He completes an ROS form while in the waiting area, and the administrative medical assistant confirms that there are no registration updates at this time. Once Michael has been brought into the exam room, you will change his appointment status to "Admitted."

1. Log in to e-Medsys®.
2. Using the steps learned in previous lessons, check the appointment schedule to ensure that the patient is listed as Arrived and Registered.
3. At the top of the screen, click on EHR, and then click on EHR Home Page from the drop-down box.

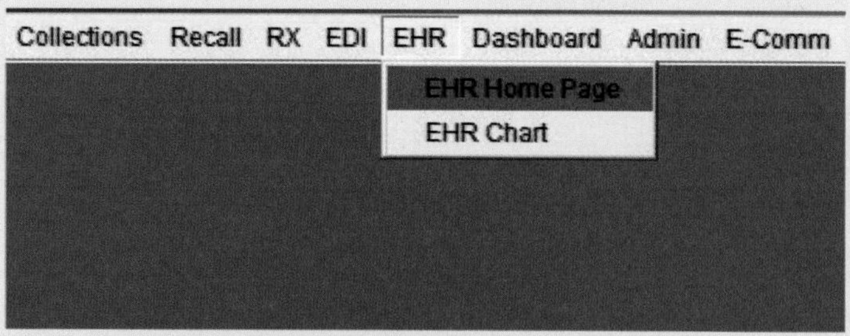

4. This opens the EHR home page in a new window.
5. On the left side of the screen, select Dixon from the list of providers.
6. Type in "08/20/12", and press the TAB button on your keyboard to find the correct date.
7. Below the calendar, be sure the radio buttons next to Cal and Col. Per are selected (this indicates that you want to view the calendar for today's date).

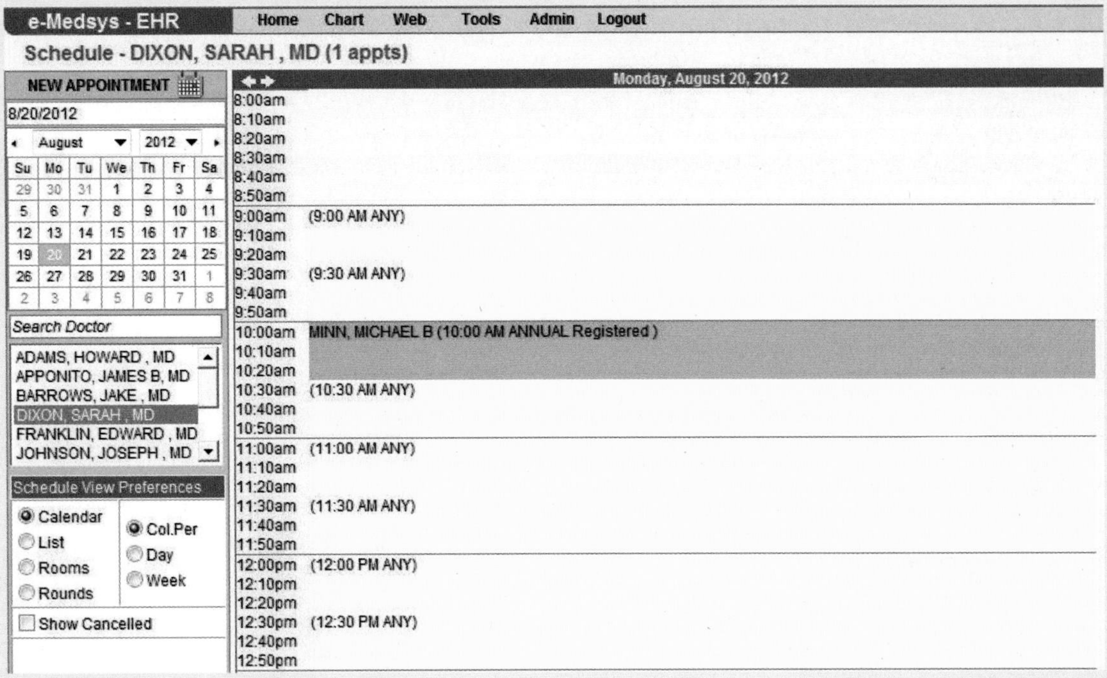

8. Dr. Dixon's schedule appears in the center of the page. You will see Michael Minn's appointment on the schedule.
9. Now, right click on Michael Minn's name on the schedule.
10. Roll your mouse over Status, and then click on Admitted. This provides a time stamp for when the patient was admitted to an exam room.

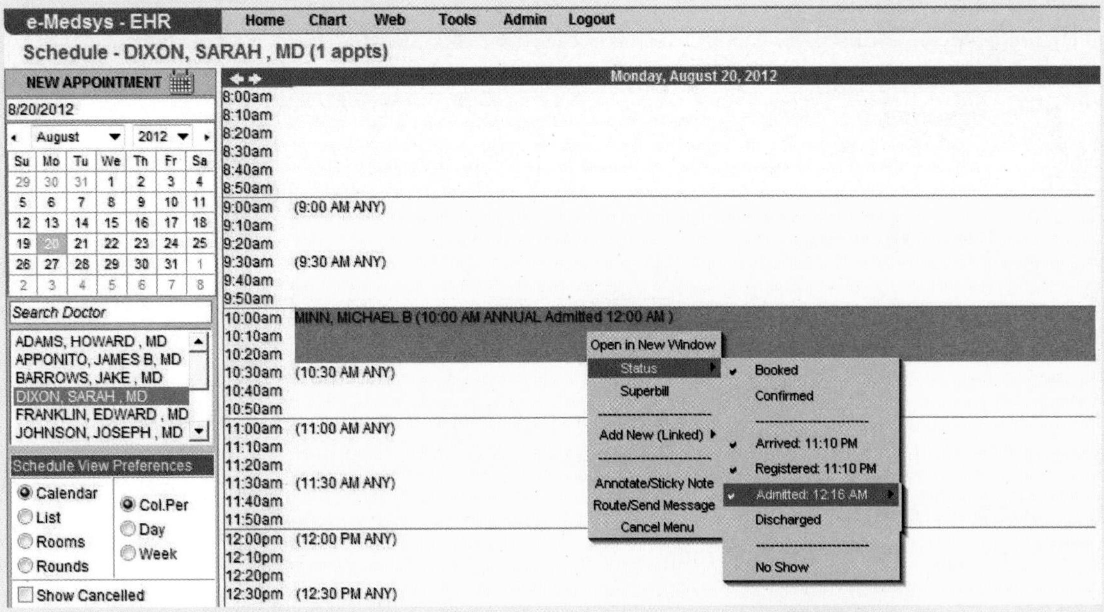

Exercise 5.2: Linking a New Annual Exam Note to a Patient Appointment and Entering Patient Data

Now that you have indicated Michael Minn has been admitted to an exam room, you will create a new patient note in his patient record.

1. While still on Dr. Dixon's schedule, right click on Michael Minn's name again.
2. This time select Add New (Linked), and then click on Patient Note from the menu.

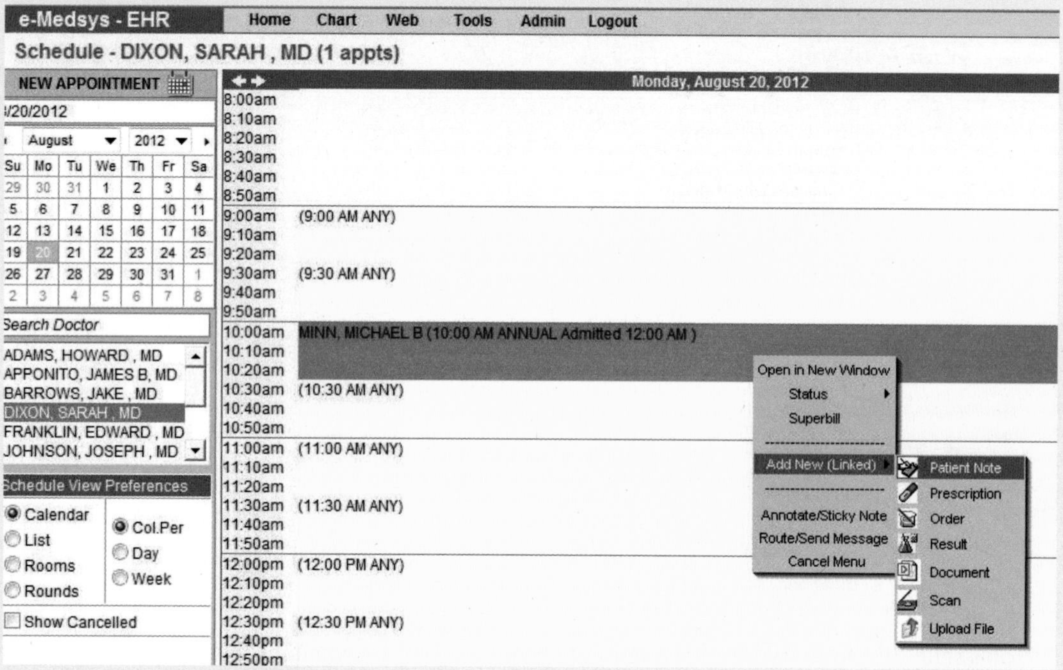

3. Now you are in the patient's individual chart, and a New Note has opened on the bottom right side of the screen. You can click on the box on the right side of the screen above the envelope icon (as shown in the following screen shot) to enlarge the New Note while you are working in it.

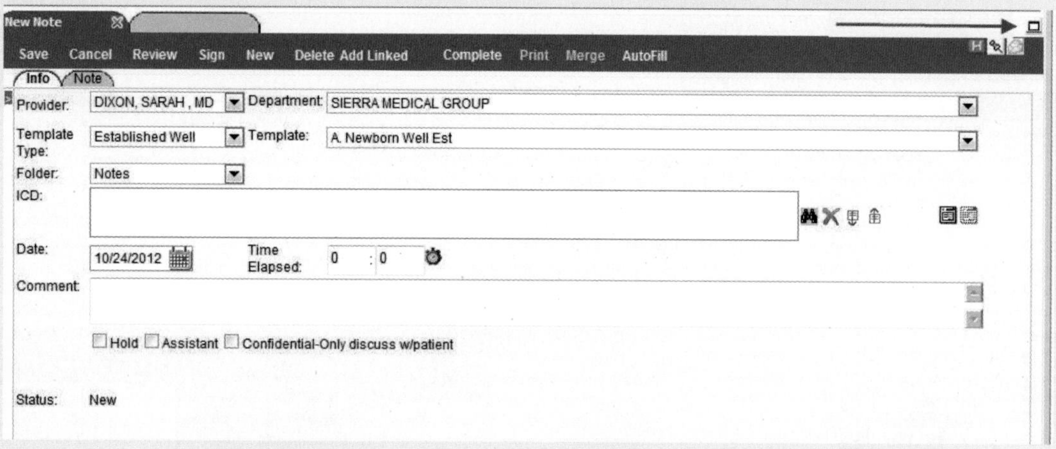

4. In the Template, match the following fields with the information provided:
   - Provider = Dixon, Sarah, MD
   - Department = Sierra Medical Group

- Template Type = Family Practice
- Template = Routine Exam Male
- Date = August 20, 2012 (*Note:* In a medical office setting, the date would be autopopulated based on today's date.)

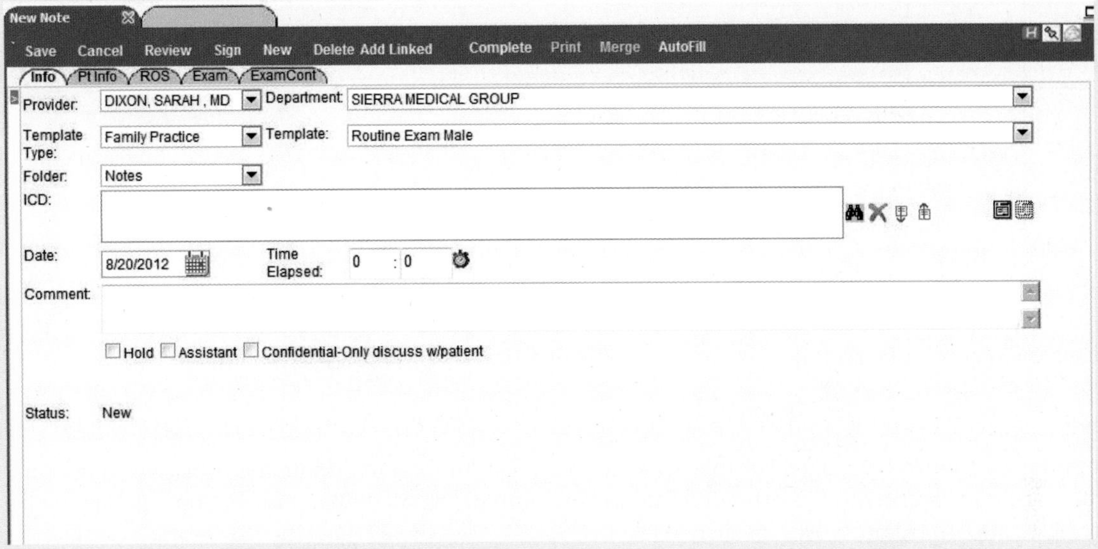

New Note
Save Cancel Review Sign New Delete Add Linked Complete Print Merge AutoFill
Info Pt Info ROS Exam ExamCont
Provider: DIXON, SARAH, MD Department: SIERRA MEDICAL GROUP
Template Type: Family Practice Template: Routine Exam Male
Folder: Notes
ICD:
Date: 8/20/2012 Time Elapsed: 0 : 0
Comment:
Hold Assistant Confidential-Only discuss w/patient
Status: New

5. Click Save, located in the upper left corner of the template.
6. Select the Pt Info Tab in the same area.
7. Change the Date of Visit field to 08/20/2012.
8. In the Chief Complaint field, choose ANNUAL PHYSICAL EXAM from the drop-down menu.

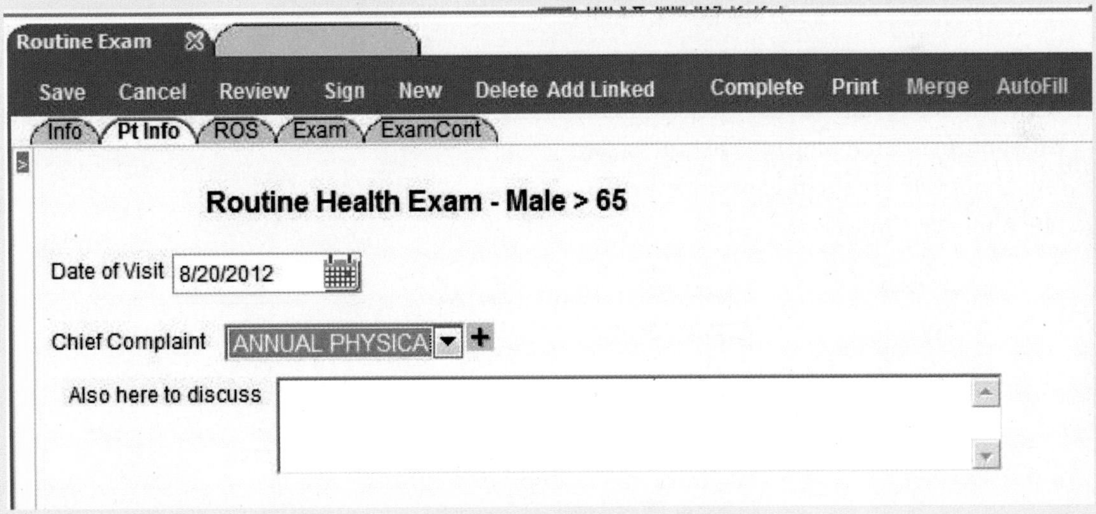

Routine Exam
Save Cancel Review Sign New Delete Add Linked Complete Print Merge AutoFill
Info Pt Info ROS Exam ExamCont
Routine Health Exam - Male > 65
Date of Visit 8/20/2012
Chief Complaint ANNUAL PHYSICA
Also here to discuss

9. In the following PMH (patient medical history) fields, enter the following:
   - Problem List: Obesity; pulmonary hypertension
   - Surgical History: Gall bladder removal
   - Family History: Mother died at age 62 of bone cancer, she also had diabetes; Father alive and well at age 84; no siblings
   - Social History: Nonsmoker, nondrinker, married, three children, worked as an investment banker for 35 years
   - Allergies: Vicodin and Latex

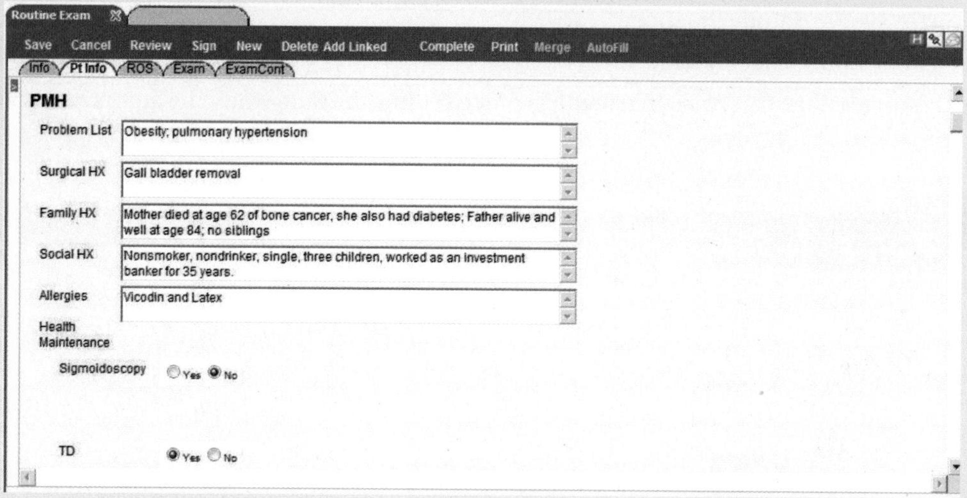

Routine Exam

Save Cancel Review Sign New Delete Add Linked Complete Print Merge AutoFill

Info Pt Info ROS Exam ExamCont

PMH

Problem List: Obesity; pulmonary hypertension

Surgical HX: Gall bladder removal

Family HX: Mother died at age 62 of bone cancer, she also had diabetes; Father alive and well at age 84; no siblings

Social HX: Nonsmoker, nondrinker, single, three children, worked as an investment banker for 35 years.

Allergies: Vicodin and Latex

Health Maintenance

Sigmoidoscopy: Yes / No (selected)

TD: Yes (selected) / No

10. Leave the rest of the screen for the provider to fill out. Click Save when you are finished.

Exercise 5.3: Entering ROS Information from a Patient Questionnaire

Recall that in the waiting area Michael completed a patient questionnaire to update the provider on his state of health. The medical assistant will enter the information into the patient's chart. All of this information will be reviewed with the patient and signed by Dr. Dixon.

1. Still in Michael Minn's New Note, select the ROS Tab. Note that the default settings are "Normal," which saves time when working in the chart. The person documenting needs to enter only remarkable or abnormal items.
2. In the first entry, Constitutional, keep the radio button set to Normal, and delete any information found in the open text box below the radio buttons.
3. Now, enter the following information for the Resp (respiratory), CV (cardiovascular), GI (gastrointestinal), GV (genitourinary), and MS (musculoskeletal) systems:
   - Resp: Abnormal; Shortness of breath
   - CV: Denies CP, palpitations, DOE, orthropea
   - GI: Abnormal; Cramping several times a day
   - GV: Abnormal; Frequent, slow urination
   - MS: Abnormal; Muscle weakness

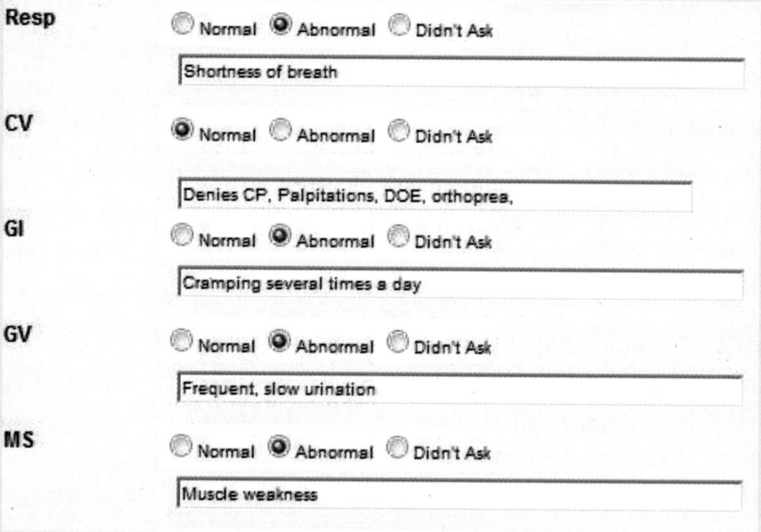

Resp: Normal / Abnormal (selected) / Didn't Ask
Shortness of breath

CV: Normal (selected) / Abnormal / Didn't Ask
Denies CP, Palpitations, DOE, orthoprea,

GI: Normal / Abnormal (selected) / Didn't Ask
Cramping several times a day

GV: Normal / Abnormal (selected) / Didn't Ask
Frequent, slow urination

MS: Normal / Abnormal (selected) / Didn't Ask
Muscle weakness

4. Click Save when you are finished.

Exercise 5.4: Entering Patient Vital Signs on a Patient Note

After taking the patient's vital signs, enter them into the New Note.

1. Still in Michael Minn's chart, select the Exam Tab.
2. Enter the following information in the appropriate fields:
    - Height: 74 inches
    - Weight: 240 pounds
    - Blood Pressure (sitting): 130/67
    - Pulse: 67
    - Respiration: 17
    - Temperature: 98.6°F

Routine Exam
Save Cancel Review Sign New Delete Add Linked Complete Print Merge AutoFill
Info Pt Info ROS Exam ExamCont

Ht	Wt	BP (sitting/standing)	BP (Supine)	Pulse	RR	Temp
74	200	130/67		67	17	98.6

Reprinted with permission of TriMed Technologies, Corp.

3. Click Save when you are finished. The provider will complete the rest of this page during the exam.
4. Now click the Print button, and select PDF Form. Print to your local printer, and label the printout as Exercise 5.4.
5. When you are done, minimize the right side of the screen by clicking on the same box on the right of the screen above the envelope icon.
6. Then click the X on the Routine Exam Tab.

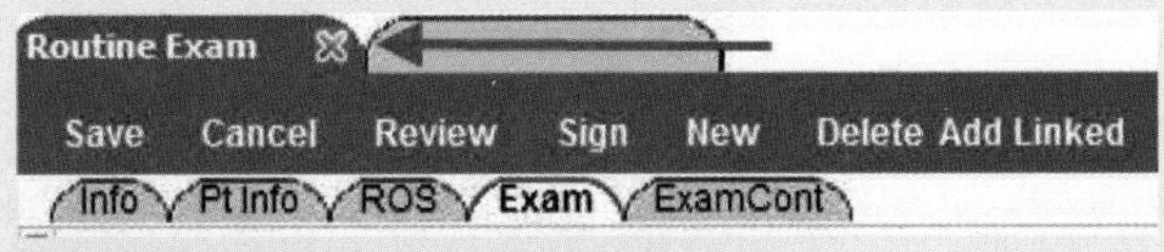

Reprinted with permission of TriMed Technologies, Corp.

Exercise 5.5: Navigating the Patient Chart Using Tree View

This exercise is designed to familiarize you with the navigation of individual patient charts. You should still be in Michael Minn's chart.

1. So far you have learned how to enter information in one area of the chart (creating a new Note). On the lower left side of the screen, you should see a group of vertical tabs. This is your left navigation bar.

My Summary
Review
Appts
Notes
Meds
Orders
Results
Docs
Scans
Other
All

Reprinted with permission of TriMed Technologies, Corp.

2. Click on the APPTS button. This will show all of the appointments that have been scheduled for Michael at the medical office. Make sure the box next to Tree is selected (the next step gives more explanation on Tree View). Make sure the box next to Appts: Inc Cancl is *not* selected. This suppresses appointments that were cancelled.

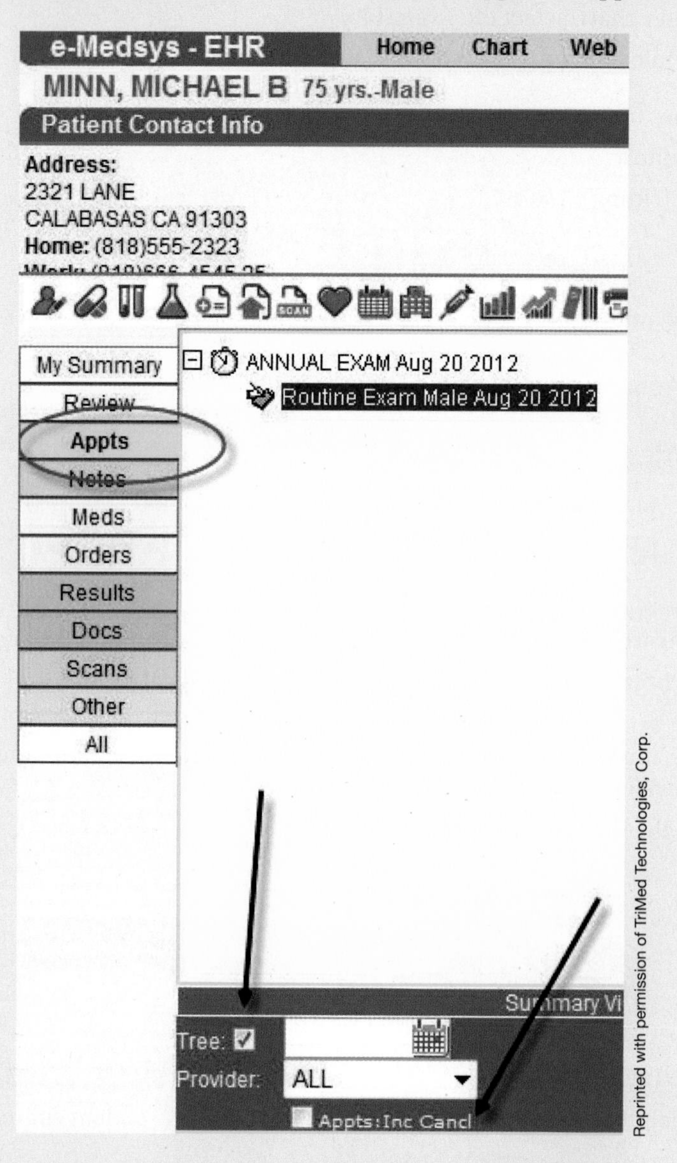

3. Tree View shows items as they are connected with one another. So, on your screen, you should see that Michael Minn has one appointment (on August 20). The August 20 appointment has a patient note associated with it. The Tree View will continue to build when additional items are added to the patient's chart during each appointment.
4. Click on the Home button at the top of the screen to return to the EHR schedule.

PUTTING IT INTO PRACTICE

Exercise 5.6: Linking a New Annual Exam Note to a Patient Appointment

Without using step-by-step instructions, as given in the previous exercises, this exercise requires you to (1) receive the patient (indicating Arrived on the schedule), (2) update patient information (indicating Registered on the schedule), (3) admit the patient using the EHR schedule, (4) link a new Note to the patient's appointment, and (5) enter information and vital signs in the new Note.

Cory Haines arrives for his appointment on August 6, 2012, at 10:00 a.m. Using the following information, enter data in his chart prior to his being seen for his annual exam with Dr. McGraw. Upon check-in, Mr. Haines indicates that he has a new work phone number, (323) 598-5252 x119, and he now has a cell phone number, (730) 658-2896. He has also advised you that his emergency contact is Sally Haines with a contact number of (730) 934-7936.

When you have finished entering the information in the patient's record, print your work and label it Exercise 5.6.

Chief Complaint	Annual Physical Exam (*Hint:* This is now in the drop-down list.)
Also here to discuss:	Sore right hip for past two weeks
Surgical History	Left knee amputation two years ago
Family History	Father's whereabouts unknown; Mother alive and well; older brother was diagnosed with juvenile diabetes at age 10
Social History	Married, has smoked a pack of cigarettes a day for five years, social drinker, no illicit drug use, minimal coffee drinker
Constitutional	Healthy appearing, no significant weight loss or gain
Gastrointestinal	Normal
Musculoskeletal	Pain in right hip, often trips over himself while walking
Neurological	Migraines (several per month)
Height	71 inches
Weight	165 pounds
Blood Pressure	118/70 (sitting)
Pulse	75
Respiration	18
Temperature	98.9

Exercise 5.7: Linking a New Multisystem Exam Note to a Patient Appointment and Entering Vital Signs

Today is June 20, 2012. You are working with Dr. Dixon today as a clinical medical assistant. Wilma Flint is a patient of Dr. Dixon and is being seen today for extreme fatigue and dizziness that have lingered for several weeks. The patient does not have registration updates today.

1. Log in to e-Medsys®.
2. Using the steps learned in previous lessons, indicate on the appointment schedule that the patient has arrived and is registered.
3. Click on EHR from the top menu, and then select EHR Home Page from the drop-down box. This opens the EHR home page in a new window.
4. Open Dr. Dixon's schedule on the EHR schedule, and navigate to today's date (remember it is June 20, 2012).
5. Find Wilma's appointment, and indicate that she has been Admitted.
6. Using the EHR schedule, right click on the patient's appointment, and link a new note to the appointment.
7. Now the patient's individual chart appears on the screen, and the lower right side of the screen has a New Note. (Recall that you can enlarge the New Note while you are working in it.) In the Template field, use the drop-down to complete the following:
   - Provider = Dr. Dixon
   - Department = Sierra Medical Group

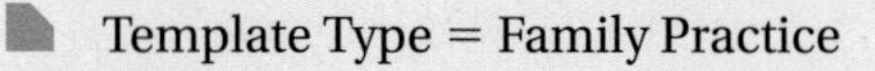

- Template Type = Family Practice
- Template = MultisystemE&M1

Change the date to 06/20/2012, and click Save.

Multisysteme

Save Cancel Review Sign New Delete Add Linked Complete Print Merge AutoFill

Info General PFSH/HPI Exam ExamCont Decision

Provider: DIXON, SARAH , MD Department: SIERRA MEDICAL GROUP

Template Type: Family Practice Template: MultisystemE&M1

Folder: Notes

ICD:

Date: 6/20/2012 Time Elapsed: 0 0

Comment:

Hold Assistant Confidential-Only discuss w/patient

8. Now, click on the General Tab. Enter the following information:

- Height: 64 inches
- Weight: 168 pounds
- Blood Pressure: 120/80 (sitting)
- Pulse: 67
- Respiration: 23
- Temperature: 101°F
- General appearance: In obvious pain and discomfort
- CC: Has had lingering fatigue and dizziness

Multisysteme

Save Cancel Review Sign New Delete Add Linked Complete Print Merge AutoFill

Info General PFSH/HPI Exam ExamCont Decision

height: 64

weight: 168

BP:(sitting/standing) 120/80

BP:(Supine)

Pulse: 67

Respiration: 23

Temperature: 101

General appearance In obvious pain and discomfort

CC: Has had lingering fatigue and dizziness

9. When you are finished entering this information, click Save.

Exercise 5.8: Entering Patient, Family, and Social History (PFSH) on a Patient Note

1. Still in the same note, click on the PFSH/HPI Tab.
2. Click on the box with the three dots next to the Social History field, select "smokes," and click on "5" and "drinks." (Clicking anywhere outside of the drop-down box will return you to the PFSH screen.)

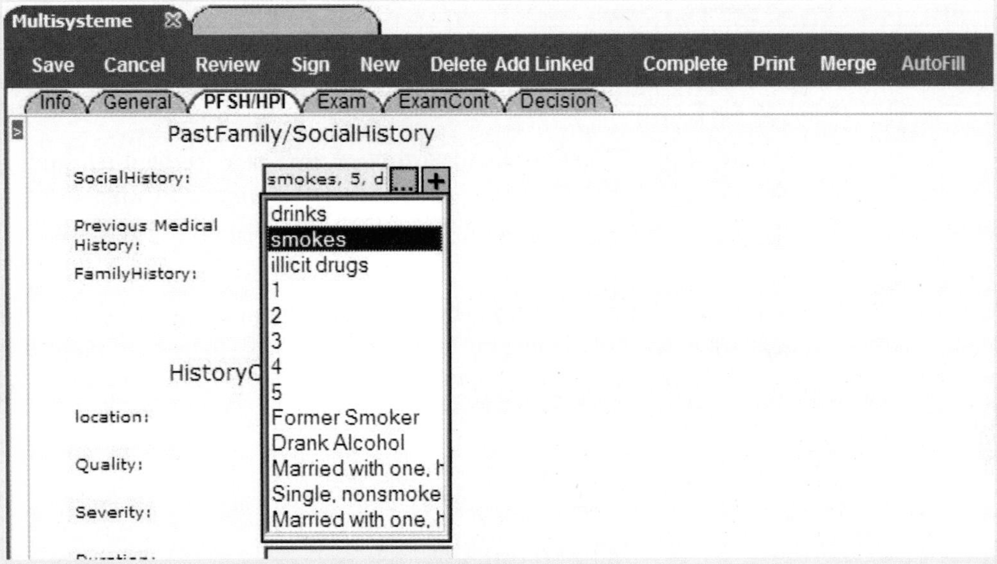

Reprinted with permission of TriMed Technologies, Corp.

3. Click on the plus sign next to Previous Medical History.
4. Enter "APPENDECTOMY" in the pop-up box, and click OK.

Reprinted with permission of TriMed Technologies, Corp.

5. Click on the box with the three dots next to Family History. Highlight Alcoholism, and hit Enter.

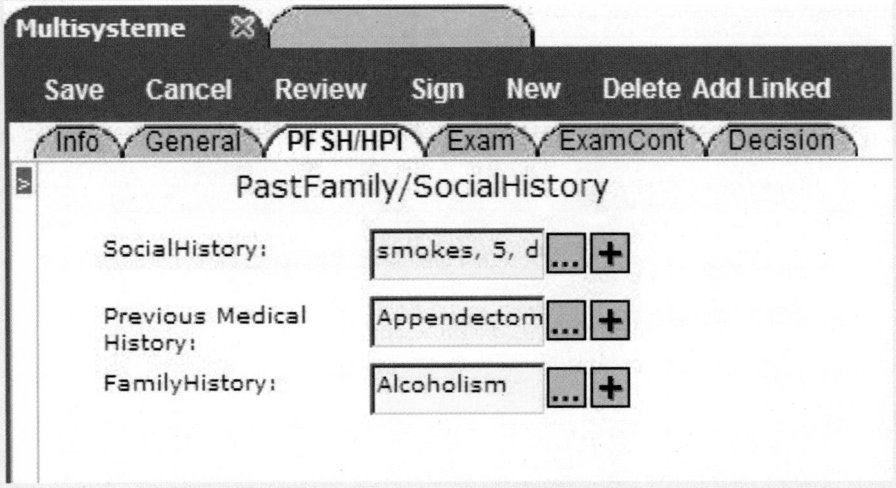

Reprinted with permission of TriMed Technologies, Corp.

6. Click Save when you have finished. The provider will complete the rest of this page during the exam.
7. Now click the Print button, and select PDF Form. Print to your local printer, and label the printout as Exercise 5.8.
8. When you are done, minimize the right side of the screen.
9. Then click the X on the MultisystemE Tab.

PUTTING IT ALL TOGETHER

Exercise 5.9: Linking New Notes to Patient Appointments and Recording Patient Information

Without using step-by-step instructions, as given in the previous exercises, this exercise requires you to (1) receive the patient (indicating Arrived on the schedule), (2) update patient information if appropriate (indicating Registered on the schedule), (3) admit the patient using the EHR schedule, (4) link a new Note to the patient's appointment, and (5) enter information and vital signs in the new Note.

Debbie Huston arrives for her appointment on July 25, 2012. She has no updates to her registration information. Using the following information, create a multisystem exam template note for Debbie Huston, who is being seen by Dr. McGraw for possible hypothyroidism. When you have finished entering the information in the patient's record, print your work, and label it Exercise 5.9.

Height	56 inches
Weight	155 pounds
Blood Pressure	110/70 (sitting)
Pulse	63
Respiration	19
Temperature	100.2°F
General Appearance	Slightly pale
Social History	Single; nonsmoker, nondrinker
Previous Medical History	Healthy
Family History	Mother deceased, diabetes with complications; Father alive—obesity; younger sister healthy

Exercise 5.10: Entering a Patient Contact Note in the EMR

Today is August 30, 2012. You are covering in the registration area over lunchtime. Sally Jones called and informed you that she is changing insurance next year and would like Dr. McGraw's office to be aware of that. Note this in her chart.

1. Log in to e-Medsys®.
2. At the top of the screen, click on EHR, and then click on the EHR Home Page from the drop-down box.
3. This opens the EHR page in a new window.
4. At the top of the screen, click on Chart to search for Sally Jones' chart.

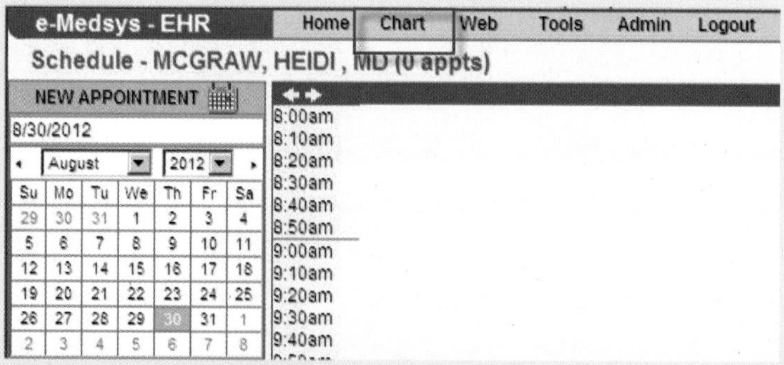

5. Next to Pat. Name, type in "JONES" and press Enter.
6. Double click on Sally's name to select her chart.
7. On the left side of the screen, click on the New Patient Note icon. A new patient note will be created.

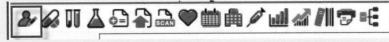

Reprinted with permission of TriMed Technologies, Corp.

8. In the Template Type field, use the drop-down to select Patient Contact. In the Template field, select Telephone Contact. In the Date field, enter "8/30/2012".
9. In the Comment field, type "Patient called today to inform us that she is changing insurances in January of next year."

New Note

Save Cancel Review Sign New Delete Add Linked Complete Print Merge AutoFill

Info Note

Provider: MCGRAW, HEIDI , MD Department: SIERRA MEDICAL GROUP

Template Type: Patient Contact Template: Telephone Contact

Folder: Notes

ICD:

Date: 8/30/2012 Time Elapsed: 0 : 0

Comment: Patient called today to inform us that she is changing insurances in January of next year.

Hold Assistant Confidential-Only discuss w/patient

Reprinted with permission of TriMed Technologies, Corp.

10. Click Save when you are finished.

TASK 6—CREATING PRESCRIPTIONS FOR PROVIDER AUTHORIZATION

Exercise 6.1: Creating a Prescription for a Patient

Today is July 25, 2012. Dr. McGraw has prescribed Synthroid (.0125 mg), 30 tablets for Debbie Huston, who has hypothyroidism. She has indicated that Debbie should take one each day for a month; the patient may have three refills.

1. Log in to e-Medsys®.
2. Using the steps learned in previous lessons, check the appointment schedule to ensure that Debbie is listed as Arrived and Registered.
3. Then open the EHR Home Page, and using the steps learned in previous lessons, check the EHR schedule to ensure that Debbie has been Admitted.
4. Now, double click on Debbie's appointment on the EHR schedule. This is a shortcut that brings you directly to Debbie's individual patient record. Your screen should look like the following screen shot.

Reprinted with permission of TriMed Technologies, Corp.

5. Right click on today's appointment.
6. This action brings up a menu similar to what you saw on the EHR schedule. Select Add New (Linked), and then click on Prescription.

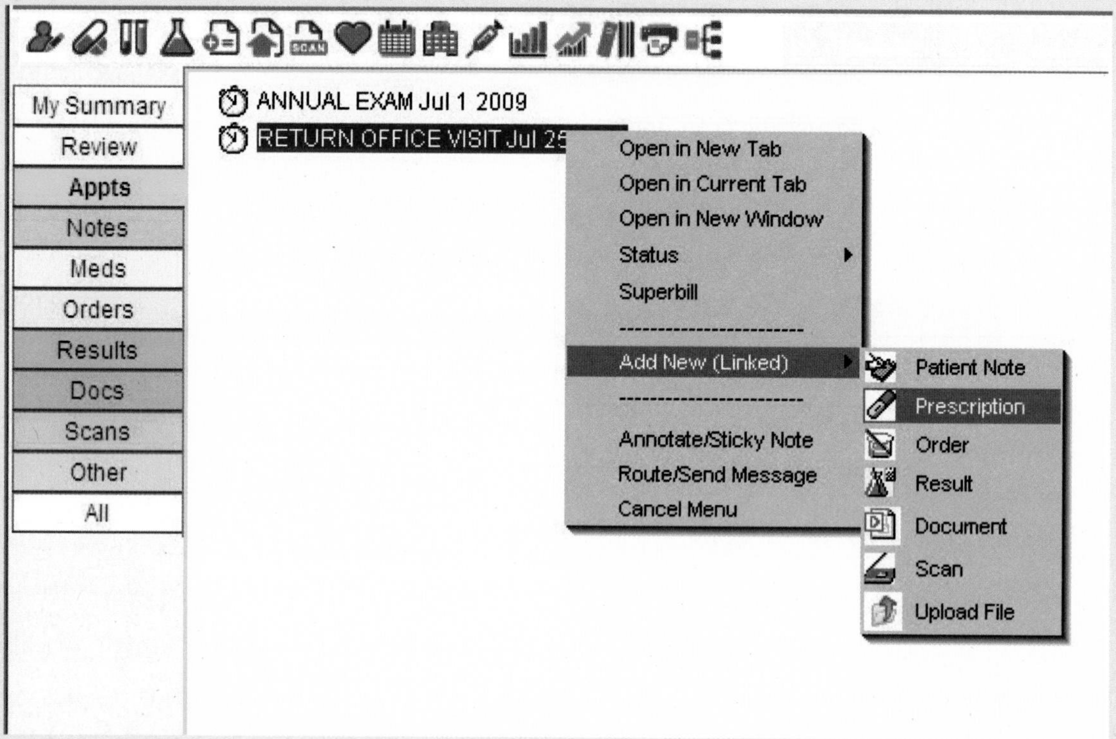

Reprinted with permission of TriMed Technologies, Corp.

7. When you select this, a new Prescription Tab opens on the bottom right side of the screen. You can enlarge the tab by clicking on the corner box.
8. Within this tab, the provider (Dr. McGraw) and the location (Sierra Medical Group) should be established. Leave the Template field blank. The Folder field is autopopulated with Meds.
9. To the right of the ICD field, click on the binoculars icon to search for the diagnosis related to the medication being prescribed.

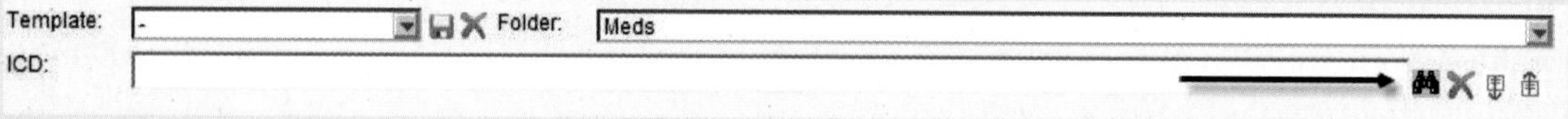

Reprinted with permission of TriMed Technologies, Corp.

10. Click on the radio button to the left of Search, type "HYPOTHYROIDISM" in the Description field, and then press Enter on your keyboard.

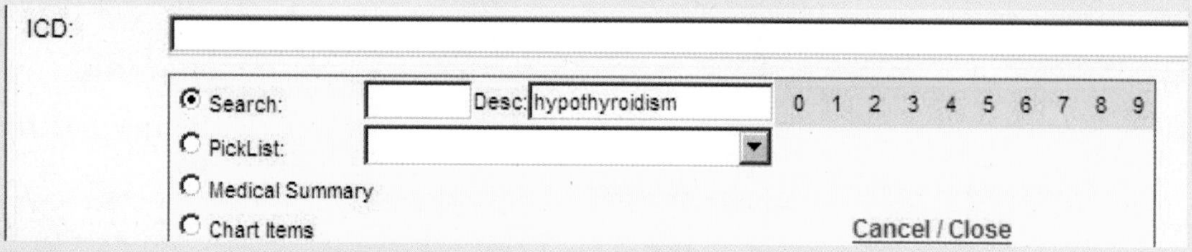

Reprinted with permission of TriMed Technologies, Corp.

11. The ICD code, 244.8, is now populated in the field for ICD.

12. Beneath the Details Tab, in the field next to Drug, enter "SYN" (the first three letters of the drug to be prescribed), and then click on the binoculars icon to the right of the field (make sure that the box to the left of Search All has a checkmark in it).

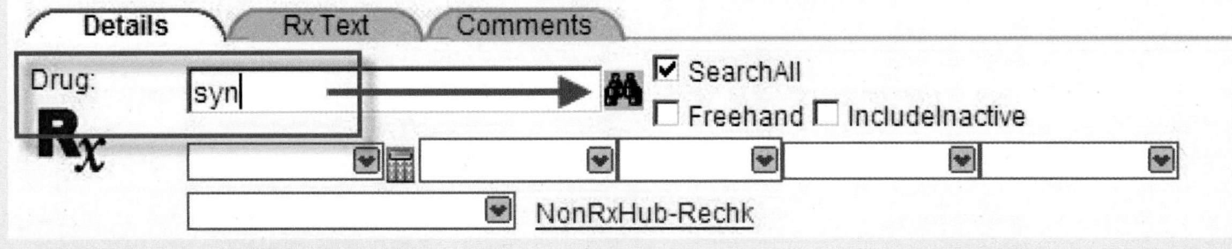

Reprinted with permission of TriMed Technologies, Corp.

13. Scroll through the resulting list until you find Synthroid 125 mcg Tab. Click on it. The frequency, the form, and the route of administration will autopopulate based on your selection. The category of the drug will also autopopulate.
14. In the Date field, type today's date, 07/25/2012.
15. In the field for Quantity, type "30." Note that when you do this, the field for Duration autopopulates.
16. In the Refills field, enter "3." This means that the patient can obtain three refills of this prescription before obtaining a new prescription.
17. Make sure the checkbox to the left of Current is selected. Check your work with the following screen shot.

Prescription
Save Cancel Review Sign New Delete Add Linked Refill/Copy Print e-Send
Provider: MCGRAW, HEIDI , MD Location: SIERRA MEDICAL GROUP
Template: - Folder: Meds
ICD: 244.8 (HYPOTHYROIDISM ACQUIRED)
Details Rx Text Comments
Drug: Synthroid SearchAll Freehand IncludeInactive
125 mcg QD Routine Tablet Oral
NonRxHub-Rechk
Interactions Leaflets Discontinued DrugID: 183683 DEAClass: 0 Drug Level: 0
Date: 7/25/2012 Category: Synthetic T4 (Thyroxine)
Quantity: 30 Tablet Dur Days: 30 Refills: 3
Current Substitution Allowed Sample Lot#:
Hold Side Effects Discussed Auto-Expire 03/25/2013
Assistant Confidential-Only discuss w/patient
Status: New

Reprinted with permission of TriMed Technologies, Corp.

18. Click on Save. Note that the new prescription now appears in the Tree View beneath today's appointment date.

Exercise 6.2: Sending a Prescription for Provider Sign-Off

1. With the prescription saved and the screen still open on it, click on the open envelope in the top right corner of the template. This action allows you to send a message informing the provider that the prescription is ready for sign-off.

Synthroid
Save Cancel Review Sign New Delete Add Linked Refill/Copy Print e-Send

Reprinted with permission of TriMed Technologies, Corp.

2. A new window will open. On the left side of the screen, beneath Select Individual Staff, highlight "Cengage Instructor." (In a real medical office, you would select the patient's provider.)

3. With the instructor entry highlighted, click on the > button.

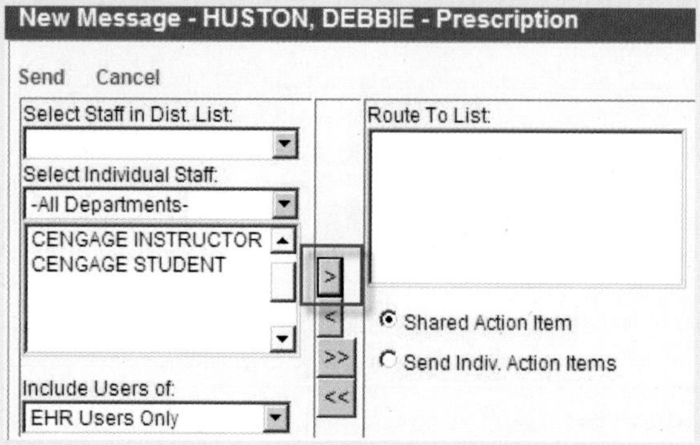

Reprinted with permission of TriMed Technologies, Corp.

4. This moves the instructor name into the Route To list. Click on this entry in the Route To list to select it.
5. Click on the radio button for Send Indiv. Action Items.
6. The Route Date and Time fields will autopopulate with the current date and time.
7. In the Action Type field, use the drop-down menu to select Sign Off.
8. Leave the Priority as Normal.
9. The Attachment/Routed Item field is autopopulated with the prescription information. Check your work with the following screen shot.

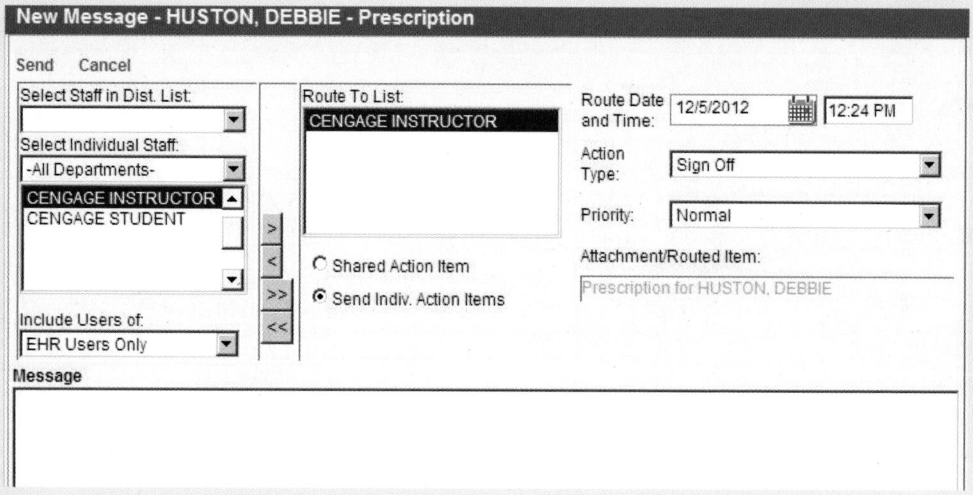

Reprinted with permission of TriMed Technologies, Corp.

10. Click Send. Now you are back on the prescription screen. Minimize the screen by clicking on that same button on the right side of the screen. Click on the X next to Synthroid to close out of the screen.
11. Click the Home button to return to the EHR schedule.

PUTTING IT INTO PRACTICE

Exercise 6.3: Creating Prescriptions and Sending Them for Provider Sign-Off

This exercise requires you to create prescriptions and send them to the provider for authorization without using step-by-step instructions, as given in the previous exercises.

Today is June 20, 2012. Wilma Flint is a patient of Dr. Dixon, who has prescribed medication for her anemia.

1. Using the steps learned in previous lessons, check the appointment schedule to ensure that the patient is listed as Arrived and Registered. (The patient has no registration updates.)

2. Then open the EHR Home Page, and using the steps learned in previous lessons, check the EHR schedule to ensure that the patient has been Admitted.
3. Create a new prescription for Ms. Flint using the following information provided by Dr. Dixon, and send it for provider approval.

- Diagnosis: Anemia (285.9)
- Medication: Ferrous Fumarate
- Dosage: 324 mg (106 mg elemental) tablets
- Frequency: Once per day
- Quantity: 30
- Refills: 12

Today is August 7, 2012. Scott McGuire is a patient of Dr. Howard Zuane, who has prescribed medication for his high blood pressure.

1. Using the steps learned in previous lessons, check the appointment schedule to ensure that the patient is listed as Arrived and Registered. (The patient has no registration updates.)
2. Then open the EHR Home Page, and using the steps learned in previous exercises, indicate on the EHR schedule that the patient has been Admitted.
3. Create a new prescription for Mr. McGuire using the following information provided by Dr. Zuane, and send it for provider approval.

- Diagnosis: Hypertension (401.9)
- Medication: Corgard
- Dosage: 20 mg tablets
- Frequency: Once per day
- Quantity: 30
- Refills: 2

TASK 7—RECORDING THERAPEUTIC INJECTIONS AND IMMUNIZATIONS

Exercise 7.1: Documenting Administration of a Therapeutic Injection

Today is July 3, 2012. Anthony Bates, a patient of Dr. Zuane's, is coming in today at 9:00 a.m. for a tetanus shot. He is seeing only the MA today; there will be no physician visit.

1. Log in to e-Medsys®.
2. In Task 4, the patient was already indicated as Arrived and Registered.
3. Open the EHR Home Page, and using the steps learned in Task 5, indicate on the EHR schedule that the patient has been Admitted.
4. Double click on Anthony's appointment on the EHR schedule to bring up Anthony's chart.
5. In Anthony's chart, on the left side of the screen, right click on today's appointment.
6. Select Add New (Linked) ▶ and then Patient Note. The new Note appears on the right side of the screen. You may enlarge the note if you prefer.

7. The Provider (Zuane), Department (Sierra Medical Group), Template Type (Family Practice), and Folder (Notes) fields may be autopopulated. Be sure that None is selected in the Template field.
8. In the ICD field, click on the binoculars to search for tetanus shot.
9. With the radio button next to Search selected, type "TETANUS" in the description field and press Enter on your keyboard. Now the ICD field is populated with the correct code.
10. Enter the date of administration, 7/3/2012.
11. In the Comments section, type "Tetanus shot administered by <*insert your name and credentials*>, per Dr. Zuane."
12. Check your work with the following screen shot, and then click Save.

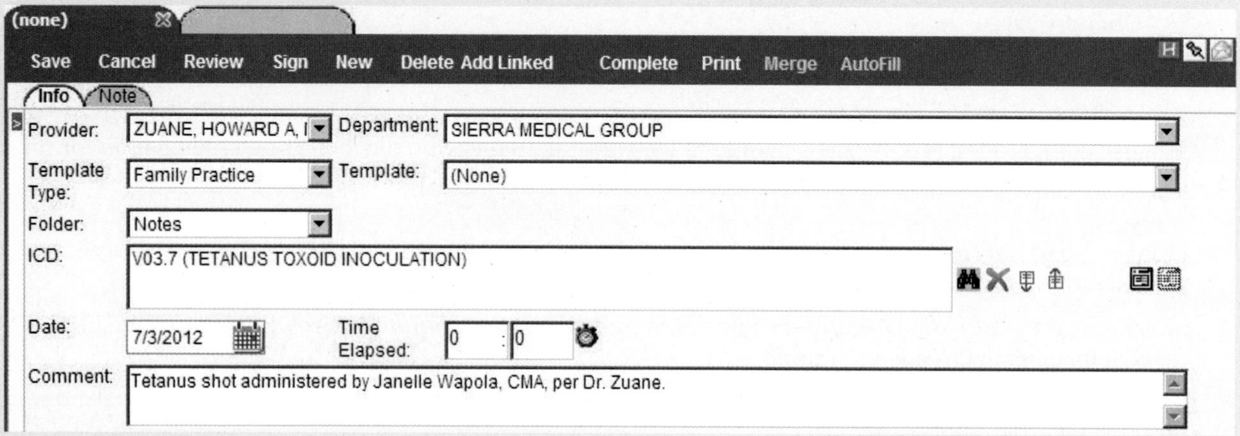

(none)
Save Cancel Review Sign New Delete Add Linked Complete Print Merge AutoFill
Info Note
Provider: ZUANE, HOWARD A, I Department: SIERRA MEDICAL GROUP
Template Type: Family Practice Template: (None)
Folder: Notes
ICD: V03.7 (TETANUS TOXOID INOCULATION)
Date: 7/3/2012 Time Elapsed: 0 : 0
Comment: Tetanus shot administered by Janelle Wapola, CMA, per Dr. Zuane.

Reprinted with permission of TriMed Technologies, Corp.

13. When you are certain that the information documented is accurate, you will sign off on this note. Click Sign.
14. A new window opens. *Your sign-off password is your user log-in* (the one that you used to log into e-Medsys®—for example, "user15"). Enter your user log-in, and click Save.

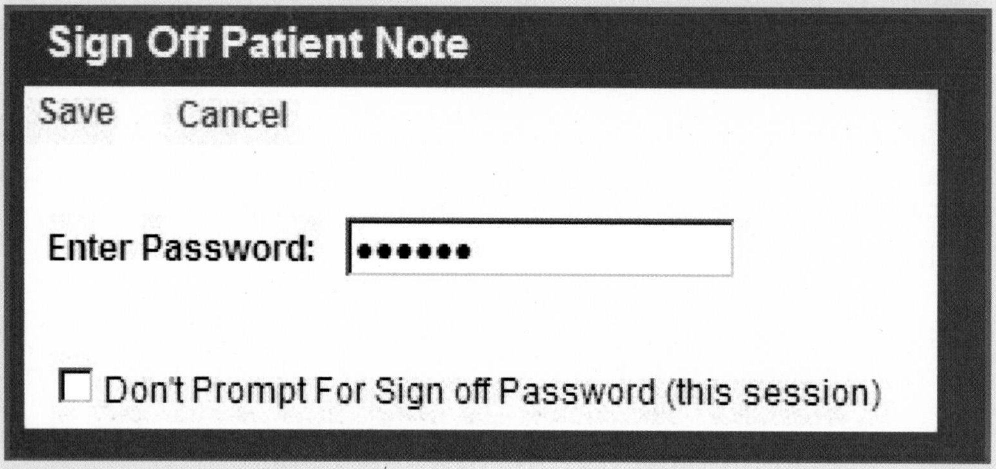

Sign Off Patient Note
Save Cancel
Enter Password: ••••••
Don't Prompt For Sign off Password (this session)

Reprinted with permission of TriMed Technologies, Corp.

15. Now, the information that you entered appears grayed out on the screen. This information is part of the patient's permanent record and cannot be further modified.

> **Note:** You must complete this exercise and sign off on the note in order to continue to Exercise 7.2.

Exercise 7.2: Completing a Superbill

Complete a superbill for Anthony Bates indicating the diagnosis of tetanus toxoid inoculation (V03.7), the administration code (90782), and the substance administration code (90703).

1. Still in Anthony Bates' chart, on the left side of the screen, click on the 7/3/2012 RETURN OFFICE VISIT appointment, highlighting it.
2. When you do this, the right side of the screen brings up more information regarding the appointment. From the right-hand corner of this screen, select the Superbill Tab.

Follow Up

07/03/2012:FOLLOW UP (ZUANE, HOWARD A, MD) — Appointment — Superbill

Provider:	ZUANE, HOWARD A, MD
Appt Date:	07/03/2012
Appt Time:	09:00 AM
Duration:	15 Minutes
Type:	FOLLOW UP
Status:	Registered
Dept:	SIERRA MEDICAL GROUP
Notes:	REASON FOR VISIT?: TETANUS SHOT
Last Updated:	11/14/2012 3:52:28 PM

Charge History (From Practice Management System):

Procedure	Description	Diag1	Diag2	Diag3	Diag4

3. The electronic superbill appears. Click on the corner box to enlarge the superbill while you are working within it.
4. Make sure that Dr. Howard Zuane's name appears in the Provider field. Leave the second provider field blank.
5. In the Date field, type today's date, 7/3/2012. The Insurance field is autopopulated based on the patient's insurance.
6. Below the Comments section, there is a section with three tabs (Ticket, Chart, and Find). The Ticket Tab is populated with some of the most common charges used in the medical office. If a charge does not appear on the Ticket Tab, you can select the Find Tab to look up a CPT code and add it to the superbill. Click on the Find Tab.

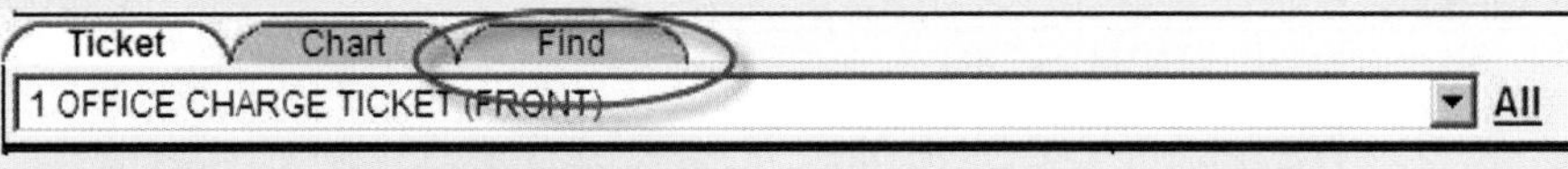

7. Type "90782" (the administration code), and then press Enter on your keyboard.
8. Now the procedure code appears below the Search field, with a box next to it. Click on the box to select it. When you do, a row at the bottom opens that indicates your selection.

Ticket — Chart — Find

PROC Code: 90782 Description: 0 1 2 3 4 5 6 7 8 9 Find

☑ 90782 INJECTION, SC/IM

Superbill

Procedure	Description	Qty	Diag1	Diag
90782	INJECTION, SC/IM	1		

9. Move your mouse into the Diag1 field. When you do, an icon of binoculars appears.

Superbill

Procedure	Description	Qty	Diag1	Diag2
90782	INJECTION, SC/IM	1		

Reprinted with permission of TriMed Technologies, Corp.

10. Click on the binoculars. Now, the cursor moves back up to the Code field. Type "TETANUS" in the Description field (to search for tetanus shot), and press Enter on your keyboard.
11. Now, the diagnosis code appears below the Search field, with a box next to it.
12. Click on the box to select it. When you do, note that the diagnosis code now appears in the Diag1 box at the bottom.
13. Click Save. Now, you are back on the Ticket Tab.
14. The next CPT code is listed on the Ticket Tab, so scroll down and select the box next to 90703 for the supply of TETANUS VACCINE, IM. Note that when you select the box, a new row appears at the bottom.

	☐ 90788 INJECTION OF ANTIBIOTIC
LABS	☑ 90703 TETANUS VACCINE, IM
☐ 81005 URINALYSIS	
☐ 81000 URINALYSIS, NONAUTO W/SCOPE	HOSPITAL VISITS
☐ 82270 TEST FOR BLOOD, FECES	☐ 99223 INITIAL HOSP Check item to add to super
☐ 36415 DRAWING BLOOD	☐ 99232 SUBSEQUENT HOSPITAL CARE

Superbill

Procedure	Description	Qty	Diag1
90782	INJECTION, SC/IM	1	V03.7
90703	TETANUS VACCINE, IM	1	

Reprinted with permission of TriMed Technologies, Corp.

15. Now, click on the triangle next to Diag1. This copies the diagnosis code that you had previously selected and enters it into the row.

Procedure	Description	Qty	Diag1
90782	INJECTION, SC/IM	1	V03.7

Reprinted with permission of TriMed Technologies, Corp.

16. Click Save.
17. When you are certain that the information documented is accurate, you will sign off on these charges. Click Sign.
18. A new window opens. *Your sign-off password is your user log-in* (the one that you used to log into e-Medsys®—for example, "user15"). Enter your user log-in, and click Save.
19. Now, the information that you entered appears grayed out on the screen, and a Lock icon appears on the Superbill Tab. This information is part of the patient's permanent record and cannot be further modified.

Note: You must complete this exercise and sign off on the superbill in order to be able to perform the exercises in Task 9.

20. Now, click Print to print a copy of the superbill. Label it Exercise 7.2. Close when finished.

Troubleshooting: Ensuring You Have Signed Off on the Superbill

If you are not sure whether you have signed off on the superbill, follow these steps:

1. Go to the EHR schedule.
2. Find Anthony Bates' appointment on the schedule. (*Hint:* Select Dr. Zuane as the provider and 7/3/2012 as the date.)
3. On the left side of the screen beneath the calendar, click on the radio button next to List.

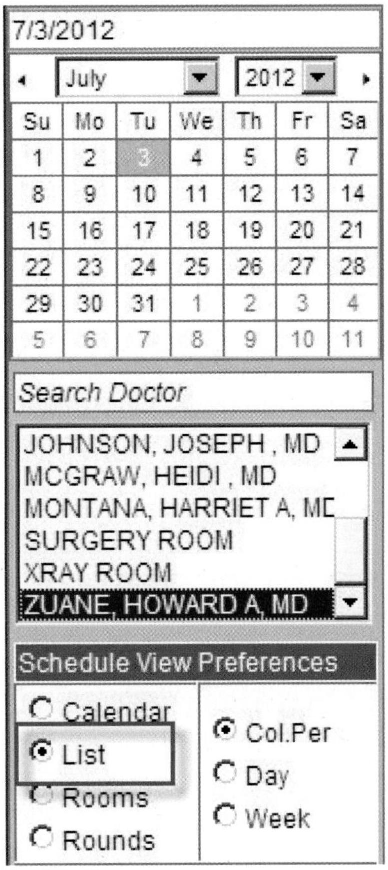

Reprinted with permission of TriMed Technologies, Corp.

4. Now, the right side of the screen brings up the schedule in List view. In this view, there is a Superbill column. In this column, the status of the superbill is indicated:
   - *Signed* means that you have signed off on the superbill.
   - *Saved* means that you have created the superbill but not signed off on it.
   - If there is nothing in this column, you have not created the superbill.
5. If you have followed the steps in Exercise 7.2, the Superbill column for Anthony Bates should indicate *Signed.*
6. If the column does not indicate *Signed,* go back into Anthony's chart. (*Hint:* Mouse over Chart on the top menu, and click on Anthony Bates from the drop-down list.) You must sign off on the superbill in order to complete Task 9.

PUTTING IT INTO PRACTICE

Exercise 7.3: Documenting Administration of a Therapeutic Injection and Creating a Superbill

Without using step-by-step instructions, as given in the previous exercises, this exercise requires you to (1) receive the patient (indicating Arrived and Registered on the schedule), (2) admit the patient using the EHR schedule, (3) create a new patient note to record the administration of an injection, and (4) create and sign off on a superbill.

Note: You must sign off on the superbill in order to complete Task 9.

On July 16, 2012, at 11:00 a.m., Lily Adams, a patient of Dr. Dixon, came in for her B-12 shot to be administered by the MA without a physician visit. Using the steps outlined in the earlier exercises and the information in the following list, document the administration of the injection and create a superbill for her. Print out the superbill, and label it Exercise 7.3.

- Diagnosis: B12 Deficiency
- Diagnosis Code: 281.1
- Administration Code: 90782
- Substance Injected Code: J3420

TASK 8—ORDERING LABORATORY TEST AND ENTERING RESULTS

Exercise 8.1: Recording a Laboratory Test Order

Today is August 31, 2012. Dr. Adams orders a glucose check for Diane Best to test for Diabetes (250.02).

1. Log in to e-Medsys®.
2. In Task 4, the patient was already indicated as Arrived and Registered.
3. Open the EHR Home Page, and using the steps learned in Task 5, indicate on the EHR schedule that the patient has been Admitted.
4. Double click on Diane's appointment on the EHR schedule to bring up her chart.
5. In Diane's chart, on the lower left side of the screen, right click on today's appointment.
6. Select Add New (Linked) ▶ and then Order.

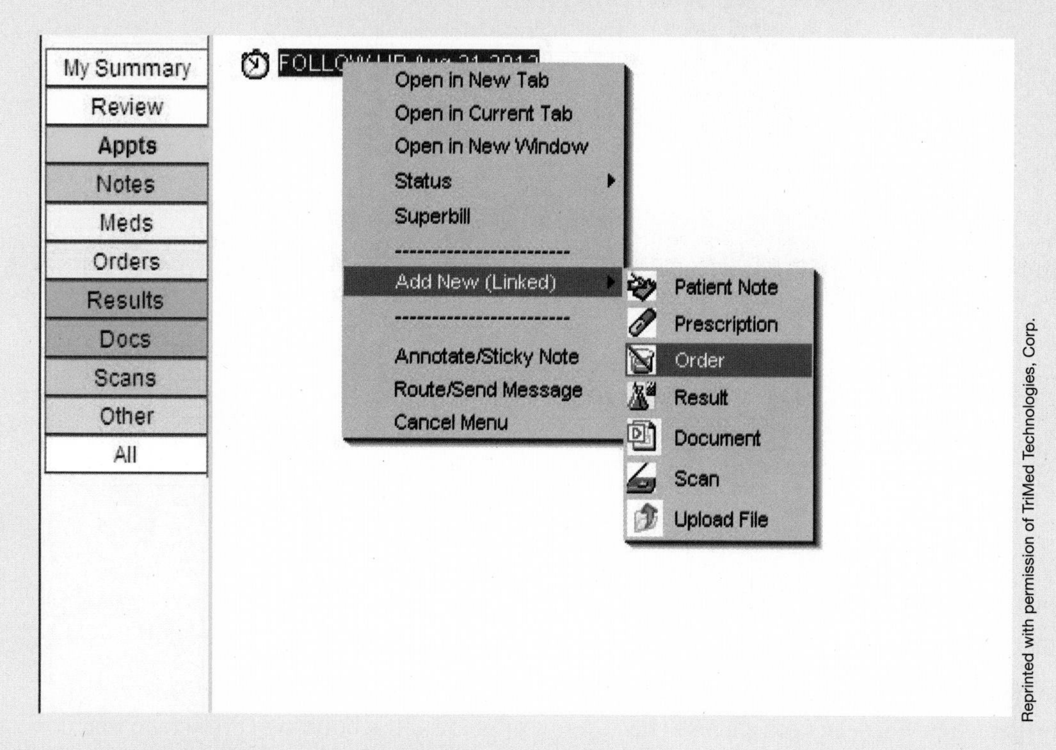

7. The new Order appears on the lower right side of the screen. The Provider (Adams), Department (Sierra Medical Group), Folder (Orders), and Insurance (Medicare) fields should be populated if they are not autopopulated.
8. In the Order Date field, enter "8/31/2012."
9. The order will be billed to the patient's insurance company, so in the Bill To option, make sure the button to the left of Insurance is selected.
10. The Priority field has various drop-down options; select Routine. The remaining fields should be left blank. Check your screen with the following screen shot.

Order-newlin

Save Cancel Review Sign New Delete Add Linked Print Word Merge Place Order

Order Tests

Order #:

Provider: ADAMS, HOWARD, MD All Dept: SIERRA MEDICAL GROUP

Folder: Orders Primary Ins: MEDICARE

Group/Policy: 365478971A

Order Date: 8/31/2012 Collection Date/Time:

Bill To: Provider Insurance Patient

Priority: Routine Secondary Ins: UNITED HEALTHCARE

CC Providers: Group/Policy: GH3215 326457874

Add CC Provider: All

Comment:

Hold Assistant Confidential-Only discuss w/patient

11. Click Save.
12. Now, click on the Tests Tab.

#1412994

Save Cancel Review Sign New Delete Add Linked Print Word

Order | Tests

Order #: 1412994

Provider: ADAMS, HOWARD , MD All

Folder: Orders

Reprinted with permission of TriMed Technologies, Corp.

13. In the Company field, select LabCorp from the drop-down menu.
14. In the Order Set field, select LabCorp Test Set From the drop-down menu.
15. Click on the Set Tests Tab and click in the box to the left of 1 HR G (Glucose, 1 hour).
16. Note that when you select the glucose check, a row appears at the bottom of the screen that indicates your selection.

Set Tests | Other Tests | ICDs | Questions

☑ 1 HR G (Glucose, 1 hour)	☐ GAMBFL (Gamma Globulin)	☐ CULTUR (Culture, Only)
	☐ GAST (Gastrin, Serum)	☐ CULBAC (Culture, Bacterial)
☐ A/G RA (A/G Ratio)	☐ HAPTOG (Haptoglobin)	☐ CULGEN (Culture, Genital)
☐ ACETLC (Acetaminophen)	☐ HAVAB (Hep A Ab, Total)	☐ CULRES (Culture, Respiratory)
☐ ACHETG (ACHE)	☐ HSV-7 (HSV CULTURE AND TYPING)	☐ SILVEP (Silver, Plasma)
☐ ADNA (Anti-DNA (DS) AB. QN)		
☐ ANSE24 (Anserine,Qn,24hr,Ur)	☐ LDH (LDH)	☐ TRIG (Triglycerides)
☐ ASPART (Aspartic acid,Qn,Am)	☐ LDL CH (LDL Cholesterol Calc)	☐ TSH (TSH)
☐ CB/D/P (CBC WITH DIFFERENTIAL/PLATELET)	☐ LP (LIPID PANEL)	☐ URE24H (Urea Nitrogen, 24hr)
	☐ LIPID (Lipid Panel w-Chol)	☐ URNALS (Urinalysis Complete)
☐ C DIFF (C DIFFICILE TOXIN A)	☐ ORANGE (F033 ORANGE)	☐ ZYGOSI (Twin Zygo. Pre/Post)
☐ CATHEP (CATHEPSIN D)		
☐ CHL UU (Chloride, Urine)	☐ PERENN (ALLERGENS, PERENNIAL)	☐ ZINC (Zinc, Serum)
☐ COMP (Complete Metabolic Panel)	☐ PREGNE (Pregnenolone)	☐ WORMWO (W005 WORMWOOD)

Test Code	Description	Diag1	Diag2	Diag3	Diag4	Order Details/Comments
1 HR G	Glucose, 1 hour					

Reprinted with permission of TriMed Technologies, Corp.

17. Now, click the ICD Tab.

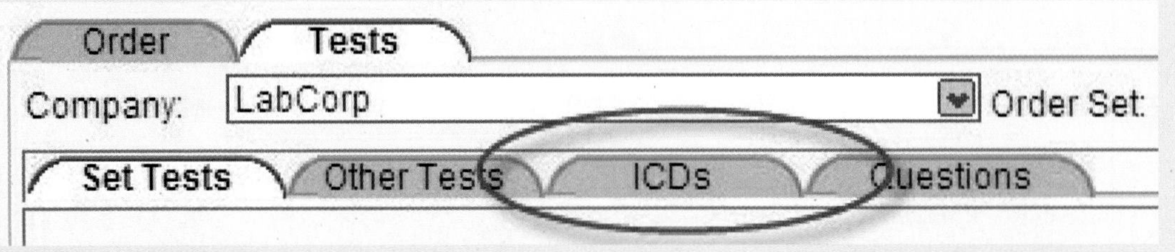

Reprinted with permission of TriMed Technologies, Corp.

18. Type "DIAB" in the Desc field, and press Enter on your keyboard. This searches for all diagnosis codes that start with these letters.

19. Click in the box to the left of 250.02 DIAB UNCOMP TYPE II UNCONTRD. Note that when you select the box, the diagnosis code appears in the row at the bottom in the Diag1 field.

20. When you are certain that the information documented, click on Save. Now, the order is ready to send to the provider for sign-off.
21. Click on the Route/Send Message icon in the upper right corner of the order screen (like you did in Task 6 for prescriptions).
22. In the Message window, select the following:

- Select Individual Staff: Choose "Cengage Instructor."
- Route To: Choose "Cengage Instructor."
- The Date and Time fields automatically populate; leave this as today's date.
- Action Type: Select Sign Off from the drop-down list.
- Priority: Select Normal from the drop-down list.

Check your work with the following screen shot.

23. Click on Send. The order has now been sent to the provider for approval. Click on the Home link at the top of the screen to return to the EHR schedule.

PUTTING IT INTO PRACTICE

Exercise 8.2: Recording a Laboratory Test Order

This exercise requires you to record a laboratory test order without using step-by-step instructions, as given in the previous exercises.

Dr. Dixon orders a urine test for Michael Minn on August 20, 2012. When you have entered the ordered test and saved it, send the order for provider sign-off.

- Company: LabCorp
- Order Set: LabCorp Test Set
- Test Ordered: URNALS
- Diagnosis: DYSURIA (788.1)

Exercise 8.3: Uploading Laboratory Test Results into a Patient Chart

Today is September 10, 2012. Diane Best's glucose check has come back from the laboratory. The results are scanned in and need to be uploaded to the patient's chart. (*Note:* In a medical office, results are often sent electronically and directly recorded to the patient's record.) Here we will simulate uploading laboratory results that were received by the office as a hard-copy fax.

Special Note: Prior to Starting Exercise 8.3

In order to complete this activity, as well as Exercise 8.4, you will need to retrieve two documents from this book's Premium Website: "Exercise 8.3: Laboratory Results" and "Exercise 8.4: Laboratory Results." Please follow these steps:

1. Go to this web site: www.cengagebrain.com.
2. Enter your access code (found on your printed access card at the front of this book) in the PrePaid Code or Access Key field. Click **Register.**
3. Register as a new user or log in as an existing user if you already have an account with Cengage Learning or cengagebrain.com.
4. Select Go to My Account.
5. Open the product from the My Account page.
6. Click on the Premium Website link on the right navigation bar.
7. Click on the file "Exercise 8.3: Laboratory Results." Save the file to a place of your choice (such as a flash drive or the desktop) where you can easily retrieve it to complete Exercise 8.3.
8. Click on the file "Exercise 8.4: Laboratory Results." Save the file to a place of your choice (such as a flash drive or the desktop) where you can easily retrieve it to complete Exercise 8.4.
9. You are ready to begin Exercise 8.3.

1. Log in to e-Medsys®.
2. Click on EHR Home Page from the drop-down box. This action opens the EHR home page in a new window. From the menu along the top of the page, click on Chart.

3. Search for Diane Best (either by typing the patient's last name and clicking Enter or by clicking the first letter of the patient's last name along the left side of the screen).
4. Double click on the patient's name to open her chart.
5. From the left navigational tab, click on APPTS. You should see Diane's appointment on 8/31/2012 as well as the order that is linked to that appointment.
6. Right click on the order from 8/31/2012. Select Add New (Linked) ▶ and then Upload File.

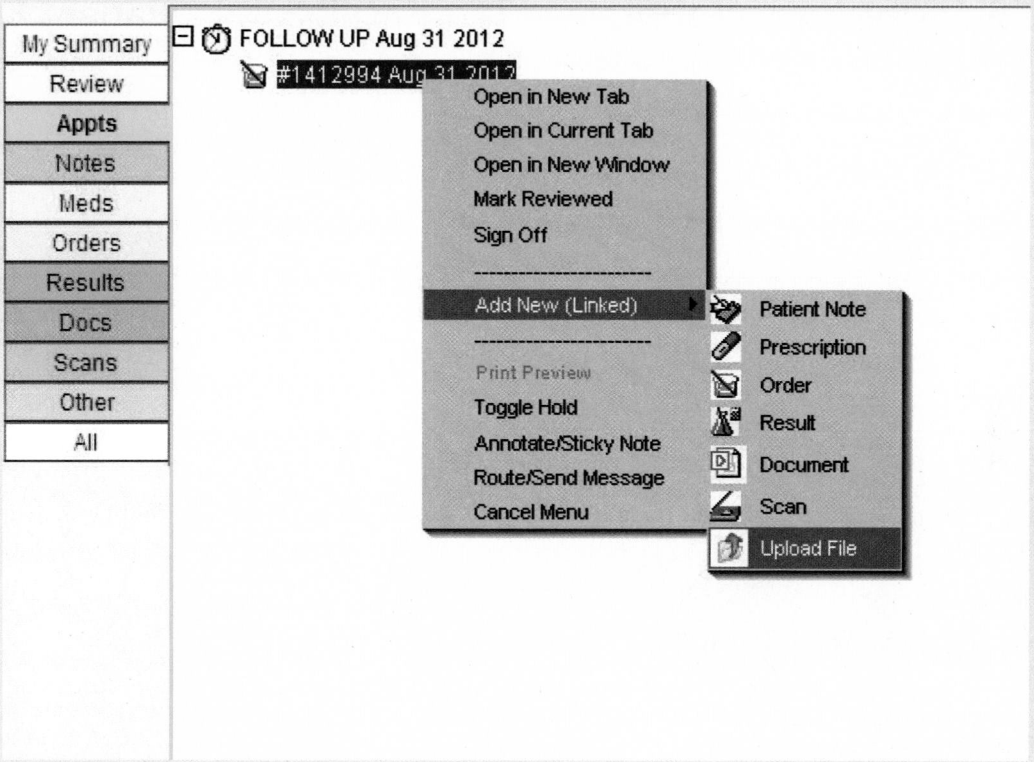
My Summary
Review
Appts
Notes
Meds
Orders
Results
Docs
Scans
Other
All
FOLLOW UP Aug 31 2012
#1412994 Aug 31 2012
Open in New Tab
Open in Current Tab
Open in New Window
Mark Reviewed
Sign Off
Add New (Linked)
Print Preview
Toggle Hold
Annotate/Sticky Note
Route/Send Message
Cancel Menu
Patient Note
Prescription
Order
Result
Document
Scan
Upload File

Reprinted with permission of TriMed Technologies, Corp.

7. The document upload appears on the right side of the screen.
8. Make sure the following fields are populated as follows - Provider: Adams, Dept: Sierra Medical Group, and Folder: Results.
9. Doc. Type: Select Lab Result Report from the drop-down menu.
10. In the ICD field, click the binoculars, and search for Diabetes (*hint:* type "diab" in the description field and press Enter). Select DIAB UNCOMP TYPE II UNCONTRD 250.02.

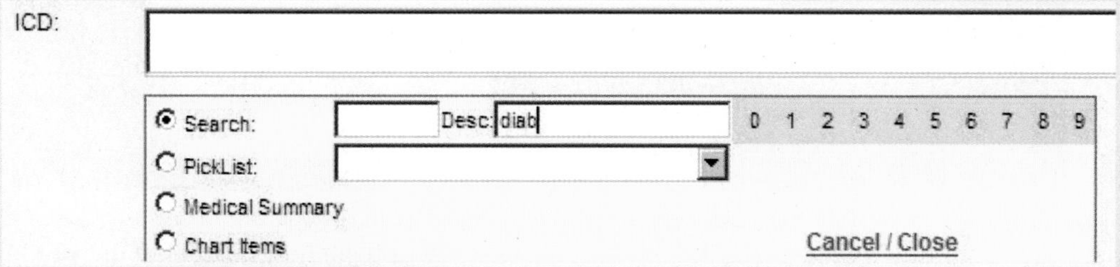
ICD:
Search:
Desc: diab
0 1 2 3 4 5 6 7 8 9
PickList:
Medical Summary
Chart Items
Cancel / Close

Reprinted with permission of TriMed Technologies, Corp.

11. Enter today's date.
12. In the Name field, enter "LAB RESULT REPORT" if it is not already populated.
13. Leave the Description field empty.
14. Next to the Document to Upload field, click Browse.
15. Locate and select the Exercise 8.3 Laboratory Results file that you downloaded from the Premium Website.

16. Click Upload to Chart.
17. Now, on the left side of the screen, the laboratory results should appear in Tree View as a submenu item beneath the 8/31/2012 Order. Click on the Home link at the top of the screen to return to the EHR schedule.

PUTTING IT INTO PRACTICE

Exercise 8.4: Uploading Laboratory Test Results into a Patient Chart

This exercise requires you to record laboratory test results without using step-by-step instructions, as given in the previous exercises.

To complete this activity, you will need to download the "Exercise 8.4 Laboratory Results" file from the Premium Website if you have not done so already. See the "Special Note" in Exercise 8.3 for directions.

Upload the laboratory results document (received today, August 30, 2012) for Michael Minn's urine test, which was performed on August 20, 2012.

TASK 9—POSTING PATIENT CHARGES AND RECORDING PAYMENTS

Exercise 9.1: Posting Charges

Today is August 13, 2012. Valerie Violet has been experiencing abdominal pain (789.00), and Dr. Zuane performed a colonoscopy (45378).

1. Log in to e-Medsys®.
2. At the top of the screen, click on Billing.
3. Click on Posting from the drop-down box and then Charge Posting from the side drop-down box. (*Note:* The keyboard shortcut for this is Ctrl + H.)

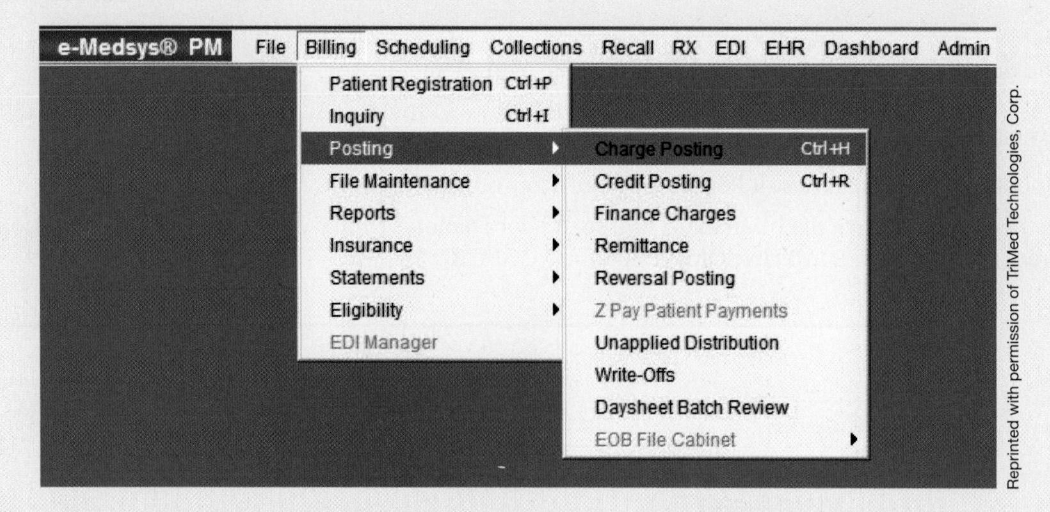

4. A Batch Posting window will appear. Click on New Batch in the top left hand corner of the window. Enter the New Batch Description: "CHARGES FOR 8/13/2012." (*Note:* Each office will have a policy for posting charges. Always follow specific office policy. For the purposes of these exercises, we will be posting procedures organized by "day.")
5. Select SIERRA MEDICAL GROUP from the drop-down list for the department. This selection indicates the location of the person entering the charges—not the location where the patient was seen. The location where the patient was seen is part of the individual charge posting. For the purposes of these exercises, you should select Sierra Medical Group as your posting location.

6. Click OK. Now the batch name appears at the top of the Charge Posting screen.
7. Type "VIOLET" (the patient's last name) in the Name field, and then click Search.

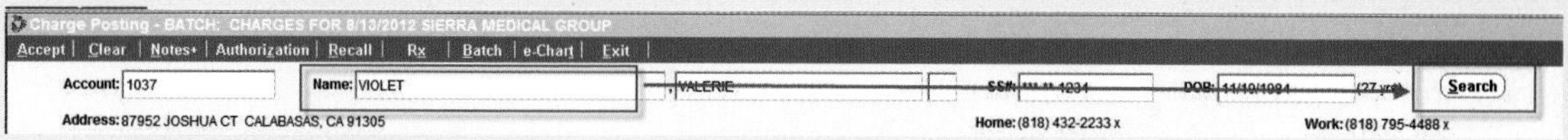

Charge Posting - BATCH: CHARGES FOR 8/13/2012 SIERRA MEDICAL GROUP

Accept | Clear | Notes+ | Authorization | Recall | Rx | Batch | e-Chart | Exit |

Account: 1037 Name: VIOLET , VALERIE SS#: ***-**-1234 DOB: 11/10/1984 (27 yrs) Search

Address: 87952 JOSHUA CT CALABASAS, CA 91305 Home: (818) 432-2233 x Work: (818) 795-4488 x

8. A charge ticket was not created for this patient, so click Cancel at the next prompt.
9. Now the cursor is at the bottom part of the window in the Charge Tab. Enter the following information:
   - Date: 08/13/2012
   - Department: Sierra Medical Group
   - Provider: Dr. Zuane
   - Primary Insurance Plan: BLUE CROSS (this is already populated from the selection in the patient registration screen)
   - Referring Provider: *Leave blank*

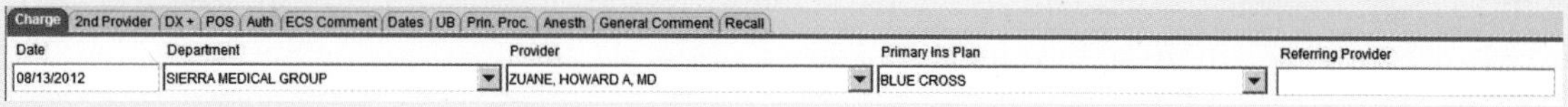

Charge | 2nd Provider | DX+ | POS | Auth | ECS Comment | Dates | UB | Prin. Proc. | Anesth | General Comment | Recall

Date	Department	Provider	Primary Ins Plan	Referring Provider
08/13/2012	SIERRA MEDICAL GROUP	ZUANE, HOWARD A, MD	BLUE CROSS	

10. In the Procedure field, type "%," and press Enter on your keyboard. This is a search function of the program and allows you to search for all procedure codes that are in the system.
11. Select 45378 from the list, and click OK.

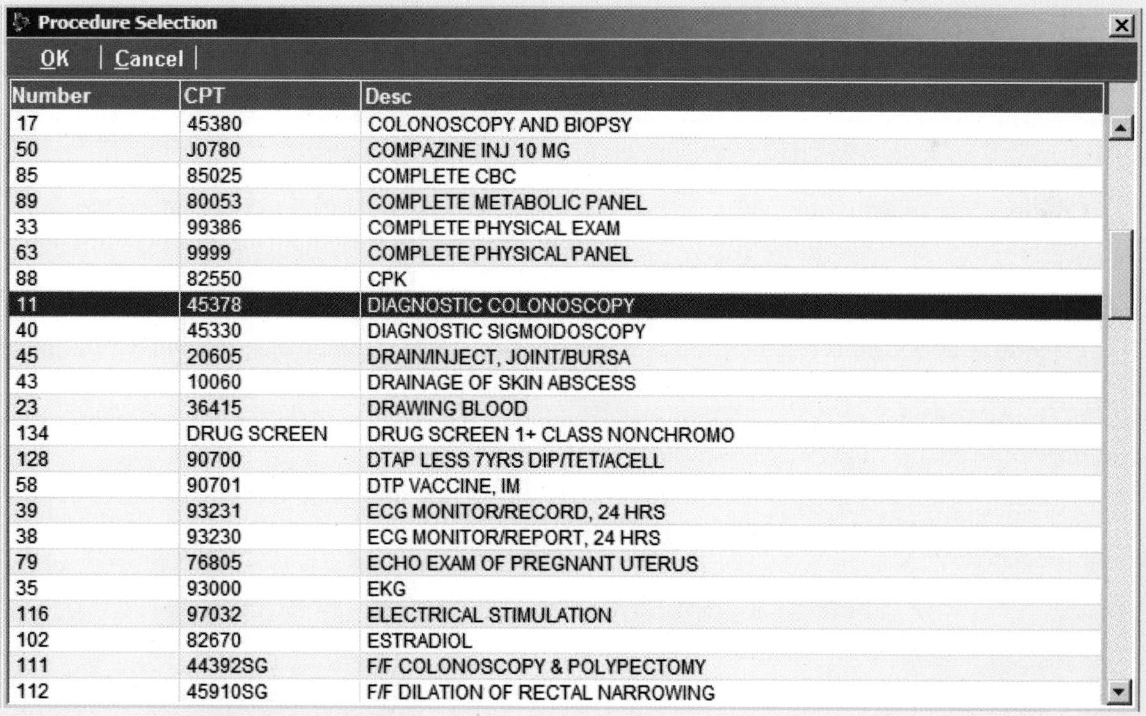

Procedure Selection

OK | Cancel |

Number	CPT	Desc
17	45380	COLONOSCOPY AND BIOPSY
50	J0780	COMPAZINE INJ 10 MG
85	85025	COMPLETE CBC
89	80053	COMPLETE METABOLIC PANEL
33	99386	COMPLETE PHYSICAL EXAM
63	9999	COMPLETE PHYSICAL PANEL
88	82550	CPK
11	45378	DIAGNOSTIC COLONOSCOPY
40	45330	DIAGNOSTIC SIGMOIDOSCOPY
45	20605	DRAIN/INJECT, JOINT/BURSA
43	10060	DRAINAGE OF SKIN ABSCESS
23	36415	DRAWING BLOOD
134	DRUG SCREEN	DRUG SCREEN 1+ CLASS NONCHROMO
128	90700	DTAP LESS 7YRS DIP/TET/ACELL
58	90701	DTP VACCINE, IM
39	93231	ECG MONITOR/RECORD, 24 HRS
38	93230	ECG MONITOR/REPORT, 24 HRS
79	76805	ECHO EXAM OF PREGNANT UTERUS
35	93000	EKG
116	97032	ELECTRICAL STIMULATION
102	82670	ESTRADIOL
111	44392SG	F/F COLONOSCOPY & POLYPECTOMY
112	45910SG	F/F DILATION OF RECTAL NARROWING

12. The program will automatically open another tab. Press Enter on your keyboard to return to the Charge Tab.
13. In the DX-1 (Diagnosis) field, type "%," and press Enter on your keyboard. Select the diagnosis 789.00, and click OK.
14. Now the program automatically opens another tab, where you can enter additional diagnosis codes (if the provider has specified these). Since there are no other diagnosis codes indicated by the provider, click the Return button.

15. You are back on the Charge Tab. Note that the POS, TOS, and Charge Amount fields have been filled in by the program, based on your code selections.
16. Keep the boxes next to STMT (Statement), INS (Insurance), and AA (Accept Assignment) checked.
17. You can leave the box next to Multiple Dates unchecked. This would be checked if you were posting multiple services done on different dates—for example, hospital charges.

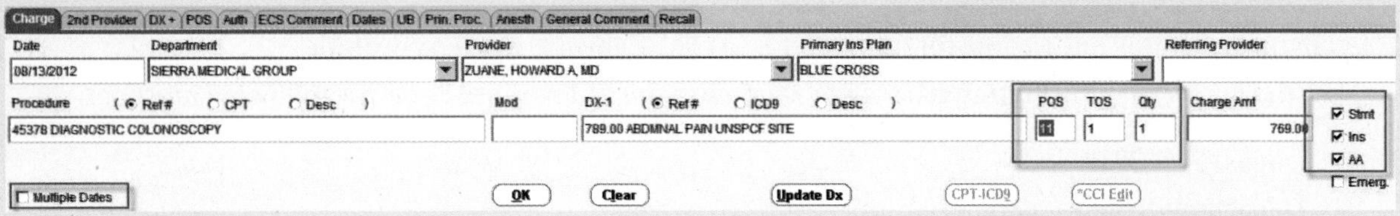

18. Click on the OK button. When you do, the information you just entered is now transferred below.

You have been working in the Charge Tab of this screen. You will note that several other tabs are available on this screen. We will discuss two additional screens. This is for your information only; you are not required to enter any data in these tabs for this exercise.

- **POS Tab:** This tab will pull forward for completion if POS is anything other than office (POS 11). This is a Table Look-Up field.
- **Auth Tab:** If an authorization has been entered for this patient for the posted procedure, this tab will display, proposing the authorization number that was entered in the authorization screen. An authorization number can be entered for this specific transaction at charge posting. Also, the Authorization button is accessible from the charge posting screen so all authorizations can be viewed.

19. Now that you have finished entering all the procedure charges for this patient, go to the bottom left corner of your screen. Check the boxes next to Credits, Prt Receipt, and Prt Claim.
    - **Credits:** Checking this box informs the system that a payment will be posted right after charges have been posted. Once the charges have been accepted, the system will automatically open the credit posting screen for this posting batch. After the payment is entered and accepted, the system will take you back to the screen you are currently on, the charge posting screen.
    - **Prt Stmt:** Checking this box informs the system that a statement should be produced for this patient after charges and payments have been posted. This box should be left unchecked.
    - **Prt Receipt:** Checking this box informs the system that a receipt should be produced for this patient (for only those charges and payments posted today).
    - **Prt Claim:** Checking this box informs the system that a claim form should be produced for this patient after charges and payments have been posted.

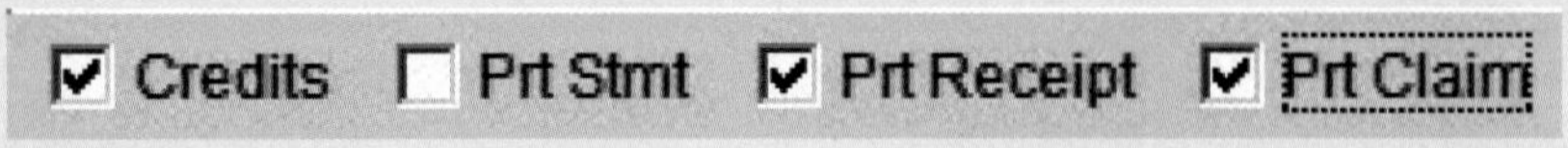

20. Now, click the Accept button on the top charge posting menu. The charges will be accepted, and the program will automatically take you to the credit posting screen. Continue to Exercise 9.2 immediately.

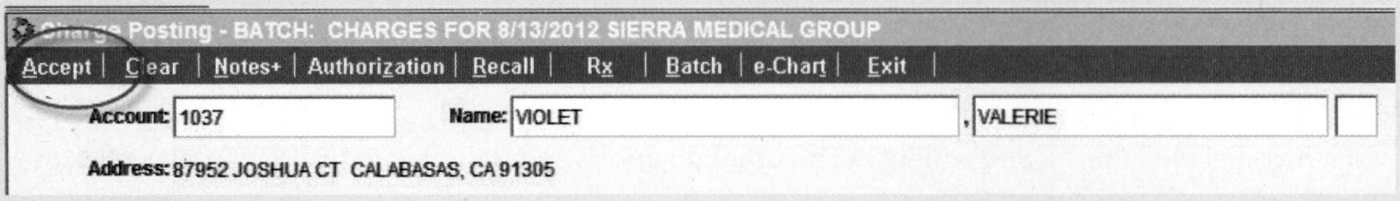

Exercise 9.2: Posting a Co-Payment

Valerie Violet's co-pay is $35, and she also has an outstanding balance of $20 in the system. She writes a check (#10589) for $55 to be applied to today's co-payment and the outstanding balance.

1. You are now working in the credit posting screen. Your cursor should be in the Credit Info Tab (which is the main screen on this page) in the Date field. The date is already populated for you.
2. Under Credit Type, use the drop-down to select Check.
3. In the Check No field, type "10589."
4. In the Amount field, type "55.00."
5. Now click the radio button next to All. When you do, three service dates appear below.

Date	Dept Prov	Proc DX	Qty	Chg Amt
03/01/2012	MSMG ZUES	99211 OFFICE/...	1	30.00
03/01/2012	MSMG ZUES	81002 URINAL...	1	10.00
08/13/2012	SMG ZUES	45378 DIAGNO...	1	769.00

Reprinted with permission of TriMed Technologies, Corp.

6. In the Applied column, enter "$15.00" in the first row, for the first 3/1/2012 charge, and "$5.00" in the second row, for the second 3/1/2012 charge. Enter "$35.00" in the third row, for today's charges.

Date	Dept Prov	Proc DX	Qty	Chg Amt	Allowed	Approved	Paid%	Applied	A
03/01/2012	MSMG ZUES	99211 OFFICE/...	1	30.00	0.00	0.00	0.00	15.00	
03/01/2012	MSMG ZUES	81002 URINAL...	1	10.00	0.00	0.00	0.00	5.00	
08/13/2012	SMG ZUES	45378 DIAGNO...	1	769.00	0.00	0.00	0.00	35.00	

Reprinted with permission of TriMed Technologies, Corp.

7. Click the Accept button in the upper left corner to apply the payments to Valerie's account. Recall that you had chosen to create a CMS-1500 form and a patient receipt in Exercise 9.1, so these files will print immediately to your local printer:
   - Label the first file (the CMS-1500 form) as Exercise 9.2A.
   - Label the second file (the patient receipt) as Exercise 9.2B.
8. When you have finished, you are back on the charge posting screen. If you had additional charges to post that day, you would continue posting. Click Exit to return to the main menu.

PUTTING IT INTO PRACTICE

Exercise 9-3: Posting Charges and Applying Co-Payments

This exercise requires you to post charges and apply co-payments for the following patients without using step-by-step instructions, as given in the previous exercises. You will print out CMS-1500 forms and patient receipts and label them as indicated below.

1. Bruce Sawtelle had an appointment with Dr. Franklin on August 8, 2012. Bruce suffers from diverticulosis (562.10), and Dr. Franklin performed a sigmoidoscopy (45330). Bruce pays his $20 co-payment with cash.
   - Label the first file (the CMS-1500 form) as Exercise 9.3-1A.
   - Label the second file (the patient receipt) as Exercise 9.3-1B.

2. Diane Best had an appointment with Dr. Adams on August 31, 2012. Dr. Adams ordered a blood glucose test (82948) to test for Diabetes (250.02). Diane does not pay a co-payment for this visit, so it is unnecessary to print a receipt for the patient. (*Hint:* Only the box next to Prt Claim will be checked.)

   - Label the CMS-1500 form as Exercise 9.3-2.

TASK 10—PUTTING IT INTO PRACTICE

CASE STUDY 10.1

Daniel Greene

Today is August 20, 2012. Daniel Greene calls today to schedule an appointment for an annual exam. He is new to the practice and would like to select Dr. Howard Adams as his primary care provider.

Exercise 1: Adding a New Patient and Scheduling an Appointment

Schedule an appointment for a new patient, Daniel Greene, on August 29, 2012, at 9:30 a.m. with Dr. Adams. You will need to add some registration information to the database prior to scheduling an appointment for the patient.

1. Open the Patient Registration screen, where you can record information from the patient. At this time, you need to record only the fields on the Patient Registration screen labeled in red. The remainder of the information will be recorded when Daniel comes into the office and completes the registration paperwork. (*Hint:* Click OK through the prompts indicating that Work and Emergency phone numbers are recommended; these fields will be completed when the patient comes into the office.)

   - Name: GREENE, DANIEL
   - Address: 52 West Palmetto Drive, Pasadena, CA 90039
   - Home Phone: (818) 555-9876
   - Social Security Number: 111-98-9800
   - Date of Birth: 03/07/1980
   - Gender: Male

2. Click on Accept. You will complete the information when the patient comes in for his appointment.
3. Daniel indicates that August 29, 2012, at 9:30 a.m. would be perfect for his annual exam. (*Hint:* Because he is a new patient, in the Visit Type field, click on the drop-down arrow, and select NP. In the Reason for Visit field on the Supplemental Information screen, type "ANNUAL EXAM.") Complete booking his appointment as you have done in previous exercises.

Exercise 2: Receiving the Patient and Completing the Registration Information

Today is August 29, 2012. Daniel Greene arrives 15 minutes early for his appointment. Indicate on the appointment schedule that Daniel has Arrived to the practice. Upon his arrival, Daniel presents the registration forms he was sent in the mail. While Daniel is waiting to see Dr. Adams, you record the information, completing his registration.

1. Find Daniel's appointment on the schedule.
2. Right click on his appointment time, and indicate that he has Arrived. The color highlighting the time slot with his name will change to show that he has arrived.
3. Find Daniel's account in the Patient Registration screen. Using the following information, complete the patient's registration.

Employer	Maddux and Sons
Work Phone	(818) 393-4002 x383
Cell Phone	(758) 343-4998
Emergency Contact	Theodore Maddux, (818) 364-5987
Marital Status	Single
Relationship to Guarantor	Self

4. Click on Accept + Ins.
5. You are now on the Insurance Tab of the Patient Registration screen. Select Add Ins from the list on the right of the screen. Enter the following information:

Insurance Plan	Blue Cross (Woodland Hills location – P O BOX 4152)
Relationship to Policyholder	Self
Effective Date	01/01/2010
Group Number	TW0819
Policy Number	08190052

6. Leave the remaining fields as they are, and click on Accept.
7. A Yes or No window will appear, asking if you want to update the patient's charges with the new insurance information you have entered. Click on Yes.
8. Click on the Guarantor Tab, verify that the information entered on previous screens has transferred correctly, and click on Accept.
9. Return to the appointment scheduling screen, and indicate on the schedule that the patient is now Registered.

Exercise 3: Linking a New Note to an Appointment and Entering Chart Information

Daniel is now taken back to an exam room.

1. Find Daniel's appointment on the EHR schedule, and indicate that he is now Admitted.
2. Right click on Daniel's appointment on the EHR schedule, and use the menu to link a New Note to his chart for today's visit (August 29, 2012).
3. On the Information Tab in the Notes, ensure that all default information is listed correctly. Use the drop-down menu to select the Routine Exam Male template. Change the date to 08/29/2012.
4. Enter the following information on the Pt Info screen, and click Save.

Chief Complaint	Annual Physical Exam
Problem List	Attention Deficit Hyperactivity Disorder
Surgical History	Emergency appendectomy at age 18
Family History	Mom alive—59 years old, healthy; Father alive–62 years old, obese; one brother in Iraq and one sister still living with his parents, healthy
Social History	Smokes one pack a day for four years, social drinker, active in recreational sports with friends, hunts, fishes

Exercise 4: Entering Information from the Patient Questionnaire

Enter the information from the patient questionnaire form that Daniel completed.

1. Still in Daniel Greene's chart, select the ROS tab.
2. Enter information for the Constitutional, HEENT, and Respiratory systems. All of this information will be reviewed with the patient and signed by Dr. Adams. Click on Save.

Constitutional	Normal
HEENT	Recent URI
Respiratory	Snores heavily

Exercise 5: Entering Patient Vital Signs

Enter the vital signs that were taken upon bringing the patient into the exam room.

1. Still in Daniel Greene's chart, select the Exam Tab.
2. Enter the vital signs in the appropriate fields, and click Save. Now click the Print button. Label this printout as Case Study 10.1A.

Height	78 inches
Weight	215 pounds
Blood Pressure	120/70 (sitting)
Pulse	65
Respiration	18
Temperature	98.6

Exercise 6: Posting Charges

You will now enter the charges for Daniel's visit.

1. Create a New Batch: "CHARGES FOR 08/29/2012." (As with other exercises, the department is listed as Sierra Medical Group.)
2. Post charges for Daniel Greene:
   - Department: Sierra Medical Group
   - Procedure Code: 99385
   - Diagnosis Code: V70.0
3. Check the box next to Prt Claim at the bottom of the screen to generate a claim form for Daniel's visit.
4. Print the CMS-1500 form, and label it Case Study 10.1B.

CASE STUDY 10.2

Julie McMurrey

Julie McMurrey is a patient of Dr. Sarah Dixon. She has been experiencing chronic abdominal pain, discomfort, bloating, and explosive diarrhea. She called today, August 13, 2012, seeking an appointment with Dr. Dixon as soon as possible. You look in Dr. Dixon's schedule and see an opening for 3:00 p.m. this afternoon.

Exercise 1: Scheduling an Appointment

Schedule an appointment (*Hint:* return office visit) for the patient at 3:00 p.m. on Monday, August 13, 2012.

Exercise 2: Receiving the Patient

It is 2:45 p.m., and Julie is in the waiting room. Indicate on the appointment schedule that the patient has Arrived at the practice. Julie indicates that there are no registration updates. Indicate that the patient is Registered on the appointment schedule.

Exercise 3: Linking a New Note to an Appointment

Indicate that the patient has been Admitted on the EHR schedule. Link a new Patient Note to the appointment. Complete the Provider (Dr. Dixon), Template Type (Family Practice), and Template (Basic SOAP) fields. (Remember to change the date on the Patient Note to 08/13/2012.)

Exercise 4: Entering Information Using a SOAP Note

On the Note Tab, enter the following information:

Subjective	The patient comes in today experiencing abdominal pain, discomfort, bloating, and explosive diarrhea. She mentions that it is worse right after she eats a large meal.
Objective	Tearful at times. She has a flat affect during the visit.
Assessment	Irritable Bowel Syndrome
Plan	Patient will have a CBC done today, and a stool sample will be collected.

Print the Patient Note and label it Case Study 10-2A.

Exercise 5: Posting Charges

Enter the charges for the patient's visit on August 13, 2012:

- Department: Sierra Medical Group
- Procedure Code: 99214 Office/Outpatient Visit, EST
- Diagnosis Code: 558.9 Noninfect Gastroenterit OT

Check the box next to Prt Claim at the bottom of the screen to generate a claim form for the patient's visit. Print the CMS-1500 form, and label it Case Study 10.2.

Exercise 6: Scheduling a Follow-Up Appointment

Dr. Dixon has indicated that she wants to see Julie in one week for a follow-up. Schedule a follow-up appointment on August 20, 2012, at 9:30 a.m.

ACRONYM GLOSSARY

ACRONYM	CHAPTER	STANDS FOR
AAAASF	4	American Association for Accreditation of Ambulatory Surgery Facilities
AAAHC	4	Accreditation Association for Ambulatory Health Care, Inc.
AAP	4	American Academy of Pediatrics
ABN	5	Advance Beneficiary Notice
ACO	1	Accountable Care Organization
ACOG	4	American College of Obstetricians and Gynecologists
AHA	11	American Hospital Association
AHIMA	4	American Health Information Management Association
AMA	11	American Medical Association
AOA	4	American Osteopathic Association
ASTM	13	American Society for Testing and Materials International
CAC	11	computer assisted coding
CCHIT	1	Certification Commission for Healthcare Information Technology
CCR	13	continuity of care record
CDT	11	Current Dental Terminology
CHPL	2	Certified Health IT Product List
CMS	1	Centers for Medicare & Medicaid Services
CoC	4	Conditions of Coverage
CoP	4	Conditions of Participation
CPOE	9	computerized physician order entry
CPT	11	Current Procedural Terminology
CPT-IV	3	Current Procedural Terminology–4th Revision
DSM-IV-TR	3	Diagnostic and Statistical Manual–Fourth Edition–Text Revision
EDI	8	electronic data interchange
EHR	1	electronic health record
EMPI	5	enterprise master patient/person index
E/M codes	11	evaluation and management codes
EMR	1	electronic medical record
EOB	11	Explanation of Benefits
EP	1	Eligible Provider
HCPCS	11	Healthcare Common Procedure Coding Systems
HEDIS	4	Health Plan Employer Data and Information Set
HIE	1	Health Information Exchange
HIPAA	3	Health Insurance Portability and Accountability Act
HITECH	1	Health Information Technology for Economic and Clinical Health Act
ICD-9-CM	3	International Classification of Diseases–9th Revision–Clinical Modification
ICD-10-CM	3	International Classification of Diseases–10th Revision–Clinical Modification
IRB	12	Institutional Review Board
JC	4	The Joint Commission
LOINC	3	Logical Observation Identifier Names and Codes
MPI	5	master patient/person index
MU	3	Meaningful Use
NANDA	3	North American Nursing Diagnosis Association
NCHS	11	National Center for Health Statistics

NCQA	4	National Committee for Quality Assurance
NCVHS	4	National Committee for Vital and Health Statistics
NDC	3	National Drug Codes
NHIN	1	National Health Information Network
NIC	3	Nursing Interventions Classification
NOC	3	Nursing Outcomes Classification
ONC	1	Office of the National Coordinator (for Health Information Technology)
PHR	13	personal health record
PMS	5	practice management system
QIO	1	Quality Improvement Organization
RA	11	remittance advice
REC	1	Regional Health Information Technology Extension Center
RFP	2	request for proposal
RHIO	1	Regional Health Information Organization
SNO	1	Sub-Network Organization
SNOMED-CT	3	Systematized Nomenclature of Medicine–Clinical Terminology
UACDS	4	Uniform Ambulatory Care Data Set

GLOSSARY

A

Accountable Care Organization (ACO): A type of network of providers that are tied not only in serving a group of patients, but also in reducing costs for that selected population while focusing on quality of care.

Accreditation Association for Ambulatory Health Care (AAAHC): One of a number of voluntary organizations providing standards for and evaluating care in ambulatory care facilities; this organization focuses entirely on various types of ambulatory care settings.

accreditation standards: Guidelines developed by independent nonprofit groups that apply to health care facilities that voluntarily choose to comply.

administrative data: Documentation in a patient's record that is not related to care or treatment provided; includes demographic, financial, and consent information.

administrative safeguards: Assignment of security management, security training, and developing policies and procedures.

Advance Beneficiary Notice (ABN): Document given to Medicare patients if it is believed that a treatment or a portion of a treatment will be considered unnecessary by Medicare and consequently will not be reimbursed.

advance directive: Document that provides guidance to practitioners about the wishes of a patient should he or she become incapacitated or no longer able to make decisions because of medical or psychiatric impairment.

alerts: Automated notices to practitioners of information that requires immediate or special attention.

allergy and adverse reaction list: Summary list of all patient allergies and adverse reactions known to the practice.

ambulatory care: The health care category of patients who are not admitted to occupy a bed but rather seek health care services usually in the provider's office setting; the patient physically moves to the provider's location in order to receive care.

American Association for Accreditation of Ambulatory Surgery Facilities (AAAASF): One of a number of voluntary organizations providing standards for and evaluating care in ambulatory surgery facilities.

American Health Information Management Association (AHIMA): A national member organization of health information management professionals that developed a core data set for ambulatory records; one of the Cooperating Party organizations that participate in recommendations regarding the content of ICD for use in the U.S.

American Hospital Association (AHA): One of the Cooperating Party organizations that participates in recommendations regarding ICD for use in the U.S.

American Medical Association (AMA): Organization that copyrights and coordinates CPT Level I codes.

American Osteopathic Association (AOA): One of a number of voluntary organizations providing standards for and evaluating care in ambulatory care facilities, laboratories, and ambulatory surgery settings.

Assignment of Benefits: Authorization by the patient for a third-party payer to reimburse the practice directly (instead of the patient) for services provided.

audit trails: Routine system tracking of all activity related to each patient's record in the EHR by user and role.

authentication protocols: Steps the EHR system requires users to take before it will accept their log-in and/or save the data they are entering.

authorization for release (disclosure) of information: Document completed and signed by the patient (or the patient's representative) to permit the sharing of confidential patient information with others for any purpose other than treatment, health care payment, or health care operations.

C

case report form: Document that summarizes research findings for a particular individual so that data can be gathered consistently across participants and statistical evaluation performed.

CCHIT Functional Criteria for Ambulatory EHRs: Standards set by the CCHIT for the tasks an EHR must perform before it is approved as meeting the processing requirements in the ambulatory care environment.

Centers for Medicare and Medicaid Services (CMS): Federal government office that oversees the Medicare and Medicaid programs.

Certification Commission for Health care Information Technology (CCHIT): An independent, non-profit organization formed to establish functional, interoperability, and security criteria and to certify HER products as meeting those criteria.

certification standards: Regulations, such as those developed by the Medicare program, that must be met in order to receive Medicare or Medicaid reimbursement; includes sections on patient records.

Certified Health IT Product List (CHPL): Official listing of EHR vendor products certified to meet the Medicare/Medicaid "Meaningful Use" functional criteria.

classification system: A system that groups similar diagnoses or procedures together for reporting purposes.

client-server architecture or client server model: One of two models for constructing a practice EHR; an annual licensing fee is paid to the EHR vendor for use of software, but all other components of the system are owned, operated, and maintained by the practice.

clinical data: Components of a patient record that relate to the care and treatment provided to the patient.

clinical trial (clinical study): Steps in the medical research process that involve humans.

code sets—coding systems: a term particularly used for those codes approved by HIPAA regulations for use in electronic transactions.

Commission for the Accreditation of Birth Centers: A voluntary organization providing standards for and evaluating care in birthing centers.

computer-assisted coding (CAC): Use of coding software that automatically generates medical codes based on documentation in the patient record.

computerized provider order entry (CPOE): A software application that allows health care providers to enter orders electronically to carry out a patient's treatment plan and electronically communicates the orders over a computer network to other individual(s) responsible for carrying out the order(s).

Conditions of Participation (CoP), or Conditions of Coverage (CoC): General name for the regulations that care providers must meet in order to participate in the Medicare/ Medicaid programs.

consent for treatment: Documentation signed by the patient giving approval to the provision of routine care.

continuity of care record (CCR): Tool for communication between authorized health care providers from different settings; includes defined sets of information from a provider's EHR database.

Cooperating Parties: Representatives from four organizations that together make recommendations for ICD code modifications and additions for use in the U.S.

Current Dental Terminology (CDT): Coding standard for dental services and the HIPAA-designated coding system for electronic transactions.

Current Procedural Terminology—4th Revision (CPT-IV): Coding nomenclature used for billing and public health reporting by ambulatory care service providers.

D

daily task list (aka "in basket"): Designation of work that needs to be completed by an employee of a practice.

data dictionary: A listing of each data field in a system; fields are defined by a unique title or label, an indication of the type of data, a functional description, and a standard format.

data field: Defined area where a specific piece of information can be entered.

data repository: Electronic holding place for data.

data-encryption protocols: System-generated scrambling of data during electronic transmission to prevent the data from being intercepted.

demographic information: Patient identifying information gathered during initial contact and patient registration.

Diagnostic and Statistical Manual—Fourth Edition— Text Revision (DSM-IV-TR): Coding classification system associated with mental disorders, personality disorders, and life events or social problems that affect people.

diagnostic trials: Type of clinical trial conducted to find better tests or procedures for diagnosing a particular disease or condition.

direct faxing: Transfer of health care provider information from one organization to another via facsimile transmission.

drop-down menu (pick list): Structured response choices presented within a data field.

drug vocabularies: National terminologies associated with pharmacy information systems to support accurate communication of prescriptions and assure correct drug labeling.

durable power of attorney for health care: Type of advance directive giving another person the right to make health care decisions for the patient.

E

EHR goals: Statements regarding desired improvements in clinical and/or office processes or in outcomes of patient care as a result of EHR implementation.

EHR project plan: Anticipated schedule and budget for selecting a vendor and completing EHR implementation.

EHR vision: A statement of the desired future state of a health care practice once the EHR is fully implemented.

electronic data interchange (EDI): Transfer of health care provider information from one organization to another electronically.

electronic health record (EHR): An electronic record of health-related information on an individual that conforms to nationally recognized interoperability standards and that can be created, managed, and consulted by authorized clinicians and staff across more than one healthcare organization.

electronic medical record (EMR): An electronic record of health-related information on an individual that can be created, gathered, managed, and consulted by authorized clinicians and staff within one health care organization.

eligible providers (EPs): Health care providers that are qualified by regulations to participate in Medicare's or Medicaid's "meaningful use" incentive programs.

e-mail and electronic text messages: Scripted messages entered on one computer, cell phone, or PDA and then sent to another computer or receiving device.

encoder: Software with current coding classification systems embedded to assist with the coding process.

encounter form: Preprinted paper template designed to record the diagnoses and procedures completed during an office visit along with their ICD or CPT codes.

enterprise master patient/ person index (EMPI): The key to locating a patient record in a health care organization with many component facilities, this listing includes patient identifying information and the assigned record number for all individuals ever receiving care by the entire organization.

evaluation and management codes (E/M codes): Part of the CPT coding system that indicates the level and complexity of an office visit.

examination protocol: Beginning with the chief complaint, a standard set of examination steps that will specifically eliminate, or specifically confirm, potential underlying causes for the chief complaint.

Explanation of Benefits (EOB) or remittance advice (RA): Communication from a third-party payer to a practice indicating payment for services, claim problems for follow-up action, or noncoverage of services.

F

flow sheet: A display of data in a time sequence, allowing care providers to see trends in areas (e.g., blood pressure, blood sugar level) they are monitoring.

free-text narrative: Unstructured documentation that allows a health care provider to dictate or key text.

functional requirements: Descriptions of the specific capabilities needed within an EHR to meet the goals of the practice.

G

graphic displays: A format for presenting numerical data that has been entered into structured (coded) data fields, showing trends in clinical data and allowing comparisons overtime.

grids: Feature that enables the entry of structured data into an EHR in a format similar to a table.

growth chart: Graphic display of the height and weight of pediatric patients comparing their data to a developmental standard for the patient's age group.

H

Health Information Exchange (HIE): National, regional, or local efforts established for electronic sharing of patient health care data among care providers; subdivisions of the NHIN that also may be referred to as SNOs.

Health Information Technology for Economic and Clinical Health Act (HITECH): Legislation authorizing a process to certify organizations to perform product reviews on behalf of the government and to award grants for further adoption of EHRs.

Health Information Technology Toolkit for Physician Offices: Developed by Stratis Health, this toolkit helps physician offices assess their readiness, plan, select, implement, make effective use of, and exchange important information about the clients they serve. The toolkit contains numerous resources, including tools for telehealth, health information exchange, and personal health records.

Health Insurance Portability and Accountability Act (HIPAA): Federal legislation establishing regulations aimed at assuring the privacy and security of protected electronic health information.

Health IT Adoption Toolbox: Developed by HHS's Health Resources and Services Administration (HRSA), this toolkit is a compilation of planning, implementation, and evaluation resources to help community health centers, other safety net providers, and ambulatory care providers implement health IT applications in their facilities. Staff from community health centers and a variety of stakeholders in the health IT arena have reviewed and contributed to the toolbox to ensure the resources are accurate, relevant, and effective in supporting health IT in health centers.

health maintenance reminder: A reminder given to a health care provider or to a patient generated with the EHR system, calling attention to some needed action related to maintaining the patient's health status.

Health Plan Employer Data and Information Set (HEDIS): Defined set of information that is found in ambulatory records outlined by the National Committee for Quality Assurance as part of a system to measure and compare quality of care across physician providers.

Healthcare Common Procedure Coding Systems (HCPCS): Coding system designated by HIPAA for electronic transactions relating to procedures performed in the ambulatory setting.

human–computer interface (user) devices: The devices practice personnel use to interact with the EHR system; examples include wall-mounted or desktop computers, laptop computers, notebook or tablet personal computers, and personal digital assistants (PDAs).

hybrid patient record: A patient record that has some electronic and some paper components.

I

icons: An image, picture, or symbol used in a computer software program to represent a function or activity.

imaged data: Digitized (digital) images.

implementation activities: A series of Interrelated steps that must be completed before a practice can "go live" with a chosen EHR system.

Institutional Review Board (IRB): Multidisciplinary group that reviews research protocols for soundness, risks to participants, safeguards, and legal and ethical issues.

integrated record: Patient record in which material is organized by type of recording.

International Classification of Diseases—10th Revision, Clinical Modification (ICD-10 CM): An international update to the ICD-9 disease classification coordinated by the World Health Organization; to be initiated in the U.S. in 2014.

International Classification of Diseases—9th Revision—Clinical Modification (ICD-9-CM): International coding classification system used for billing and public health reporting in all types of health care facilities.

International Classification of Diseases—9th Revision—Clinical Modification (ICD- 10-CM): International coding classification system used for billing and public health reporting in all types of health care facilities, which will replace ICD-9-CM effective October 1, 2013.

interoperability: The capacity of systems to communicate and exchange information with one another.

L

legal source legend: A grid that describes where and how to find specific documents that constitute the hybrid health record.

licensure standards: Regulations established by each state for health care providers or facilities desiring to operate within the state's borders.

living will: Type of advance directive that outlines the wishes of the patient in relation to medical care in life threatening situations; it also can name a representative.

Logical Observation Identifier Names and Codes (LOINC): Terminology that supports electronic transmission of laboratory test orders and results.

M

mapping: The linking of content from one terminology or classification system to another.

master patient/person index (MPI): The key to locating a patient record, this listing includes patient identifying information and the assigned record number for all individuals ever receiving care by an organization.

meaningful use: Relates to the actual ways that the EHR must be used to support patient care and specific ways that quality of care must be measured to receive incentive payments from Medicare and Medicaid Services as determined by the federal HITECH Act.

MEDCIN: Point-of-care terminology that is fully mapped to the SNOMED-CT terminology.

Medicaid: A joint state- and federal-funded program providing health care benefits to populations below a defined income level.

Medicare: National program to provide federally funded health care assistance to the elderly in the United States.

Medicare/Medicaid EHR Certification Standards for "Meaningful Use": Standards set by the National Institute for Standards and Technology (NIST) for the tasks an EHR must perform before it is approved as meeting the Medicare/ Medicaid "meaningful use" requirements in the ambulatory care environment.

Medicare qualifying trial: Clinical trial meeting Medicare's criteria as an approved study so that the routine costs of care and associated costs from medical complications it may produce can be reimbursed.

medication (drug) alerts and reminders: Messages sent to a health care provider that call attention to any potential adverse effects that could result if the intended medication order is carried out.

medication (drug) reference information: Published texts that provide details on drugs approved for use in the United States; often available in hard copy or via software.

medication list: Summary list of all the medications a patient has taken or currently is taking.

menu (navigator) bar: The first bar of icons across the top of a computer screen that (when chosen via a mouse click) allow standard functions of the software to be performed, making it easier to move through the system.

N

narrative text data: A form of unstructured data not reflected in the EHR's data dictionary.

National Center for Health Statistics (NCHS): One of the Cooperating Party organizations that participates in recommendations regarding ICD for use in the U.S.

National Committee for Quality Assurance (NCQA): One of a number of voluntary organizations providing standards for and evaluating care in managed care organizations.

National Committee for Vital and Health Statistics (NCVHS) Core Content of the Healthcare Provider Dimension: An update of the Uniform Ambulatory Care Data Set providing a list of elements to be found in health care provider patient records.

National Drug Codes (NDC): Federally recognized standard for naming and identifying drugs; used by pharmacies for communicating prescriptions and assuring correct drug labeling.

National Health Information Network (NHIN): National system underdevelopment that will permit electronic sharing of healthcare data among those involved in care provision across the United States.

natural-language processing: Software that applies artificial intelligence to narrative text in order to extract terms and data.

nomenclature: A listing of coding terms.

North American Nursing Diagnosis Association (NANDA): Nursing terminology standard applied to nursing diagnoses.

Notice of Exclusions from Medicare Benefits: Document provided to a Medicare patient if the provider knows that a particular service will not be covered by Medicare; allows the provider to bill the patient for the services.

Notice of Privacy Practices: Information that HIPAA requires be provided to patients about the use and disclosure of information by the practice, patient rights and responsibilities in relation to the record, and contact information if questions arise.

Nursing Interventions Classification (NIC): Nursing terminology standard applied to nursing interventions.

Nursing Outcomes Classification (NOC): Nursing terminology standard applied to patient outcomes.

O

Office of the National Coordinator for Health Information Technology (ONC): Federal government office introduced to lead and coordinate efforts toward a National Health Information Network.

ONC-ATCB (Authorized Testing and Certification Body): Organization authorized to perform Complete EHR and EHR Module testing in order to certify them as being able to support health care organizations in their efforts to achieve "meaningful use" of their EHR systems as defined in the CMS Meaningful Use Incentive Payment Program.

order details: Specific items that must be entered by a health care provider to make an order complete.

order entry templates: The format of structured data-entry items required to complete a medical order.

order format and details (order sentence): General sequence for the detailed information passed from the prescribing provider to the pharmacy.

P

patient portal: Secure Internet connection to a practice for communication and access to practice databases by patients.

personal health record (PHR): Documentation system that allows consumers to gather, store, access, and coordinate their health information.

physical safeguards: Mechanisms that protect the equipment and the data associated with the EHR system.

placebo: Substance with no treatment value given to some participants in a research study to compare results with those individuals who receive the product under investigation.

point of care: The time at which treatment is being provided.

practice management system (PMS): System that supports the financial and administrative functions of a practice; usually includes patient demographics, appointment scheduling, charge capture and billing, and report generation.

prevention trials: Type of clinical trial that looks for better ways to prevent a disease in people who have never had it or to prevent a disease from recurring.

principal investigator: Member of a research team who serves as its leader.

Privacy Board: Multidisciplinary group of individuals from a health care setting that reviews a research protocol for compliance with HIPAA privacy regulations.

problem list: Summary list of all the major diagnoses that a patient has experienced and been treated for by a health care practice.

problem-oriented record: Patient record organized by patient problems numbered in order as they are identified, where all recording refers back to the specific problem through documentation of its number.

procedure notes template: Structured format documentation by a health care provider describing the patient encounter.

protocol: Detailed plan for a research study.

Q

Quality Improvement Organization (QIO): An organization that contracts with the federal government to perform tasks on its behalf under the Medicare program, focusing especially on quality and necessity of care issues.

quality-of-life trials: Type of clinical trial that explores ways to improve comfort and the quality of life for individuals with a chronic disease.

R

readiness assessment: Evaluation of a practice's work, workflow, existing technologies, applications, hardware, etc., to determine its status in preparation for EHR implementation.

referral letter: Request from one health care provider to another to provide specialized services to a patient; includes the transfer of information from one practice to another.

Regional Health Information Organizations (RHIOs): Network of regional healthcare providers established for electronic sharing of patient health care data.

Regional Health Information Technology Extension Centers (RECs): Regional centers that offer technical assistance, guidance, and information on best practices to support and accelerate healthcare providers' efforts to become meaningful users of Electronic Health Records.

Regional HIT Extension Centers (RECs): Regional centers that offer technical assistance, guidance, and information on best practices to support and accelerate health care providers' efforts to become meaningful users of Electronic Health Records.

reminders: Automated notices to practitioners or patients regarding actions that need to be taken.

reportable events: Medical diagnoses or disorders that a government entity has mandated be reported for public health or safety reasons.

request for proposal (RFP): An RFP is a document constructed by an organization and used by the organization to solicit bids from potential vendors for a product or service.

results reporting: Communication of the findings associated with a completed diagnostic-test order.

risk analysis: An assessment of the potential risks and vulnerabilities to the confidentiality, integrity, and availability of electronic protected health information that is maintained by the health care organization

RxNorm: Federally recognized standard for naming and identifying drugs; used by pharmacies for communicating prescriptions and assuring correct drug labeling.

S

screening trials: Type of clinical trial that tests the best way to detect certain diseases or health conditions.

scrubber: Software developed to review claims for discrepancies or errors and to validate compliance with regulatory mandates prior to submission to third-party payers.

secure e-mail: An e-mail message sent via the Internet that has been encrypted to make it unreadable during transit.

smart card: Patient-held portable summary of important health information digitized on a medium the size of a credit card.

software-as-a-service (SaaS) model: The second model for constructing a practice EHR. With the SaaS approach, the practice purchases the hardware devices (computer terminals, laptops, etc.)

and telecommunications system. The EHR product vendor continues to own, support, and maintain the servers, database software, and application software at the core of the EHR system.

source-oriented record: Patient record in which content is organized by the type of health professional entering data.

standards organizations: Government agencies, voluntary groups, and industry associations involved in establishing guidelines to assist in bringing uniformity to business processes or products.

structured (discrete) data: Data fields where either numbers or dates must be entered or in which a selection from a defined list of options must be made.

Sub-Network Organizations (SNOs): National, regional, or local efforts established for electronic sharing of patient health care data among care providers.

summary lists: Lists of significant diagnoses, procedures, drug allergies, and medications that the Joint Commission requires ambulatory patient records to contain.

Systematized Nomenclature of Medicine—Clinical Terminology (SNOMED-CT): Medical vocabulary approved by the federal government as a standard for the EHR.

T

technical safeguards: Automated processes that limit who is able to access the EHR and what they are able to do within the system.

telemonitoring: Using telecommunications technology to gather physiologic or diagnostic data and transmit it to a health care provider who can evaluate patients who are located a distance from the care provider setting.

telephone (voice mail) patient messages: Messages recorded by voice over the telephone when the person or practice called cannot or does not answer the call.

templates: Preformatted data collection screens containing specific structured or free-text data fields and designed to support efficient and complete documentation.

The Joint Commission (JC): One of a number of voluntary organizations providing standards for and evaluating care in ambulatory care facilities; this organization provides these services to a wide variety of types of health care settings in addition to ambulatory care facilities.

The Joint Commission's "Do Not Use" Abbreviation List: The Joint Commission's list of medical abbreviations that cause errors in interpretation and hence should not be found in the patient documentation of facilities that desire their accreditation.

toolbar: The second bar of icons across the top of a computer screen that (when chosen via a mouse click) allow standard functions of the software to be performed, making moving through the system easier.

treatment notes or procedure notes: Unstructured writing by a health care provider describing the patient encounter.

treatment plan: A final component of an assessment which specifies any number and variety of actions needed to appropriately address the patient's health care problem(s). In a SOAP note it is the content in the "P" section of the documentation.

treatment protocols: Established guidelines for treatment of specific diseases.

treatment trials: Type of clinical trial that tests experimental treatments, new combinations of drugs, or new approaches to surgery or radiation therapy.

U

Uniform Ambulatory Care Data Set (UACDS): Basic list of information that should be found in ambulatory patient records, as initially approved in 1989 by the National Committee on Vital and Health Statistics.

unit record: One longitudinal record for each individual no matter how many times the individual has been seen by an organization (or organizations).

unstructured (text) data: Data fields that allow a user to enter data in free-text or narrative form.

user- and role-based access controls: Limitations on what a user can view and do within a patient's EHR.

V

vendor selection: The process of developing a request for proposal, receiving vendor responses, and evaluating them against established criteria in order to determine a specific EHR product for implementation.

VistA-Office EHR: A component of the Veterans Administration's electronic health record system available for use in non-VA ambulatory care settings.

INDEX

Italics indicate tables or figures.

A

D

E

F

G

H

I

J

L

M

N

O

S

T

U

V

W